D1566273

METHODS IN CANCER RESEARCH

Volume XX

TUMOR MARKERS

Contributors to This Volume

REBECCA BYRD
STEFAN CARREL
NICOLAS DE TRIBOLET
DAVID M. GOLDENBERG
CURTIS C. HARRIS
J. FRANK HENDERSON
M. HOSOKAWA
IH-CHANG HSU
DAREL HUNTING
ZDENKA L. JONAK
ROGER H. KENNETT
H. KOBAYASHI
HILARY KOPROWSKI
JEAN-PIERRE MACH
JOHN A. MANNICK
PAUL K. NAKANE
F. JAMES PRIMUS
ARNOLD E. REIF
GLENN STEELE, JR.
ZENON STEPLEWSKI
BOSCO S. WANG
ROBERT H. YOLKEN

METHODS IN CANCER RESEARCH
Volume XX

TUMOR MARKERS

Edited by

HARRIS BUSCH

DEPARTMENT OF PHARMACOLOGY
BAYLOR COLLEGE OF MEDICINE
TEXAS MEDICAL CENTER
HOUSTON, TEXAS

and

LYNN C. YEOMAN

DEPARTMENT OF PHARMACOLOGY
BAYLOR COLLEGE OF MEDICINE
TEXAS MEDICAL CENTER
HOUSTON, TEXAS

1982

ACADEMIC PRESS
A Subsidiary of Harcourt Brace Jovanovich, Publishers

New York   London
Paris   San Diego   San Francisco   São Paulo   Sydney   Tokyo   Toronto

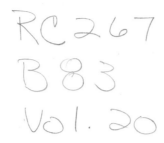

ACADEMIC PRESS, INC.
111 Fifth Avenue, New York, New York 10003

United Kingdom Edition published by
ACADEMIC PRESS, INC. (LONDON) LTD.
24/28 Oval Road, London NW1 7DX

LIBRARY OF CONGRESS CATALOG CARD NUMBER: 66–29495

ISBN 0–12–147680–4

PRINTED IN THE UNITED STATES OF AMERICA

82 83 84 85   9 8 7 6 5 4 3 2 1

Contents

TUMOR IMMUNOGENICITY AND CELLULAR IMMUNITY

CHAPTER I.   **Antigenicity of Tumors: A Comprehensive
System of Measurement**

Arnold E. Reif

CHAPTER II.   **Allogeneic Cell Immunity**

M. Hosokawa and H. Kobayashi

CHAPTER VII.   **Methods for the Determination of Deoxyribonucleoside Triphosphate Concentrations**

Darel Hunting and J. Frank Henderson

MONOCLONAL ANTIBODIES AND THE TUMOR CELL SURFACE

CHAPTER VIII.   **Monoclonal Antibody Development in the Study of Colorectal Carcinoma-Associated Antigens**

Zenon Steplewski and Hilary Koprowski

CHAPTER IX.   **Human Melanoma- and Glioma-Associated Antigen(s) Identified by Monoclonal Antibodies**

Stefan Carrel, Nicolas de Tribolet, and Jean-Pierre Mach

CHAPTER X. **Cell Surface Changes in Malignancy**

Roger H. Kennett, Zdenka L. Jonak, and Rebecca Byrd

Contributors

Numbers in parentheses indicate the pages on which the authors' contributions begin.

REBECCA BYRD (355), Division of Oncology, Children's Hospital of Philadelphia and Department of Human Genetics, University of Pennsylvania School of Medicine, Philadelphia, Pennsylvania 19104

STEFAN CARREL (317), Ludwig Institute for Cancer Research, Division de Lausanne, Ch. des Boveresses, CH-1066 Epalinges S/Lausanne, Switzerland

NICOLAS DE TRIBOLET (317), Ludwig Institute for Cancer Research, Division de Lausanne, Ch. des Boveresses, CH-1066 Epalinges S/Lausanne, Switzerland

DAVID M. GOLDENBERG (139), Division of Experimental Pathology, Department of Pathology, University of Kentucky College of Medicine, Lexington, Kentucky 40536

CURTIS C. HARRIS (213), Laboratory of Human Carcinogenesis, National Cancer Institute, National Institutes of Health, Bethesda, Maryland 20205

J. FRANK HENDERSON (245), Cancer Research Unit (McEachern Laboratory) and Department of Biochemistry, University of Alberta, Edmonton, Alberta, Canada T6G 2H7

M. HOSOKAWA (85), Laboratory of Pathology, Cancer Institute, Hokkaido University School of Medicine, Sapporo 060, Japan

IH-CHANG HSU* (213), Department of Pediatrics, The Johns Hopkins University School of Medicine, Baltimore, Maryland 21205

DAREL HUNTING[†] (245), Cancer Research Unit (McEachern Laboratory) and Department of Biochemistry, University of Alberta, Edmonton, Alberta, Canada T6G 2H7

ZDENKA L. JONAK (355), Department of Human Genetics, University of Pennsylvania School of Medicine, Philadelphia, Pennsylvania 19104

*Present address: Department of Pathology, University of Maryland School of Medicine, Baltimore, Maryland 21201

[†]Present address: Department of Pathology, Washington University School of Medicine, St. Louis, Missouri 63110

ROGER H. KENNETT (355), Department of Human Genetics, University of Pennsylvania School of Medicine, Philadelphia, Pennsylvania 19104

H. KOBAYASHI (85), Laboratory of Pathology, Cancer Institute, Hokkaido University School of Medicine, Sapporo 060, Japan

HILARY KOPROWSKI (285), The Wistar Institute, Philadelphia, Pennsylvania 19104

JEAN-PIERRE MACH (317), Ludwig Institute for Cancer Research, Division de Lausanne, Ch. des Boveresses, CH-1066 Epalinges S/Lausanne, Switzerland

JOHN A. MANNICK (107), Department of Surgery, Brigham and Women's Hospital, Harvard Medical School, Boston, Massachusetts 02115

PAUL K. NAKANE (183), Department of Pathology, University of Colorado Health Sciences Center, Denver, Colorado 80262

F. JAMES PRIMUS (139), Division of Experimental Pathology, Department of Pathology, University of Kentucky College of Medicine, Lexington, Kentucky 40536

ARNOLD E. REIF (3), Mallory Institute of Pathology, Boston University School of Medicine, Boston City Hospital, Boston, Massachusetts 02118

GLENN STEELE, JR. (107), Department of Surgery, Brigham and Women's Hospital, Harvard Medical School, Boston, Massachusetts 02115

ZENON STEPLEWSKI (285), The Wistar Institute, Philadelphia, Pennsylvania 19104

BOSCO S. WANG (107), Department of Surgery, Brigham and Women's Hospital, Harvard Medical School, Boston, Massachusetts 02115

ROBERT H. YOLKEN (213), Laboratory of Human Carcinogenesis, National Cancer Institute, National Institutes of Health, Bethesda, Maryland 20205

Preface

The subject of "tumor markers" is becoming of great interest to oncologists. A number of opportunities exist in this area, particularly for diagnosis of cancer and assessment of body burden either by direct interactions between antigens of cancer cells and specific antibodies or by the products produced in cancer cells that may exhibit sufficiently distinctive features for clinical utility.

Beginning with Volume II, this treatise has dealt with immunology and special products of cancer cells. Volumes XIX and XX are specifically related to newer information on tumor markers. In Volume XX the first section addresses tumor immunogenicity and cellular immunity, and includes sections on antigenicity, cell immunity, and cytolysis. The second section deals with immunochemical assays and antigen localization by histopathology, electron microscopy, and immunoassay. The third section concerns monoclonal antibodies and their use in the evaluation of colorectal carcinomas, melanomas, and gliomas. The volume concludes with a chapter on cell surface changes in malignancy.

It is our hope that the topics presented are timely and useful to investigators in these and related fields.

HARRIS BUSCH

Contents of Other Volumes

VOLUME XIX: Tumor Markers

Cell Surface Markers for Neoplasia

Antigen Markers of Tumor Cells and Nuclei

Models and Methods for Diagnosis and Therapy

TUMOR IMMUNOGENICITY AND CELLULAR IMMUNITY

CHAPTER I

ANTIGENICITY OF TUMORS: A COMPREHENSIVE SYSTEM OF MEASUREMENT*

ARNOLD E. REIF

* This work was supported by USPHS Research Grant CA 15952 from the National Cancer Institute, DHHS.

I. Introduction

Mathé (1978) has said that tumor immunology is at best haltingly emerging from the Middle Ages. Perhaps the single most important parameter in tumor immunology is the "antigenic strength" of a tumor. Until a unified quantitative system for the measurement of tumor antigenicity is used, Mathé's assessment could be right on the mark.

The beginning of modern tumor immunology can be assigned to 1943 (Rapp, 1979) when Gross published the first unequivocal evidence that tumors induced by a chemical carcinogen possess tumor-associated transplantation antigens (Gross, 1943). During the subsequent four decades, no comprehensive system for measuring the antigenicity of tumors appears to have been suggested or used. Each investigator has felt free to use his own version of a tumor antigenicity assay, and as a result a comparison of the antigenicity of tumors used by different investigators is difficult, except in a very rough manner. This usually takes the form of assigning the tumor empirically to classes such as the following: undetectable antigenicity (−), questionable or weak antigenicity (±), antigenicity (+), strong antigenicity (+ +), and very strong antigenicity (+ + +).

Why has a comprehensive quantitative assay system for tumor antigenicity not been proposed previously? The answer is that there are many difficulties. First, experimental tumors possess a wide range of antigenicities. A single assay that spans the entire range has not yet been discovered. Therefore, several assays may be necessary. Second, a choice must be made of what types of assays are to be used. Third, the conditions of the assays must be defined precisely. Details regarding the methods of immunization and challenge require standardization. Even the approximate number of mice in each assay group must be decided upon, since the statistical validity of the results obtained varies greatly with changes in this number. Fourth, a choice must be made regarding the method for scoring the results of the assay. Fifth, guidelines are required to accommodate common unavoidable deviations from the recommended procedure. Sixth, flexibility must be incorporated into the protocol to permit future modifications and extensions.

Sufficient work has now been done by different investigators to permit *reasonable* choices to be made regarding standardization of a comprehensive assay for tumor antigenicity. The accent is on "reasonable," for the conditions chosen represent a compromise between what an investigator with strictly limited resources can perform easily, and what might be optimal. The scoring system chosen spans the entire range of antigenicity of experimental tumors, from nonantigenic to extremely antigenic. While only the central range of tumor antigenicity has been investigated by the writer, guidelines are given that enable investigators to determine antigenicities outside the main range, for tumors with very low or with very high antigenicities. Further, a suggestion is made regarding how the present system could be applied to measure the antigenicity of human tumors. An outline of the system, and of its application to radiation-induced, chemically induced, and spontaneous tumors has already been presented (Reif and Tomas, 1980; Argyris and Reif, 1981; Reif, 1981; Cataldo and Reif, 1982).

II. Considerations Relevant for Choice of an Assay System

A. NOMENCLATURE

Specialized disciplines often possess their own vocabularies: immunology and its subspecialty, cancer immunology, are no exception. However, as time progresses the meanings of technical words can change, as has happened in cancer immunology. It is therefore relevant to clarify the sense of words vital for an understanding of the present subject.

1. Antigen

The adjective is "antigenic." An outmoded definition of antigen is still given by the Task Force on Immunology and Disease (1977): "a substance that elicits a specific immune response when introduced into the tissues of the body." This definition is now reserved for an immunogen (see Section II,A,4). The current definition of antigen (Thaler et al., 1977), slightly modified, is "a molecular entity that can be bound by antibody."

2. Antigenic Tumor*

In the older literature (Klein, 1968), an antigenic tumor is depicted as "able to stimulate an immune response inferred to be relevant for tumor rejection (whether in a favorable or in an unfavorable direction) in the au-

---

* Sulitzeanu and Weiss (1981) suggest that a tumor should be called "antigenic" if it can initiate a response that is indifferent (or of unknown value) to host resistance against a tumor, or "immunogenic" if it can elicit a response known to affect resistance (whether in favorable or in unfavorable directions). The problem with this definition is that it imputes far more than is obvious or historically denoted by these expressions. Only "insiders" conversant with definitions could hope to understand them. By adding the term "immunorejective strength" to the vocabulary, the need to define antigenicity in more than the classical sense is avoided here.

tologous or isogenic host." This is the present redefinition of what was not stated explicitly. Because this definition of antigenicity is an umbrella term that may include the interaction between the immunogenicity and the immunosensitivity of a tumor (see Sections II,A,6 and 7) and covers the host responses both of tumor rejection and of enhancement, it is retained in its original meaning and frequently used in the present paper.*

3. Autochthonous, Autologous: "Self-same"

A tumor in its autochthonous host is in the host in which it arose.

4. Immunogen

The adjective is "immunogenic": "able to elicit cellular immunization or antibody formation" (slightly modified from Humphrey and White, 1970).

5. Immunogenic Tumor

This is "a tumor that can elicit an immune response in the autochthonous or isogenic host." In contradistinction to an antigenic tumor, which must elicit a response that is relevant to the growth of the tumor, the type of response is not specified. Therefore, all antigenic tumors are immunogenic, though the reverse is not true.

6. Immunoinsensitivity

The adjective is "immunoinsensitive" (synonym: "immunoresistive"): "insensitive to damage by immunological agents, whether cellular or humoral."

7. Immunoinsensitive Tumor

"This is a tumor that is insensitive to damage by immune cells or humoral factors in autochthonous or isogenic hosts."

8. Immunosensitivity

The adjective is "immunosensitive": as defined above, with "insensitive" replaced by "sensitive."

---

* Under certain conditions of immunization, an enhancement rather than an inhibition of growth may be obtained. For this reason, the definition includes a statement that recognizes that an antigenic tumor may elicit either a rejection or an enhancement response in its host.

9. Immunorejectivity

The adjective is "immunorejective," suggested here to indicate "rejection by an immune mechanism."

10. Isogenic, Isogeneic, Isologous, Syngeneic

These terms denote "within its own inbred strain of animal." An isogenic transplant is made from one member of an inbred strain to another member of the same strain.

11. Negative (or Promotional) Antigenicity

This is a type of antigenicity that produces tolerance rather than rejection. When applied to a tumor, negative antigenicity indicates that an increase (enhancement or promotion) of tumor growth rather than an inhibition is obtained under the stated conditions of immunization.

12. Relative Antigenic Strength (RAS)

This is "a comparative measure of the tumor's ability to stimulate an immune response inferred to be relevant for tumor rejection in its autologous or isogenic host."

13. Relative Immunorejective Strength (RIS)

This is "a comparative measure of the tumor's ability to stimulate an immune rejection response in its autologous or isogenic host."

Other specialized words are used as defined by Humphrey and White (1970), Thaler et al. (1977), or the Task Force on Immunology and Disease (1977).

B. TOWARD A MEANINGFUL DEFINITION OF TUMOR ANTIGENICITY

We are presently beginning to appreciate the complexities of the host response to a tumor. We are becoming aware of the existence of a variety of immune response mechanisms, of the fine structure of their cellular orchestration, and of the multiplicity of humoral factors involved. Considering all these intricacies, is anything useful to be gained by work on an assay that depends upon the interplay of so many different mechanisms, cell types, and factors?

The authors of reviews on tumor immunology and tumor antigenicity published during the 1960s and early 1970s had no problem in choosing the most relevant parameter of tumor antigenicity (Old and Boyse, 1964;

Hattler and Amos, 1966; Klein, 1968, 1969; Law, 1969; Prager and Baechtel, 1973; Prager, 1975). Although implied rather than stated, this parameter was the relative strength with which an immunized host could reject either its autochthonous tumor or an isogenic transplant (isograft) of a tumor. Perhaps the most important validation of this concept is the rough correlation between the immunorejective strengths of tumors and our ability to cure these tumors by various modalities of therapy (Reif, 1978, 1979). Further, when oncologists involved in the treatment of patients talk about the antigenicity of tumors (Fisher, 1975; Order, 1975), they define it as the property of the tumor that mediates tumor rejection. For these reasons, the immunorejective strength of a tumor is chosen here as the most meaningful measure of the antigenicity of tumors.

Is there any evidence that immunorejective strength is really an inherent property of a tumor which can be measured with consistency? It could be argued correctly that tumors contain a variety of host cells, including macrophages, lymphocytes, polymorphs, and mesenchymal cells. Is it possible that the transfer of these normal cells, as much or more than the transfer of tumor cells, is responsible for activation of the host effector cells that are involved in tumor rejection? Certainly, removal of macrophages from a tumor transplant can cause more rapid growth of the transplanted tumor cells (Wood and Gellespie, 1975).

Lawler et al. (1981) concluded that the relative immunogenicities of tumors were characteristics of the tumors themselves and not artifacts due to the immunization or challenge procedures used. This conclusion was reached after studying three methods of immunization and two methods of challenge for a dozen or more methylcholanthrene-induced tumors. Immunogenicity was measured by the decrease in the mean diameter of tumors in immunized as compared to control mice; the same measurement is also used in the present paper as an index of immunorejective strength. Thus, there is evidence that tumors possess characteristic immunorejective strengths in isogenic hosts, and that the measurement of this parameter can be performed with consistency. Furthermore, the complement of normal cells present in a tumor is another inherent property of a given tumor. Therefore, it is not surprising that removal of this complement may alter the immunorejective strength of the tumor. After all, other treatments of tumor cells, for instance incubation with neuraminidase, may increase the immunogenicity of a tumor (Prager and Baechtel, 1973).

Still, the elaboration of suppressor cells, which oppose the action or proliferation of host cells cytotoxic to the tumor cells, represents a complexity that is not taken into account in the measurement of immunorejective strength. Further, the relationship between the host's production of cytotoxic cells and of suppressor cells would have to be determined be-fore a concrete proposal could be made regarding a suitable protocol for immunization and challenge of the host with tumor cells. Argyris and Reif (1981) have found that the property of being able to induce suppressor cells both in an autochthonous and in an isogenic host is a characteristic property of the tumor. In this sense, a tumor's ability to induce suppres-sor cells is as characteristic a property as its ability to stimulate the host to produce lymphokines or T-cell factors.

The objection could be raised that some tumors can stimulate the host to promote (enhance or accelerate) tumor growth rather than to inhibit (re-tard) it, at least under certain conditions of immunization and challenge. The ample body of evidence accumulated by tumor immunologists (see Section III) now permits a rational choice to be made as to the number of immunizations that should be used and the time interval between them in order to achieve an adequate representation of host response to immuni-zation with a given tumor. If the chosen conditions prove to promote tumor growth rather than to retard it, then this finding is valid when taken at face value. It would indicate that the tumor demonstrates "negative" or "promotional" antigenicity under the conditions chosen, and serve warning that the more usual immunization protocols may produce en-hancement rather than inhibition of tumor growth. Such a finding does not imply that more favorable conditions of immunization, as perhaps at-tained by addition of an inhibitor of suppressor cells such as cimetidine (Osband *et al.*, 1981), positive rather than negative antigenicity might not be displayed by the tumor.

In summary, tumor antigenicity is here defined as the tumor's ability to stimulate a response meaningful for its rejection by its autochthonous or isogenic host. Past evidence suggests that the results of immunorejection assays have meaning with regard to antitumor response in the autochtho-nous or isogenic host. The definition does not imply that the tumor might not behave very differently when different conditions of immunization are used against it.

C. REASONS FOR STANDARDIZATION OF AN ASSAY SYSTEM

Why do immunologists adhere closely to methods for preparation of specific antisera, yet tend to use their own adaptations of the many methods already described to measure tumor antigenicity? There appear to be many reasons for this discrepancy. While serological specificity has its roots in quantitative differences, these are often so large as to give the impression that they are really qualitative differences. In contrast, "tumor antigenicity" is in part dependent upon its definition. Prior to the present attempt, no proposal seems to have been made for a comprehensive quantitative assay system, which by analogy would represent the "reagent" necessary for standardization. Usually investigators have been satisfied to use their own method for determining tumor antigenicity or that facet of antigenicity in which they were interested, for their purpose was to obtain a comparative ranking of the tumors that they were using rather than a comparison of their tumors with those used by other research workers.

Even though the assay most commonly employed to measure the antigenicity of tumors has been *in vivo* immunorejection, the immunization protocols show a great deal of variation (see Section III). Taken together with other *in vivo* and *in vitro* assays that measure some particular facet of tumor antigenicity, what emerges is a veritable tower of Babel. This makes it difficult or impossible to fit the work performed by different investigators into a common framework from which meaningful conclusions can be drawn. Only when investigators are willing to impose sufficient discipline upon themselves to run a standardized assay for tumor antigenicity as routinely as they would use serological reagents to characterize their tumors will meaningful advances in tumor immunology be possible.

It is important to appreciate that a standardized assay for tumor antigenicity need not discourage investigators from using any other assay in addition. On the contrary, a full understanding of what such an assay measures can be gained only if other types of assays, and measurements of other facets of tumor antigenicity (such as the separate determination of immunogenicity and immunosensitivity), are run alongside. The ideal time to decide upon the details of a standardized assay would doubtless be at a tumor immunology workshop set up with this goal in mind; but until such a workshop has convened, investigators are urged to use the present system as a beginning on the road toward standardization of tumor antigenicity.

III. Past Work on Tumor Antigenicity

Tests related to the various facets of tumor antigenicity can be divided into two main groups: *in vivo* and *in vitro* assays. In this section, *in vivo* assays have been subdivided into those based on active immunization followed by challenge with viable tumor cells (prophylactic immunorejection tests), since this is the most common type of test performed in animals (Section III,A), and all other types of *in vivo* assays (Section III,B). For the present purpose, our interest in *in vitro* tests is confined to those that appear related to the immunogenicity of tumors, and only such tests are considered here (Section III,C).

A. *In Vivo* Tests of Immunorejective Strength

Such tests are based on immunization of an experimental group of animals with growth-inactivated tumor, or tumor extract, followed by challenge with viable tumor (Table I). Some of the conclusions that may be drawn from this past work are set out below. However, there are so many different types of tumors that it seems likely that some will be found to act differently, and that some of the conclusions will be invalid. Additional new data from our laboratory are given in Section VI.

1. Choice of Tumor Vaccine

As Prager (1975) has stated, tumor cells modified for use as a vaccine must (a) be immunogenic in autochthonous or isogenic hosts, (b) elicit an immune response that cross-reacts with the unmodified tumor cells, and (c) produce effects sufficiently rapid to be of value. To these three precepts can be added the following: (d) treatment of the tumor cells for use in immunization must growth inactivate them—it must prevent them from being able to grow into a tumor when inoculated into the host that is to be immunized, and (e) treatment of the tumor cells for use in immunization must not introduce an agent that will threaten the life of the host into which the treated cells are to be introduced.

It used to be thought that the most effective method for immunizing a relevant (autochthonous or isogenic) host* was by implantation of a tumor, followed by its excision. The most recent work by Prehn's group (Lawler *et al.*, 1981) indicates that a single inoculum of tumor X-irradiated with 15,000 rad and given by sc dorsal injection can be equally or more effective. In contrast, treatment of the cells with mitomycin C was somewhat less successful.

For the purpose of determining the relative antigenic strength of a tumor in the main range B (see Section V), the most effective method that introduces minimal extraneous agents seems appropriate. These considerations rule out the use of chemical or viral modification of the tumor cells, or the use of immune adjuvants or immunostimulants within this range. According to the above experiments (Lawler *et al.*, 1981), irradiation is the treatment of choice for growth inactivation of the tumor cells that are to be used as vaccine.

---

* Only autochthonous or isogenic hosts represent relevant test systems for tumor-associated antigens, since allogeneic or xenogeneic (heterologous) hosts recognize antigens on the tumor cell surface that are related to a disparity in normal tissue antigens between themselves and the host in which the tumor originated.

TABLE I

EXPERIMENTAL CONDITIONS AND RESULTS OF TESTS OF TUMOR ANTIGENICITY USING *in Vivo* ASSAYS OF TUMOR REJECTION (PROPHYLAXIS)

Induction or type of tumor	Host	Details of immunization — Treatment of tumor, number of injections, and route[a]	Details of challenge — Time interval, inoculum, route, and end point[b]	Further details and results	Reference
Chemical, sarcomas	Mice	Excision of growing tumor	0–7 days, 10–20 mg, sc, with or without 450 rad whole-body irradiation to recipients; antigenicity ratio = tumor size in controls/tumor size in immunized mice	There is an inverse relationship between latent period and antigenic strength which is due to immuno-selection during tumor development	Bartlett (1972a)
Various	Various			Parallel to skin graft rejection	Kahan (1972)
Various	Mice, rats	Ionizing radiation or UV used to prevent tumor takes, immunizations given 1–10 times	Various	Review of literature to 1972 regarding tumor rejection assays to measure antigenic strength; modification of cells to increase antigenicity is covered	Prager and Baechtel (1973)
Various	Various	Excision of growing tumor or injection of irradiated tumor given one to several times by sc or ip route	0–7 days after last immunization, challenge by trocar implant, ip, or iv; best end point is TD_{50}[c]	Detailed instructions for tumor rejection assays and review of the literature; full coverage of tumor transplantation, including definitions	Vaage (1973)
Various	Various	Not specified in detail	Not specified	Review that comments on low antigenicity of tumors, especially of spontaneous tumors; antigenicity determined by a virus does not prove viral etiology of the tumor	G. Klein (1975)

Lymphomas	Mice	Irradiation, sonication, chemical modification, adjuvant use; immunization 1–12 times, in various doses, by different routes	1 to 2 weeks after immunization seems optimal	Review of the various parameters that influence the results of tumor rejection assays to measure antigenic strength of tumors with or without antigenic modification; detailed discussion of methodology	Prager (1975)
Chemical, fibrosarcomas	Mice	Extraction of antigens, one injection with a range of doses	10 days after immunization, by iv or sc route	Review of methods to demonstrate the immunogenicity of soluble tumor antigens effective for tumor rejection	Pellis and Kahan (1976)
Various	Various	Not specified in detail	Not specified	Review that includes discussion of the immunogenicity of tumors, and of immune reactions to tumors	Harris and Sinkovics (1976)
Chemical, carcinomas	Mice	Allowed to regress in untreated mice	Thymectomy plus total-body irradiation necessary for takes	Antigenic strength of tumor was increased by tissue culture	Jamasbi and Nettesheim (1977)
Chemical, fibrosarcomas	Mice	43.5°C or 10,000 rad used to prevent takes; three immunizations given first sc, then ip	14–27 days after immunization, challenge with graded doses of tumor cells to determine TD_{50}^c	X-irradiation is more effective than heat treatment for preparation of a tumor cell vaccine that will not give tumor takes	Suit et al. (1977)
Spontaneous, leukemias	Guinea pigs	Viable or mitomycin C-treated tumor cells emulsified in complete Freund's adjuvant given in footpad, boosted 14 days later by id route	14–21 days after immunization, challenged with 3 × 10^5 or 5 × 10^6 cells; survivors recorded	Good immunoprotection obtained	Murphy et al. (1977)

(continued)

13

TABLE I (*continued*)

Induction or type of tumor	Host	Details of immunization — Treatment of tumor, number of injections, and route[a]	Details of challenge — Time interval, inoculum, route, and end point[b]	Further details and results	Reference
Spontaneous, chemical	Rats	Admixture of viable tumor with or without *C. parvum* injected only once	30–40 days later challenge sc; tumor growth or rejection noted	*Corynebacterium parvum* must be admixed with tumor cells to produce a beneficial effect when used as described	Pimm and Baldwin (1977)
Spontaneous, chemical	Rats	MuLV infection, 6000 rad, 0.2% formalin, or ligation all used to treat tumor cells and immunize host with one injection of 10^7 cells	3 days later, challenge with 10^3, 10^4, 10^5, 10^6, 10^7, or 10^8 tumor cells	Tumors artificially infected with MuLV provide much better protection against challenge than do the other treatments of the tumor cells used to immunize the host	Kobayashi *et al.* (1977, 1978)
Spontaneous, mammary carcinomas	Mice	Excision of 1 mm³ of tumor inoculum when grown to 8- to 10-mm size	0–7 days later, sc on side opposite to side immunized, or else ip	Tested in different transplant generations, most tumors were stable in antigenicity, but 3/100 lost immunosensitivity and 2/100 gained immunogenicity and/or immunosensitivity	Vaage (1978)
Spontaneous, mammary carcinomas	Mice	Excision of 1 mm³ of tumor inoculum when grown to 8- to 10-mm size	0 days later, sc implant of 5×10^5 cells at two sites; evaluated from tumor size measurements in immunized and control groups	Early appearance of tumors following immunization and challenge was related to presence of MTV-S and host genetics; end point of assay was the tumor growth value (average tumor size × percentage of incidence) in immunized and controls	Vaage and Medina (1978)

14

mammary tumors		tumor inoculum when grown to 8- to 10-mm size	10^5 cells; end point: tumor size in immunized and control groups	genicity were paralleled by in vitro results in a microcytotoxicity test of lymph node cells from immunized mice against tumor cells as targets	(1978)
Chemical, hepatomas	Rats	15,000 rad to tumor, one or three sc or ip injections of 10^4, 10^5, 10^6, 10^7, or 10^8 tumor cells	7–13 days after last immunization, challenge sc with 10^4 or 5×10^5 cells; determine tumor takes or rejections	Three immunizations were far more effective than one immunization, and the ip route better than sc immunization; tumor extracts prepared with 3 M KCl were only weakly effective within a restricted dose range	Price et al. (1978)
Chemical, respiratory tract tumors	Rats	Amputation of tumor-bearing leg 30–40 days after implantation	7 days later, im challenge with $10 \times TD_{50}$ cell dose	The tumors most able to metastasize were the least immunogenic	Jamasbi et al. (1978)
Chemical, cell cultures	Rats	15,000 rad to tumor, 10^6 cells injected im three times at three sites, or excision of tumors 20 mm in size two or three times	7 days later, with $5 \times TD_{50}$	Cultured tumor cells showed an increase in immunogenicity, apparently due to preexisting antigens rather than acquisition of antigens such as viruses, mycoplasmas, or serum proteins during culture	Jamasbi and Nettesheim (1979)
Spontaneous, mammary tumors	Mice	One injection of 10^4 mitomycin C-treated tumor cells given ip	14 days later, sc challenge with 5×10^5 cells	Tumor rejection is dependent upon specific recognition of tumor membrane antigens	Forni et al. (1979)
Spontaneous, mammary carcinomas	Mice	Excision of 1 mm^3 of tumor inoculum when grown to 8- to 10-mm size	0 days later, sc implant of 5×10^5 cells at two sites; evaluated from tumor size measurements in immunized and control groups	Total-body irradiation of the host prior to tumor implantation increases tumor growth *unrelated* to immunogenicity of the tumor	Vaage (1979)

(continued)

15

TABLE I (*continued*)

Induction or type of tumor	Host	Details of immunization — Treatment of tumor, number of injections, and route[a]	Details of challenge — Time interval, inoculum, route, and end point[b]	Further details and results	Reference
Spontaneous, mammary carcinomas	Mice	Excision of 1 mm³ of tumor inoculum when grown to 8- to 10-mm size	0 days later, sc implant of 5×10^5 cells at two sites; evaluated from tumor size measurements in immunized and control groups	Progression of tumors on repeated transplantation to acquire growth in lungs on iv challenge was related to acquisition of increased growth rate, not to loss of immunogenicity	Vaage (1980)
Various	Various	General description only	Not specified	Review that includes immunogenicity	Weiss (1980)
Chemical, viral	Mice	Soluble antigens injected twice, 10 days apart	10 days later, challenged with 2×10^4 cells; end point: percentage of tumor volume relative to the control group	Review on solubilized antigens of tumors effective for tumor rejection	Law et al. (1980)
Chemical, lymphosarcomas	Mice	One to three ip injections of cell membranes	4 days later, ip challenge with 5×10^4 to 10^6 tumor cells	Protection was achieved with cell membrane preparations; positive effect of pertussis vaccine and concanavalin A	McCollester (1980)
Chemical, fibrosarcomas	Mice	One sc injection of various doses of tumor cell extract	10 days later, sc challenge with 10^4 cells; end point by tumor size measurement	Extracts of tumor cells prepared with 2.5% butanol provide better protection against tumor challenge than obtained with 3 M KCl extraction	LeGrue et al. (1980)

16

Viral	Hamsters	One to three weekly immunizations with 10^4–10^7 5000-rad-treated cells given sc or ip	7–10 days later, challenge with 10^3 or 10^4 tumor cells; tumor takes or tumor diameter measurements noted	Results of tumor rejection assays were reproducible, evidenced by a lower number of tumor takes or inhibition of tumor growth	Mousawy et al. (1980)
Various	Various	Details not given	Not specified	Review: tumor-specific antigens demonstrated in a few instances	Old (1981)
Spontaneous	Rats	Four or five injections of 15,000-rad-, mitomycin C-, or formalin-treated tumor by trocar or, when trypsinized, ip or im at 2-week intervals	7 days after the last injection, challenge with minimum dose for tumor takes, or graded doses, or trocar injection of a 1- to 2-mm graft of tumor tissue	In no case was immunogenicity observed with 28 tumors of various types; concomitant immunity was also negative, except in one instance	Middle and Embleton (1981)
Chemical, sarcomas	Mice	Excision of a growing tumor 2- to 8-mm diameter, or 10^6 single cells, mitomycin C treated or 15,000 rad irradiated	20 days later, all mice received 350 rad whole-body radiation, challenged 1 day later with 5×10^4 and 5×10^5 cells or a 2-mm trocar piece	Trocar challenge was as sensitive a measure of antitumor response as challenge with a single cell suspension; three different methods of immunization and two methods of challenge gave comparable results	Lawler et al. (1981)
Various	Mice, rats	Details not given	Not specified	Review of antigenicity of tumor cells and its alteration by irradiation, other physical treatments, effect of chemicals, viruses, and hybridization of tumor cells	Kobayashi (1982)

[a] sc, Subcutaneously; ip, intraperitoneally; iv, intravenously; im, intramuscularly; id, intradermally. Immunizations are performed in such a manner that the tumor cannot grow to kill the host.

[b] Challenges are performed with viable tumor cells at a dose at which the majority or all of the mice in control groups die of tumor.

[c] TD_{50} is the tumor dose that causes 50% of injected mice to die from tumors.

17

2. Storage of Tumor Cells

Relatively few data are available on how storing cells affects their efficacy for use as tumor vaccines. Experiments with mouse lymphoma cells modified with iodoacetamide suggested that storage in the refrigerator as well as frozen storage was permissible. In the latter case, treatment with iodoacetamide had to be performed prior to freezing the cells rather than after thawing (Prager, 1975). An attempt to store guinea pig hepatoma cells L10 in liquid nitrogen at $-196°C$ proved unsuccessful: the thawed cells were not effective for immunoprophylaxis, despite the fact that 50% of the cells excluded trypan blue (Bartlett et al., 1977). However, Leibo (1978) has commented that Bartlett et al. incorrectly equated exclusion of trypan blue with cell viability. In fact, viability can be far lower than indicated by this test (Reif and Norris, 1960). Leibo suggested that the application of the precise techniques of modern cryobiology should make it possible to devise techniques for freezing and thawing single cell suspensions of tumors that will preserve intact both cell viability and cell immunogenicity. Leibo seems to have been correct, for Peters et al. (1979) reported that frozen L10 cells are as effective as freshly harvested L10 cells, but only as long as they are cryobiologically frozen, stored, and thawed, with a final vital-stain membrane integrity (after X-irradiation) approximately equal to that of freshly harvested L10 cells. When Peters' use of vital staining is examined in terms of Leibo's comments, it can be judged adequate, with the interpretation that even a slight drop in exclusion of vital stain might indicate a large loss in cell viability, which was paralleled by a large loss in cell immunogenicity (Peters et al., 1979).

3. Quantity of Tumor Tissue

There is agreement that, in general, the larger the dose of immunizing cells injected, the stronger the immunorejection response (Vaage, 1973; Prager, 1975; Price et al., 1978). There may well exist an optimal quantity beyond which injection of tumor will produce "high dose tolerance" and decrease rather than increase the response. This consideration appears particularly relevant for immunotherapy experiments, which contrast with the immunoprophylactic experiments in that the host already bears a growing mass of viable tumor prior to immunization. High dose tolerance could also be a problem when tumor extracts or purified tumor antigens are used, for then the quantity of immunogen available may be far higher than when whole cells are employed. For the purpose of measuring the relative antigenic strength of a tumor in the main range B (see Section V), use of whole tumor cells rather than of extracts or purified antigens seems preferable. This ensures that basic properties of tumor cells are measured, rather than those properties altered by the efficacy of the extraction procedure. For the purpose of making the assay convenient and easy for wide use, it seems more important to chose quantities of tumor cells for immunization that are conveniently obtainable, rather than to chose a cell dose that will provide optimal sensitization, especially since this dose may vary from tumor to tumor.

4. Number and Time Sequence of Injections

There is agreement that several injections are more effective than one or two (Vaage, 1973; Prager, 1975; Price et al., 1978). As many as 12 consecutive immunizations have been used (Prager, 1975). While most investigators have used an interval of 1 week between injections (Table I), 2 to 3 weeks have also been used (Middle and Embleton, 1981).

5. Route of Immunization Injections

While immunizations can be effective by many different routes, Price et al. (1978) have found that the ip route is superior to sc immunization. However, most work has been done using the sc route (Table I).

6. Time Interval between Last Immunization and Challenge

Most investigators have used 7 to 10 days for this time interval (Table I). However, as few as 0 to 6 days, or as many as 20 and 27 days, have been used also. For the present purpose, use of 7 days appears to be both appropriate and convenient.

7. Form of Challenge Cells

According to Lawler et al. (1981), challenge with explants of tumor tissue can be as sensitive as use of a single cell suspension. However, when a single cell suspension can be prepared, this has the great advantage that precise enumeration of the number of cells used for challenge is possible.

For tumor cells that are not already in ascites form, a conversion to ascites form is sometimes possible. This can be attempted by preparing a single cell suspension of the tumor and injecting it (10^7–10^8 cells) into the peritoneal cavity of a suitable number of mice. Once success in peritoneal conversion has been attained, the tumor can be passaged in ascites form.

The simplest method of preparing a single cell suspension of a solid tumor is by mechanical disruption. The tumor can be minced and passed through a stainless-steel mesh (Lawler et al., 1981). Further details are given in Sections V,B and VII,B,2,b.

Many tumors do not produce single cell suspensions of high viability when mechanical disruption is used. In that case, a variety of enzyme treatments may be used to disrupt the tumor (Vaage, 1973). A recent survey of these methods by Peters and co-workers (1979) suggests that use of collagenase I exhibited the greatest potential in dissociation with the least destruction of tumor cell surface antigens. However, different enzymes may be optimal for different types of tumors (see p. 41).

8. Cell Dose for Challenge Inoculum

Preliminary experiments are necessary to determine the TD_{50} dose (the dose of tumor cells at which 50% of injected animals die from tumor) and its reproducibility. Most investigators have used a challenge dose that is just above the TD_{50}; this is called the minimum lethal dose (MLD). More commonly, challenges have been performed at one or more multiples (such as 3, 10, 15, or 100 times) of the TD_{50} value (Table I). Trocar injection of fragments has also been used.

9. Route of Challenge Injections

For ascites tumors, the ip route is generally used for challenge. For solid tumors, sc, id, im, and iv routes have been employed. For injection by routes that localize the inoculum at a single anatomical site, the one invariable precept is that this site has not been injected previously during immunization.

10. End Point of Assay

The most usual observation that summarizes the results of the assay is the number of animals that develop tumors per total number challenged in each group. The experiment is generally continued sufficiently long to permit all animals that would eventually contract tumors due to the challenge injection to do so. The result cannot be used to differentiate between immunized and control mice challenged with the same inoculum if all or nearly all animals develop tumors. In that case, the mean day of death may provide a statistically significant difference between immunized and control mice. Measurement of tumor diameter is also used to differentiate such groups in situations where most animals, both in immunized and in control groups, develop tumors. Tumor diameters may either be measured when tumors in the control group have reached a preselected diameter, or serially with time, so that a convenient time point for analysis may be picked; or, all the results may be utilized. In many studies, the results obtained in immunized animals are compared to those obtained in their corresponding control group by use of an appropriate index (Table I). Invariably, statistical methods are employed to test whether observed differences between experimental and control groups are significant.

B. *In Vivo* Tests Not Based on Active Immunization and Challenge

In contrast to the tests listed in Table I, not all those listed in Table II can be used for quantitative determination of tumor antigenicity. To be sure that such tests have meaning with regard to the existence or relative strength of tumor-associated antigens, all must be performed either in autologous or in isogenic systems. With this restriction, qualitative evidence for the existence of tumor-associated antigens can be obtained from passive immunization with antisera, *in situ* tumor immunity (especially if this involved the testing *in vitro* of antibodies or of host cells separated from tumor grown *in vivo*), immunotherapy by nonspecific immunopotentiators, immunotherapy by active specific immunization (as long as this does not involve xenogenization by viral infection, since the viral infection could probably involve even the uninfected tumor used for challenge, as the host might become infected with virus during immunization with virus-infected tumor), specific adoptive immunotherapy, and instructional methods of immunotherapy. Quantitative information on the relative strength of tumor-associated antigens could be obtained from suitable adaptations of tests such as adoptive immunization, the Winn test, concomitant immunity, the delayed cutaneous hypersensitivity (DCH) reaction, and the passive delayed cutaneous hypersensitivity (PDCH) reaction (Table II).

C. *In Vitro* Tests That Involve Tumor Antigenicity

Positive results for any of the *in vitro* tests set out in Table III denote the presence of tumor-associated antigens only when obtained in autologous or isogenic systems. The various tests (Table III) differ in terms of their relevance, effort and time requirements, chance of success, sensitivity, reproducibility, and ease of quantification. There usually exist several modifications for each of the tests listed, and these tend to have different strengths and weaknesses.

For detection of antibody to tumor-associated antigens (Table III,A), neither precipitation, simple agglutination, or antibody-dependent cellular cytoxicity (ADCC) are used commonly. In contrast, radioimmunoassay (RIA), enzyme-linked immunosorbent assay (ELISA), fluorescent anti-

TABLE II

In Vivo TESTS OF TUMOR ANTIGENICITY (EXCLUDING
PROPHYLAXIS) AND OF IMMUNOTHERAPY

Name of test	Description of *in vivo* assay method	Reference
Passive immunization with alloantiserum	Alloantiserum, prepared by injecting mice of different strains with C57BL leukemia EL-4, suppressed the temporary growth of this leukemia in C57BL mice. This suggested the presence of the X antigen on EL4 cells	Gorer and Amos (1956)
Passive immunization with isogenic antiserum	Autoantiserum or isogenic antiserum were prepared by injection of growth-inabled tumor cells into their respectively autochthonous or isogenic host. If antiserum will either inhibit or enhance the growth of the tumor cells in isogenic hosts, this indicates the presence of tumor-associated antigen	Old and Boyse (1964); Klein (1968)
Passive immunization with "specific" antibodies	Antibodies with varying degrees of specificity may be prepared in allogeneic or xenogeneic hosts, or monoclonal antibodies may be prepared by allogeneic or xenogeneic hybridomas. The immunogens used to prepare these antibodies have included whole cells, membranes, extracts, or purified antigens of tumor cells. A variety of methods have been used in attempts to remove antibodies directed against normal rather than tumor-associated antigens. If it can be shown that the purified antibodies are specific for the tumor in question, then the possibility arises that these antibodies indicate the presence of tumor-associated antigens, which might be immunogenic in autochthonous or isogenic hosts	Nadler *et al.* (1980); Davis and Preston (1981)
Adoptive immunization	Transfer of lymphoid cells from host immunized with autochthonous or isogenic tumor to another isogenic mouse which either bears this tumor or is simultaneously or subsequently challenged with it; the references cite reviews on this subject	Snell (1963); Hellström and Möller (1965); Vaage (1973)
Winn test	Lymphoid cells taken from mice immunized with autochthonous or isogenic tumor are briefly incubated with a small proportion of viable tumor cells, then the mixture is injected into normal autochthonous or isogenic mice; the outgrowth of tumor cells may be inhibited relative to controls, for which the lymphoid cells are taken from unimmunized mice	Winn (1961); Pellis and Kahan (1976)

TABLE II (*continued*)

Name of test	Description of *in vivo* assay method	Reference
Concomitant immunity	Patients with progressively growing tumors may possess concomitant immunity, being able to reject their own tumor if injected sc in small quantity	Southam *et al.* (1966)
Repopulation of lethally irradi-ated mice	Repopulation with lymphoid cells from isogenic mice, irrespective of whether normal or immunized, inhibits the growth of primary or transplanted tumors which they bear; this represents *nonspecific* cellular cytotoxicity to tumor-associated antigen	Basombrio and Prehn (1972)
Delayed cutaneous hypersensi-tivity (DCH) reaction	If guinea pigs immunized against an isologous tumor are challenged id with viable tumor cells, they may develop a typical DCH reaction at the site of challenge, and this may prevent tumor growth; DCH reactions tend to be much weaker in mice, but if the mouse's footpad is used as the injection site, a DH reaction marked by footpad swelling may occur	Churchill *et al.* (1968); Bartlett (1972)
Passive delayed cutaneous hypersensi-tivity (PDCH) reaction	Lymphoid cells taken from a donor immunized with isologous tumor are mixed with a small proportion of viable tumor cells, briefly incubated, and injected id (rather than sc as in the Winn test) into a normal isogenic host; they may cause a typical PDCH reaction, which may prevent tumor growth	Kronman *et al.* (1969a); Bartlett (1972b)
In situ tumor immunity	Immune reactions that occur at the site of the tumor in the tumor-bearing host may, depend-ing upon their type, be classified either as *in vivo* or *in vitro* reactions against tumor-associated antigens	Witz and Hanna (1980)
Immunotherapy	Immunotherapy differs from immunoprophylaxis (Table I) in that the time sequence of the immunizations and the challenge are reversed. Since the challenge is given first, the subse-quent immunizations must act swiftly relative to tumor growth, or they will prove ineffective. Immunotherapy can be viewed as an attempt to enhance the immune response to tumor-associated antigens. In that case, the degree of its success may be related to the strength of tumor-associated antigens. References refer mainly to reviews	Gilbert (1972); Southam and Friedman (1976); Green *et al.* (1977); Hersh and Sinkovics (1978); Terry and Windhorst (1978); Reif (1979); Woodruff (1980)

(*continued*)

TABLE II (*continued*)

Name of test	Description of *in vivo* assay method	Reference
Immunotherapy by nonspecific immunopotentiation	A form of immunotherapy in which presumably nonspecific stimulants of immune reactivity are injected into the tumor-bearing host. Active agents include certain bacterial toxins, BCG, *C. parvum*, levanisole, tuftsin, and others. In the case of BCG, optimal affects are obtained when this adjuvant is mixed with or injected into tumor	See references under Immunotherapy; Crispen (1976)
Immunotherapy by active specific immunization	Active specific immunization can be performed with unaltered, aged, or irradiated cells, as well as with cell membranes, extracts, purified antigens, chemically altered cells or cell products, enzyme-treated cells, cells xenogenized by viral infection, and cell hybrids of which the tumor is a partner	See references under Immunotherapy; Prager (1975); Murthy (1976); Jami *et al.* (1976); Baumal and Marks (1981)
Specific adoptive immunotherapy	Specific adoptive methods of immunotherapy refer to transfer of specifically immunized lymphoid cells to the tumor-bearing host. In animal systems, the immunization can be performed isogenically, so that the sensitization is directed against tumor-associated antigens	See references under Immunotherapy
Passive immunotherapy with "specific" antibodics	Preparation of such antibodies has already been discussed at the start of this table. Antibodies may be used without further modification, with or without addition of complement (C), which is required for direct lysis of cells by antibody. Antibodies can be made more toxic by attachment of a radioisotope such as ^{131}I, or of various toxins or chemotherapeutic agents. One of the sources of difficulty is the frequent presence of tumor-associated antigens in the circulation	Reif *et al.* (1974); Rosenberg and Terry (1977); Goldenberg (1980)
Instructional methods of immunotherapy	Instructional methods include the passive injection of transfer factor, immune RNA, thymosin, and interferon. In each case where a positive effect on tumor growth has been obtained, it appears to depend upon strengthening the immune response to tumor-associated antigens	See references under Immunotherapy; Crane *et al.* (1978); Gunby (1981)

TABLE II (*continued*)

Name of test	Description of *in vivo* assay method	Reference
Elimination of suppressor cells	Certain types of tumors can stimulate the host to produce suppressor cells that switch off some of the immune responses against tumor cells. The drugs busulfan and cimetidine appear to inhibit suppressor cell activity nonspecifically. Methods for specific inhibition of suppressor cells that frustrate immune responses to tumor cells have not yet been found	Broder and Waldmann (1978a,b); Mizushima *et al.* (1981); Osband *et al.* (1981)
Immunosorption of tumor-associated antigen–antibody complexes	The immune response against tumor-associated antigens may be rendered ineffective by the presence of antigen–antibody complexes between tumor-associated antigens and host antibodies against them. Extracorporeal (*ex vivo*) adsorption of immune complexes by a nonspecific immunosorbent such as *Staphylococcus aureus* has produced dramatic therapeutic results in feline leukemia, and initial trials in human breast cancer have given encouraging results. While the treatment may protect the host's own tumor-specific antibodies by removal of circulating immune complexes that contain tumor antigens, the true mechanism is still obscure	Jones *et al.* (1980); Terman *et al.* (1981)

body (FA), and immune adherence (IA) are widely used and extremely sensitive tests for antibody. Compared to RIA, ELISA has the advantage that the conjugated antibody reagent has a long shelf life, and that expensive equipment for measurement of radioisotopes is not required. Fluorescent antibody is used for localization of antigens on histologic sections. Immune adherence has been used to detect antibodies in melanoma patients (Shiku *et al.*, 1976), and can even utilize formalin-fixed cells (Müller and Sorg, 1975).

With regard to the assays that involve immune lymphoid cells (Table III, B), use of the Millipore chamber is now outdated, and the colony inhibition (CI) test has largely been abandoned in favor of the microcytotoxicity (MC) test. Although use of the MC test and of lymphocyte transformation is common, both tests suffer from a high level of control reactivity and a high variability in results. The choice of concentrations of antigens used in these tests has been criticized on the basis that it is made to produce the expected results (Hager and Heppner, 1978). Similar considerations

TABLE III

In Vitro TESTS THAT INVOLVE TUMOR IMMUNOGENICITY AND/OR
IMMUNOSENSITIVITY WHEN USED IN AUTOLOGOUS OR ISOGENIC SITUATIONS

Name of assay	Description of *in vitro* assay	Reference
A. Antibody Precipitation	Immune precipitation has been used for α-fetoprotein, but not using autologous or isogenic sera	Abelev *et al.* (1979)
Agglutination	Tumor cells can be agglutinated by antisera. However, end points are far more difficult to quantify than for assays such as immune cytolysis (see below). Tumor cells are more easily agglutinated by plant lectins than are normal cells. Use of subthreshold levels of lectins to enhance antibody-mediated agglutination does not seem to have been studied	Shields (1975)
Radioimmuno- assay	Autologous production of IgM antibody against carcinoembryonic antigen (CEA) has been demonstrated by this method	Gold *et al.* (1978)
Enzyme- linked im- munosorbent assay	An adaptation of solid-phase RIA in which an enzyme is used as immunoglobulin marker instead of a radioisotope	Voller and Bidwell (1980)
Fluorescent antibody	Commonly used to demonstrate antitumor antibodies; however, quantitative measurements are more easily performed using RIA	Möller (1961); Klein and Klein (1964)
Immune cytolysis	Lysis of cells by antibody in the presence of complement; a precise method that uses an end point of 50% cytolysis; restricted to tumors with a high concentration of surface antigens, such as leukemias and lymphomas	Reif and Kim (1971); Vaage and Agarwal (1978)
Complement fixation	This laborious method has the advantage that it can be applied to nonviable tumor cells and their extracts. Quantification may be improved by use of tumor antigen to inhibit C fixation	Eilber and Morton (1970); Humphrey *et al.* (1974)
Immune adherence	This sensitive method uses indicator cells (primate erythrocytes or nonprimate platelets) to attach to antigen–antibody complexes by means of their C3 receptor. Binding of indicator cells is observed under the microscope or by reading hemagglutination patterns. It can be used to detect tumor-associated antigen (whether on cells, biopsy material, or cell membranes) or tumor-directed antibody. Quantification is imprecise	Nelson (1953); Hager and Heppner (1978)

TABLE III (*continued*)

Name of assay	Description of *in vitro* assay	Reference
Antibody-dependent cellular cytotoxicity	Normal lymphoid cells can be directed to attack tumor target cells by the addition of antitumor antibody. Most commonly employed with allogeneic or xenogeneic antibody	Perlmann and Perlmann (1970); Zichelboim et al. (1973)
Additional methods that involve antibodies	These methods include inhibition of tumor cell motility, the mixed antiglobulin reaction, and the related mixed hemadsorption test.	Woodruff (1980); Harris and Sinkovics (1976)
B. Immune lymphoid cells		
Cell-mediated immunity	Thoracic duct lymphocytes from mice immunized with tumor are mixed with viable tumor cells and placed in Millipore chambers in the peritoneal cavities of isogenic hosts; cytotoxicity to tumor cells is observed	Hattler and Amos (1966)
Colony inhibition test	An adaptation of the above test. Tumor cells are plated in Petri dishes, and sensitized lymphoid cells are added. Inhibition in outgrowth of the tumor cells relative to controls represents a positive result. Test requires multiple controls, and can be difficult to quantify. "Serum blocking" of the colony inhibition test occurs when addition of serum from a tumor-bearing host to the Petri dishes reverses the inhibition of colony formation effected by the immune lymphocytes. Serum blocking is attributed to the presence of tumor antigens, or of immune complexes composed of tumor antigens and host antibodies	Hellström and Hellström (1971); Kaiser and Reif (1975)
Microcytotoxicity test	A microadaptation of the colony inhibition test in which the total number of tumor cells rather than the colonies are determined following incubation with sensitized tumor cells. Microculture wells rather than Petri dishes are used. In long-term tests, incubation for 2 or 3 days at 37°C is used while in short-term assays, incubation for 4–8 hours is employed. A far more reliable estimate of the loss of tumor cells is obtained when they are radiolabeled. Use of ^{51}Cr for this purpose is only useful for short-term assays, whereas [^{125}I]iodo-2'-deoxyuridine is more sensitive for 1-day assays and [^{3}H]proline for 2-day assays. Technetium-99m (^{99m}Tc) appears to be at least as effective as [^{125}I]iododeoxyuridine	Brunner et al. (1968); Takasugi and Klein (1970); Barth et al. (1972); Oldham et al. (1977)

(*continued*)

TABLE III (*continued*)

Name of assay	Description of *in vitro* assay	Reference
Lymphocyte binding	A simple test that depends on the adherence of sensitized lymphocytes to the tumor cells used for sensitization. Test is scored following incubation for 1 hour under tissue culture conditions	Lavrovsky and Viksler (1980)
Leukocyte adherence inhibition	Peritoneal cells from mice immunized against a chemically induced tumor were inhibited from adhering to glass by addition of soluble antigen obtained from the tumor used for immunization. The response was specific for each of several tumors induced by the same carcinogen. The method has been used to show a specific reaction against human tumors, and claimed to correlate with the clinical state of tumor patients	Halliday and Miller (1972); Gibson and Martin (1978); Schmidt *et al.* (1981)
Lymphocyte transformation (blastogenesis)	When sensitized lymphocytes are exposed in tissue culture to an antigen to which they have been sensitized, a proportion may transform into lymphoblasts. This transformation is accompanied by an increased uptake of [^{3}H]thymidine which can be used as an index of lymphocyte transformation	Bach *et al.* (1969); Golub (1975)
Generation of cytotoxic lymphocytes *in vitro*	Following primary immunization *in vivo*, secondary induction of cytotoxic lymphocytes against virally induced tumors is possible in tissue culture	Wagner and Rollinghoff (1973); Alaba and Law (1978); Yefenof *et al.* (1980)
C. Lymphokines Migration inhibition factor (indirect MIF assay)	Macrophages placed in a capillary tube will normally migrate outward onto glass. However, migration stops when macrophages encounter MIF, which is released when lymphocytes meet the antigen to which they have been immunized. Thus, if tumor-sensitized lymphocytes and normal macrophages are mixed and placed in a capillary tube, the degree to which macrophages are inhibited from migrating outward measures lymphocyte sensitization to the tumor cells. Assay is simple and requires only one day	Kronman *et al.* (1969b)

TABLE III (*continued*)

Name of assay	Description of *in vitro* assay	Reference
Leukocyte migration inhibition (direct LMI assay)	More successful than the "indirect" MIF assay has been use of the "direct" LMI assay in which leukocytes from cancer patients are tested for migration from capillary tubes in the presence and absence of extracts of the patient's tumor, or tumors of similar histologic type. It is not known whether the lymphokines involved in the MIF and LMI assays are identical	Andersen *et al.* (1970); Rivera *et al.* (1979)
Other lymphokine assays	At last count, the different soluble factors produced by activated lymphocytes were capable of inducing at least 56 biologic activities; most of these seemed unrelated to immunity. As far as specific immune response to tumor-associated antigens is concerned, only immune lymphokines seem to be relevant. Some of the assays described above, including LAI, may depend on the action of immune lymphokines.	Bloom (1980)

apply to the leukocyte adherence inhibition (LAI) test, which also suffers from the disadvantage that the level of response is often low. Lymphocyte binding appears to be a simple test that has not yet been explored in depth.

Lymphokine assays (Table III,C) have the advantage of simplicity when compared to long-term MC tests. While the antigens used in the leukocyte migration inhibition (LMI) test are usually soluble extracts of tumor cells, cryostat sections of tumors have also been used (Black *et al.*, 1974). Capillary tube assays can be performed in 3 hours, which is a great advantage (Urist *et al.*, 1976). Relatively little work seems to have been done with LMI in autologous systems (Hager and Heppner, 1978). An adaptation has been described in which soluble antigens are used to inhibit the spreading of monocytes from tumor patients (Mazuran *et al.*, 1976).

IV. Choice of Assay Conditions

The fact that widely different assay conditions can be justified is attested by the variety of conditions chosen by investigators to measure tumor antigenicity. The present purpose is to discuss what is optimal and what is practical for each of the choices that must be made for assay conditions. Certainly, a compromise must be made between what is optimal and what is practical.

As a result of this discussion, recommendations are made as to what are desirable values, what are acceptable limits, and what constitutes undesirable conditions for assay. The intent is to suggest guidelines for future investigators. While it is hoped that they will choose desirable values, the most important point about their assay is that they specify succinctly what conditions they have chosen. The advantage in the choice of assay conditions that are in reasonable agreement with those of a standardized assay, such as the present one, is that other investigators are able to relate the results obtained to a common standard of tumor antigenicity.

A. TYPE, SEX, AND NUMBER OF ANIMALS IN EACH GROUP

The proper strain for tests of antigenic strength is the inbred strain in which the tumor under consideration arose. Less ideal is use of F_1 hybrids, one parent of which is the strain in which the tumor arose. In theory, all histocompatibility antigens are dominantly inherited and therefore expressed in F_1 hybrids, which are heterozygous for the genes involved. However, a few minor histocompatibility antigens may be inherited recessively and only expressed when the genes are inherited in homozygous form. In that case, an F_1 hybrid would recognize as foreign a weak antigen, coded by such genes, which would be present on the tumor cell (which was derived from the parent homozygous strain) but absent from the hybrid. In practice, an F_1 hybrid effect can be observed only when low doses of tumor cells are used for challenge, and is quite weak (J. Klein, 1975).

Regarding the sex of mice, the hormonal balance may affect the "takes" and growth of some types of tumors. Therefore, it seems wise to confine all work to one sex. Since females fight less than males and seldom die due to this cause, use of female mice is recommended.

The number of mice chosen for experimental and control groups has a surprisingly strong impact on the likelihood that the results obtained will prove to be statistically significant. The entire system suggested here for scoring antigenic strength rests upon whether or not the results of a given assay show statistically significant differences between experimental and control groups. Therefore, it has been necessary to determine how many animals are necessary in order to demonstrate a statistically significant difference between the results obtained for experimental and control groups (Appendix, Section VII,A). The results indicate that the larger the

TABLE IV

RECOMMENDED CONDITIONS FOR IMMUNOREJECTION ASSAY OF ANTIGENIC STRENGTH

Item	Most desirable choice	Less desirable choice, notes
Strain of animal	Inbred strain of origin of the tumor	F_1 hybrid, with strain of origin of tumor as one parent
Sex and age of mice	Females 9–24 weeks old	Males 9–24 weeks old. Sex should not be interchanged
Number of animals per group	Eight	Seven or nine
Vaccine and its treatment	Freshly harvested tumor, irradiated with 12,000 rad	Frozen tumor if tested for equivalence with fresh tumor
Route for vaccine injections	ip for ascites tumors, sc for solid tumors	ip for all types of tumors
Quantity of tumor injected per mouse	5 million ascites tumor cells, or 25 mg wet weight of minced solid tumor	3–10 million ascites cells, or 10–30 mg solid tumor
Number of injections	6 weekly injections, or both 4 and 6 weekly injections	4 weekly injections
Addition of C. parvum	4 weekly injections of tumor admixed with 20 μg C. parvum[a]	Omit this trial
Time to challenge	One week after last immunization	5–10 days after last immunization
Form of tumor cells used for challenge	Single cell suspension prepared under mild conditions	Mince loaded into syringe with stirrer method, kept in suspension during injections
Tumor cell dose used for challenge	$3 \times LD_{50}$, $10 \times LD_{50}$, and $100 \times LD_{50}$, plus controls at each of these levels and at $1 \times LD_{50}$, $0.3 \times LD_{50}$, and $0.1 \times LD_{50}$	For highly antigenic tumors, substitute $1000 \times LD_{50}$ for $3 \times LD_{50}$
Route of challenge injections	ip for ascites tumors, sc for solid tumors, on side opposite to that used for immunizations	ip for all types of tumors
Total number of separate groups of animals	For *each* of the three doses used for challenge, add groups immunized 6×, 4× + C. Parvum or BCC[a], 2×, and 0× (controls). Add also three control groups for challenge at low LD_{50} (see Table XII)	For *each* of the three doses used for challenge, add groups immunized 4× and 0× (controls). Add also three control groups for challenge at low LD_{50}

(*continued*)

TABLE IV (*continued*)

Item	Most desirable choice	Less desirable choice, notes
Data determined for each group of mice	Number of survivors/tumor deaths, days from challenge to tumor death, tumor diameters at 3- to 7-day intervals (for solid tumors only)	Omit determination of tumor diameters for solid tumors
Evaluation of data	Use statistical methods described in Appendix, Section VII	Same
Further tests and scoring of tumor antigenicity	See text and Tables IX and X	Same

[a] *Corynebacterium parvum* is purchased from Wellcome Fine Chemicals, 3030 Cornwallis Road, Research Triangle Park, North Carolina 27709 and used at 20 μg admixed with 25 mg minced tumor or 5 million viable cells of a single cell suspension of tumor for each of the four injections of each mouse. Instead of *C. parvum*, BCG (ITR, Biochemical Research, 904 West Adams Street, Chicago, Illinois 60607) may be used at 1×10^6 viable organisms.

number of animals chosen, the lower the difference in results obtained for experimental and control groups that prove to have statistical significance. Still, if one investigator uses a different number of animals per group than other investigators, the results of his assay will be atypical, irrespective of whether he has used fewer or more animals. Therefore, a range of desirable numbers of animals is suggested (Table IV). Also included in Table IV are limits between which less desirable values can be suggested.

B. TUMOR VACCINE

A consideration of the data discussed in Section III,A,1–3 suggests that freshly harvested tumor X-irradiated with approximately 12,000 rad be used in otherwise untreated hosts. With regard to the quantity of the irradiated tumor, it is important to realize that convenient rather than optimal conditions have been chosen (Table IV). While higher quantities may produce stronger immunity, adequate results are obtained under the conditions chosen.

C. NUMBER OF IMMUNIZATIONS

Regarding how many immunizations are necessary, the work discussed in Section III,A,4 as well as experiments performed in our laboratory indicate that extensive immunization is necessary to obtain positive results with some types of tumors. For instance, six successive weekly immunizations with the L1210 subline L/Ha produced statistically significant survival after challenge with 1.5×10^6 tumor cells, while four successive weekly immunizations (begun 2 weeks later, to permit simultaneous challenge 1 week after the last immunization) did not have a statistically significant effect (Table V). A similar experiment performed with the L1210 subline L-W showed that six weekly immunizations produced four survivors in all treatment groups, while four weekly immunizations produced only one survivor (Table VI). While these differences are not statistically significant, the mean time of survival of the group of mice immunized six times was 24.1 ± 7.7 days, compared to 14.7 ± 5.1 days for the group immunized four times, when challenged with 30,000 tumor cells. These survival times are significantly different when tested by the one-way analysis of variance ($p < 0.01$), indicating that six immunizations were more protective (see Appendix, Section VII,A,2).

TABLE V

RESULTS OF CHALLENGE WITH VIABLE TUMOR: EFFECT OF VARIATION IN NUMBER
OF IMMUNIZATIONS AND POTENTIATION WITH BCG AND *C. parvum*
ON IMMUNOREJECTION ASSAY WITH L1210-L/HA[a]

Challenge dose of L1210-L/Ha cells (number)	Number of weekly immunizations with 5×10^6 irradiated L1210-L/Ha cells									
	0×		6×		4×		4× +BCG[b]		4× + C. parvum[c]	
	S[d]	D	S	D	S	D	S	D	S	D
5	2	7								
50	1	8								
15,000	0	7	7	0	7	0	7	0	7	0
150,000	—		5	2	6	1	7	0	6	0
1,500,000	—		5	2	3	3	6	0	7	0
15,000,000	—		3	3	1	6	6	1	2	4

[a] DBF₁ hybrid females were immunized as indicated and challenged with viable cells of the L/Ha subline of L1210 leukemia, at cell doses 30-fold lower than those shown, 1 week after the last immunization. All immunized mice survived this challenge. These mice, plus fresh mice to serve as controls, were rechallenged with the stated numbers of viable L/Ha cells 4 weeks after the first challenge. Because the protocol for RAS determination was not followed, the results cannot be used to assess a RAS score.

[b] One million viable BCG organisms were mixed with the irradiated tumor cells injected into each mouse. See footnote *a* of Table IV for source of BCG.

[c] Twenty micrograms *C. parvum* were mixed with the irradiated tumor cells injected into each mouse. See footnote *a* of Table IV for source of *C. parvum*.

[d] S, Survivors; D, tumor deaths.

TABLE VI

RESULTS OF CHALLENGE WITH VIABLE TUMOR: EFFECT OF VARIATION IN NUMBER OF IMMUNIZATIONS AND POTENTIATION WITH BCG AND C. parvum ON IMMUNOREJECTION ASSAY WITH L1210-L-W[a]

| Challenge dose of L1210-L-W cells (number) | Number of weekly immunizations with 5×10^6 irradiated L1210-L-W cells | | | | | | | | | |
| | 0× | | 6× | | 4× | | 4× + BCG[a] | | 4× + C. parvum[b] | |
	S[c]	D	S	D	S	D	S	D	S	D
5	5	4								
30	1	8								
300	0	9								
3,000	0	9	3	6	1	8	6	2	9	0
30,000	0	9	0	7	0	9	7	2	9	0
300,000	0	8	1	6	0	9	6	3	6	2
3,000,000	0	9	0	7	0	9	3	6	4	4
30,000,000	0	9	0	8	0	9	0	9	2	7

[a] L-W subline of L1210 leukemia used for challenge of DBF_1 hybrid females 18 weeks old at the time of challenge. Experiment performed in two portions on the same day to reduce the total time required between sacrifice of a tumor-bearing mouse and the last use of its cells to challenge mice to less than 2.5 hours for each portion of the experiment.

[b] See footnotes b and c of Table V for details regarding BCG and C. parvum.

[c] S, Survivors; D, tumor deaths.

Similar data were obtained when solid tumors rather than ascites tumors were tested. For the chemically induced carcinoma SMx-E, challenge with 5.0 mg per mouse gave survivors/tumor deaths ratios of 7/2 for the group immunized with six injections, compared to 0/9 or 1/8 for the groups immunized four or three times, respectively (Table VII). The results for the latter two immunizations are significantly less prophylactic than those for the former ($p < 0.01$) when tested by Fisher's exact probability test (see Appendix, Section VII,A,1 and Table XXVII) (Fisher, 1946). For the chemically induced sarcoma SMx-F, which has weak antigenicity in its transplant generation 51, there was no difference in survivors/tumor deaths for mice immunized either six or four times (Table VIII). However, tumor diameter measurements made on 9 different days at 3- or 4-day intervals showed that the mean size of tumors was significantly smaller ($p < 0.01$) for mice immunized six times than for those immunized four times when the data were tested statistically (see Appendix, Section VII,A,3).

All of the above data, obtained with four different tumors, indicate that six immunizations produce a higher degree of immunity than four immuni-

TABLE VII

RESULTS OF CHALLENGE WITH VIABLE TUMOR: EFFECT OF VARIATION IN NUMBER
OF IMMUNIZATIONS ON IMMUNOREJECTION ASSAY WITH TUMOR SMx-E[a]

Challenge dose of SMx-E cells (mg)	Number of weekly immunizations with 25 mg irradiated SMx-E cells									
	0×		2×		3×		4×		6×	
	S[b]	D	S	D	S	D	S	D	S	D
0.8	8	1								
2	0	9								
5	3	6	2	7	1	8	0	9	7	2
12	2	7	3	6	0	9	1	8	1	8
30	0	9	0	9	0	8	0	9	0	9
75	0	9	0	9	0	8	0	9	0	8

[a] Challenges were performed with transplant generation 39 of carcinoma SMx-E, induced with DMBA in the submaxillary glands of a C57BL/6J mouse, in which strain this tumor is carried (Cataldo and Reif, 1982). The mice used here were DBF$_1$ hybrid females 16 weeks old on the day of challenge. At any one dose of minced challenge cells, the order in which groups were injected was 6×, 4×, 3×, 2×, and 0×. Thus, the control group was injected last to avoid spurious positive results due to progressive loss of viability of the cells. Experiment done in four portions on same day, with sacrifice of a tumor-bearing mouse for each portion of the experiment.
[b] S, Survivors; D, tumor deaths.

zations. Further, in some instances (Tables VI and VII) no substantial increase in survivors/tumor deaths was achieved unless six immunizations were given. While the length of time required to perform six successive weekly immunizations constitutes a serious disadvantage, the data speak for themselves.

D. ROUTE OF IMMUNIZATIONS AND CHALLENGE INJECTIONS

In our work, we have used the ip route both for immunization and for challenge with ascites tumors, but use the sc route for work with solid tumors. As indicated in Section III,A,5, the ip route may be superior for all types of tumors. Lacking definitive data, it is suggested that investigators retain the above distinction in routes of injection (Table IV).

E. CONDITIONS FOR CHALLENGE INJECTIONS

For choice of a time interval between the last immunization and challenge, data are relatively sparse (Section III,A,6). With reqard to the form

TABLE VIII

RESULTS OF CHALLENGE WITH VIABLE TUMOR: EFFECT OF VARIATION IN NUMBER OF
IMMUNIZATIONS AND POTENTIATION WITH BCG AND C. parvum ON
IMMUNOREJECTION ASSAY WITH TUMOR SMx-F[a]

Challenge dose of SMx-F cells (mg)	Number of weekly immunizations with 25 mg irradiated SMx-F cells										
	0×		6×		4×		4× + BCG		4× + C. parvum		4× + both[b]
	S[c]	D	S	D	S	D	S	D	S	D	S	D
0.03	7	2										
0.3	3	6	4	4	4	5	6	3	8	1	8	0
3.0	0	9	0	9	0	8	0	9	2	7	2	7

[a] Challenges performed with transplant generation 51 of sarcoma SMx-F, induced with DMBA in the submaxillary glands of a C57BL/6J mouse, in which strain this tumor is carried (Cataldo and Reif, 1982). The mice used here were DBF₁ hybrid females 15 weeks old on the day of challenge. The experiment was performed in two portions on the same day, with sacrifice of a tumor-bearing mouse for each portion. The order of injection of groups at each of the two cell doses was from right to left of the groups recorded above.

[b] See footnotes b and c of Table V for details regarding BCG and C. parvum. The last group (extreme right of this table) was injected with both BCG and with C. parvum admixed with tumor.

[c] S, Survivors; D, tumor deaths.

of challenge cells (Section III,A,7), single cell suspensions are preferable to minced tumor if their viability is high. The ideal cell dose for challenge to obtain the most sensitive distinction between an immunized and a control group is the dose at which 100% or close to 100% of the control mice develop tumors, while also being the minimum challenge dose that will permit this result. To achieve inclusion of one pair of experimental and control groups for which this ideal dose is realized, it may be necessary to straddle the dose at which this result is expected from preliminary experiments. If the tumor is expected to be highly antigenic, pairs of groups challenged at much higher doses should be included in the experiment.

The most meaningful end point of the assay (see Section III,A,10) is provided by data on survivors/tumor deaths, since these data indicate whether or not prophylactic immunizations can be used to prevent the development of tumor. The data are easily tested for significance by Fisher's exact probability test (Appendix, Section VII,A,1). Additional data, which require little effort for collection, are the number of days between challenge and death of each tumor-bearing mouse. The mean day of death for mice from different groups can then be compared by one-way analysis of variance (AOV) (Appendix, Section VII,A,2). Far more laborious is the measurement of the length and breadth of tumors on 5 or more different days. However, when such data are treated by modern statistical methods (Appendix, Section VII,A,3), significant differences between immunized and control groups are sometimes found in the absence of significant differences in data on survivors/tumor deaths or of the mean day of death from tumor.

V. Comprehensive System for Measurement of Tumor Antigenicity

The system outlined below has already been described, although in a more rudimentary form (Reif and Tomas, 1980; Argyris and Reif, 1981; Reif, 1981). Here, changes and refinements are presented. Suggestions are also made for the extension of the classification from experimental to human tumors.

A. RELATIVE RANGES OF TUMOR ANTIGENICITY AND SCORING

Ranges that cover the entire spectrum of tumor antigenicity can be assigned in a manner that takes into account some of the basic differences in the immunobiological behavior of tumors (Table IX). Range A includes tumors that are rejected by isogenic hosts unless the hosts are immunosuppressed; some of the tumors induced by UV light (Kripke, 1980) fall in this range. Range B encompasses tumors with sufficiently high antigenic strength that immunization with irradiated tumor cells provides significant protection against tumor challenge; some chemically and virally induced tumors belong in this range. Range C includes tumors that are sufficiently weakly antigenic to fail the tests of range B, yet are capable of tumor rejection provided that either the isogenic host or the tumor immunogen are treated appropriately. Also included in range C are tumors that fail to provide protection against tumor "takes" in range B, yet delay or retard tumor growth when used for immunization. Range D includes tumors which are sufficiently weakly antigenic that they fail to give positive results for the tests of ranges B and C, yet show significant immunogenicity or immunosensitivity *in vitro*. Finally, tumors that fail to react positively in range B, C, and D are assigned to class E, indicating minimal relative antigenicity.

More detailed treatment of the above classification scheme is presented in Table X. Many of the ranges outlined in Table IX can be subdivided into subranges. These subranges comprise tests that can be run either alone or together with those of another subrange. Examples of the use of some of these tests are given later.

TABLE IX
OVERVIEW OF RANGES OF RELATIVE ANTIGENIC STRENGTH[a]

Range	RAS score	Reason for assignment to range
A	9.0–10	Tumor will not take in normal isogenic hosts
B	1.0–8.9	Immunization with irradiated tumor provides protection against death from tumor
C	0.1–0.9	Immunization with tumor will only provide protection if immune modification of host or tumor is performed, or else will only delay or inhibit the tumor growth rate
D	0.01–0.09	Tests in ranges B and C are negative, but in vitro tests of immunogenicity or of immunosensitivity give positive results
E	<0.01	Assays in ranges B, C, and D are all negative

[a] Tests are run in the direction from A to D. One stops as soon as a statistically significant result is obtained. Tests for a tumor that fails to give significant results can be stopped at any point, and the RAS score reported as less than the lowest score for the lowest range tested.

Under certain conditions, immunization with some tumors can cause enhancement of (increase in) tumor takes. In general, the conditions of tests in ranges B and C have been chosen to make this eventuality unlikely. Nevertheless, if statistically significant results of enhancement are obtained in tests in these two ranges, the RAS score that would have been assigned had the results been in the opposite (positive) direction are recorded with a negative sign (−) placed in front of them.

The assignment of scores for specific tests in the various ranges of RAS is relatively simple and straightforward (Table XI). Tests are performed in order from range A to range D. As soon as positive results in any one range are obtained, no further tests are run in lower ranges. Scoring in ranges B and C is illustrated below by typical results obtained in our laboratory. For scoring in ranges A2 and D, investigators should feel free to make their own score assignments using the values in Table XI and the examples for ranges B and C as guidelines.

B. PRELIMINARY EXPERIMENTS

Preliminary experiments are vital to answer the following questions:

1. What method will produce a single cell suspension of high viability?
2. What medium will maintain the viability of the tumor cell suspension for a period of 90 to 120 minutes?
3. Having chosen the method and medium, what is the LD_{10}, LD_{50}, and LD_{90} cell dose with their use for the tumor in question?

4. How variable are the LD_{10}, LD_{50}, and LD_{90} when redetermined with tissue of the same tumor harvested from a different animal transplanted with the same generation of the tumor?

TABLE X

DETAILS OF RANGES OF RELATIVE ANTIGENIC STRENGTH

Range	RAS score[a]	Conditions for assignment to range
A1	10.0	Tumor cannot be transplanted isogenically even into immuno-suppressed hosts
A2	9.0–9.9	Tumor can be transplanted isogenically only into immunosuppressed animals, even if up to 25 mg fresh minced tumor or 25 million cells of a single cell suspension are used
B1	5.0–8.9	Two standardized immunizations protect significantly against death from tumor following challenge
B2	1.0–4.9	Six standardized immunizations protect significantly against death from tumor following challenge, while two injections are ineffective
C1	0.5–0.95	Assays in range B2 give negative results for protection against death from tumor, but statistically significant protection is provided if both experimental and control groups receive immune modification, or if immunopotentiation of the immunizing inoculum or of the challenge tumor cells is performed
C2	0.2–0.49	Assays in ranges B2 and C1 give negative results for survivors/tumor deaths, but tests B1 or B2 provide statistically significant data for survival days before death from tumor following challenge, or for measurements of tumor diameter
C3	0.1–0.19	Assays in ranges B, C1, and C2 are negative, but test C1 provides positive results analogous to those set out in section C2 for the data of tests B1 and B2
D1	0.05–0.09	Assays in ranges A, B, and C give negative results. Positive results are obtained in an *in vitro* test or tests both of tumor immunogenicity and of tumor immunosensitivity
D2	0.02–0.049	Assays in ranges A, B, C, and D1 give negative results. Positive results are obtained in an *in vitro* test of tumor immunogenicity
D3	0.01–0.019	Assays in ranges A, B, C, D1, and D2 give negative results. Positive results are obtained in an *in vitro* test of tumor immunosensitivity
E	<0.01	Assays in ranges A, B, C, and D all give negative results

[a] If a tumor can be transplanted into normal isogenic recipients, tests in range A do not apply. Negative values of RAS scores denote statistically significant enhancement rather than inhibition of tumor growth in a given test.

TABLE XI

Assignment of Scores for Tests of Relative Antigenic Strength

RAS range	Score for first significant result	Maximum score for range	Additional scores for a difference between results for a single (or several pooled) experimental groups and a control group at a single challenge dose level[a]	
			$p \leq 0.05$	$p \leq 0.01$
A1	10.0	10.0		
A2	9.0	9.9	0.2	0.3
B1	5.0	8.9	1.0	1.5
B2	1.0	4.9	1.0	1.5
C1	0.5	0.95	0.10	0.15
C2	0.2	0.49	0.05	0.07
C3	0.10	0.19	0.02	0.03
D1	0.05	0.09	0.01	0.015
D2	0.02	0.049	0.005	0.007
D3	0.01	0.019	0.002	0.003

[a] If more than one challenge level yields statistically significant differences between experimental (immunized) and control groups, then the scores obtained at other dose levels are added to the score obtained for the first significant result. Only one score at each dose level may be used to arrive at the aggregate score for the relative antigenic strength of a tumor in a given test range. If at any single challenge level there is no significant difference between results for an experimental and a control group, then results obtained at that dose level for several experimental groups (for instance, for groups immunized $2\times$ and $6\times$) can be pooled for statistical comparison with the control group. If no significant differences are obtained at any dose level, corresponding experimental groups at different dose levels may be pooled for comparison with similarly pooled control groups. Whenever pooled data are used for statistical comparisons, a positive result merits assignment of the score $p \leq 0.05$, even when at the level of $p \leq 0.01$. When the score for the first significant result is earned for a comparison between an experimental and a control group, then if this comparison is significant at $p \leq 0.01$, a "bonus" score is added that corresponds to the difference between the score for $p \leq 0.05$ and the score for $p \leq 0.01$ for that particular RAS range. The above scoring system has been changed somewhat from its original form (Reif and Tomas, 1980; Argyris and Reif, 1981; Reif, 1981).

Past work on the preparation of a single cell suspension of tumors is reviewed in Section III,A,7. Mechanical disruption should be investigated first (Vaage and Agarwal, 1978; Fidler, 1978; Peters et al., 1979). The tumor is minced in a simple tissue culture medium such as Medium 99 or Medium 199 (Difco). If desired, one may add to the medium 5% fetal calf serum, as long as the fetal calf serum is only injected once into each mouse: namely, at the time of challenge with tumor. It usually takes 10–15 minutes to mince 250 mg of tumor sufficiently finely in 5 ml of medium to permit its uptake into a syringe equipped with an 18-gauge needle. The tumor suspension is successively poured through stainless-steel screens of 20, 40, 60, and 100 mesh size presterilized by dipping in ethanol and flaming in a Bunsen burner. At this point, the cell concentration and the percentage of cells that will not stain with vital dye are determined in a hemacytometer chamber (see Appendix, Section VII,B,2,a). Only if the cell suspension prepared by such mechanical disruption is inadequate is there need to choose one of the methods for enzymatic dissociation of tumors discussed in Section III,A,7 (Vaage and Argalwal, 1978; Fidler, 1978; Peters *et al.*, 1979; Lawler *et al.*, 1981; Talmadge *et al.*, 1981). If neither mechanical nor enzymatic dissociation gives an adequate cell suspension, then a suspension of minced tumor tissue may be used as described in the Appendix, Sections VII,B,2,b and c. Further details on the performance of preliminary experiments and the performance of challenge experiments are given in the Appendix, Section VII,B,2.

C. Tests of Relative Antigenic Strengths in Ranges A, B, and C

1. Range A

If up to 25 mg of fresh minced tumor or of a suspension of 25 million tumor cells will not produce tumor takes in isogenic hosts, then the relative antigenic strength of the tumor lies in range A (see conditions for assignment to ranges A1 and A2 in Table X). If the tumor cannot be transplanted at the above-mentioned high doses even into strongly immunosuppressed isogenic hosts, it merits assignment to range A1 (RAS score 10.0). If it can be transplanted into isogenic hosts immunosuppressed by a standardized regimen, it is assigned to range A2 (RAS scores 9.0–9.9). If it is desired to compare the RAS of several tumors within the range A2, the same preliminary experiments used for tumors that take in normal isogenic hosts must be performed (Section V,B), but using isogenic hosts immunosuppressed by a method that is held constant throughout all experiments. Thereafter, the same experiments are done as described below for range B1, using two prophylactic immunizations with standardized amounts of irradiated tumor cells. Assignment of scores in range A2 is indicated in Table XI. In the case of range A2, these scores apply only to data of survivors/tumor deaths obtained in the immunorejection assay described in this section. If two prophylactic immunizations will not produce significant differences between immunized and control groups, then the standardized immunosuppression method should be modified to permit performance of the prophylactic immunizations *before* immunosuppression is begun. If two immunizations still produce no significant effect, then the tumor is assigned the minimum score of 9.0 for range A2 (see footnote *a*, Table XI).

2. Ranges B and C

An overview of tests in ranges B and C is given in Table X. Tests in the ranges B1, B2, and C1 are immunorejection assays that are scored for statistically significant differences in survivors/tumor deaths. These immunorejection assays can provide the data required for the assignment of tumors to ranges C2 and C3, provided these data are collected during performance of the immunorejection assays. This requires that in the days between challenge and death from tumor for each mouse in the experiment, tumor diameter measurements are performed at 3- to 7-day intervals from the time of the first appearance of the tumors, for a total of five to seven separate times. Thus, the entire ranges B and C, with all their subgroups, can be covered in a single comprehensive experiment.

Reasons for the choice of the numbers of experimental animals in each group are discussed in detail in the Appendix, Section VII,A. The number actually suggested in Table IV is 8 ± 1. This table also makes suggestions for other choices that must be made before doing an immunorejection experiment to cover ranges B and C. Further details of the design of an experiment that will cover entirely ranges B and C are given in Table XII. Groups are listed in the order in which they should be challenged at any single challenge dose, reading from left to right across the table. Immunizations must be initiated at suitable time intervals, since all mice must be challenged on a single day. If the tumor in question is suspected of having a relatively high RAS score, then the groups immunized four times with the addition of either *Corynebacterium parvum* or bacillus Calmette-Guérin(BCG; footnote *a*, Table IV), and groups immunized six times can be omitted in a first experiment, so that only the three groups immunized two times and the six control groups need to be run. If, on the other hand, the tumor is expected to be relatively low in RAS, then the three groups immunized two times could be omitted. However, unless it is certain that there will be no need to obtain the data necessary for classification in ranges C2 and C3 (see Table X), the data that must be accumulated in such an experiment (Table XII) include not only survivors/tumor deaths and mean day of death from tumor for each group of mice, but also (except for ip or iv challenges with tumor) measurements of tumor length and breadth performed on 5–7 separate days at 3- to 7-day intervals following

TABLE XII

PLAN FOR COMPREHENSIVE IMMUNOREJECTION ASSAY TO COVER RAS RANGES B AND C[a]

Challenge dose of tumor in LD$_{50}$ units[b]	Number of weekly immunizations with irradiated tumor cells[c]			
	4× + C. parvum[d]	6×	2×	0×
0.1				8[e]
0.3				8
1.0				8
3.0[f]	8	8	8	8
10.0	8	8	8	8
100.0[g]	8	8	8	8

[a] Further details are given in Table IV.

[b] Preliminary experiments are done to determine the LD$_{50}$ cell dose. The stated numbers represent multiples of this LD$_{50}$ dose. Challenges may be performed in two portions on a single day, with fresh tumor used each time (see text).

[c] For ascites tumors, 5 million cells per mouse per ip injection; for solid tumors, 25 mg minced tumor per mouse per sc injection.

[d] Instead of C. parvum, BCG can be used: see footnote a of Table IV.

[e] Number of mice in group.

[f] For tumors expected to have a high RAS score, use 1000.0 instead of 3.0.

[g] For tumors expected to have a low RAS score, use 30.0 instead of 100.0.

tne appearance of palpable tumors. Further details are given in Section IV and in the Appendix, Sections VII,A and B.

D. TESTS OF RELATIVE ANTIGENIC STRENGTHS IN RANGES D AND E

1. Range D1

Tests of RAS need be extended to range D only if tests in ranges B and C are negative, and it is essential to go beyond the answer that the RAS score is <0.1. It has been claimed that the results of in vitro immunogenicity assays can predict both qualitatively and quantitatively the results of in vivo tests (Ruppert et al., 1978). Further, there is a positive correlation between humoral immunity and the success of chemotherapy–immunotherapy for leukemia L1210 (Cantrell et al., 1976). Therefore, there is justification for extension of RAS tests to carefully chosen in vitro assays if the need for tests in this low range should ever arise.

The two in vitro tests used by Ruppert et al. (1978) to arrive at their important conclusion were cell-mediated inhibition (CMI) and microcytotoxicity, which are further described in Table III. These assays involve relevant facets both of immunogenicity, since the effector cells are lymphoid cells taken from animals immunized *in vivo* with the specific tumor in question, and of immunosensitivity, since statistically significant inhibition of tumor growth is required. Therefore, CMI and MC represent assays for RAS range D1 (see Table X). In each case, Ruppert *et al.* (1978) used the tests to obtain a yes-or-no answer to the question of whether specific immunity to the particular tumor could be demonstrated. For affirmative answers, the score that would be assigned in this situation is listed as 0.05 under the heading, "score for the first significant result," in Table XI. Assignment of this score would be valid only if the tumors had failed to provide statistically significant results when tested in RAS ranges A, B, or C. While tests in these ranges were not performed according to the present suggestions (Table XII), the *in vivo* tests that were done suggest that tumors which reacted positively *in vitro* would also have reacted positively *in vivo* in the RAS ranges of B or C.

Suppose several tumors under consideration had RAS scores in the range D1. How could the above assays be modified to permit a quantitative differentiation in the relative antigenic strengths of these tumors within this range? The tests employed above (Ruppert *et al.*, 1978) could be run with lymphoid cells harvested from mice immunized a different number of times, or with different ratios of effector lymphoid cells/target tumor cells. In either case, the investigator could assign scores in line with those suggested in Table XI, in analogous fashion to those employed in the examples given for ranges B and C, to quantify scores in range D1.

2. Range D2

Range D2 is assigned to tumors that fail to react in ranges A, B, C, and D1, yet give positive results when immunogenicity alone is tested *in vitro*. Surprisingly, many of the methods listed in Table III qualify in this regard. All methods listed under "antibody" in this table are acceptable, as long as the antibody was raised either in autochthonous or in isogenic animals and does not involve immune cytolysis or ADCC, since results for these tests rate in range D1 (see Greenberg *et al.*, 1981). In addition, methods that qualify include tests of cell-mediated immunity such as lymphocyte binding, leukocyte adherence inhibition, and lymphocyte transformation, as well as lymphokine assays such as migration inhibition factor (MIF) and LMI (Table III). As in the case of tests in range D1, a yes-or-no answer to a given test in range D2 merits assignment of the score of 0.02 for the first significant result (Table XI). Quantification to distinguish between the RAS of several tumors in range D2 is accomplished using the score assignment suggested in Table XI in analogous fashion to that described in the previous paragraph for range D1.

3. Range D3

Range D3 is assigned to tumors that fail to give statistically significant results in ranges A to D2, yet react positively in tests of immunosensitivity that do not include facets of immunogenicity specific for the tumor under consideration. Assays that could be argued to qualify as tests of immunosensitivity alone include (1) lysis by "natural" antibody (such as serum taken from normal isogenic animals), and (2) cellular cytotoxicity mediated by isogenic lymphoid cells nonspecifically activated either *in vivo* or *in vitro*, for instance with phytohemagglutinin (PHA). Scoring of RAS in this range would be performed in line with the above outline and merit the scores listed in Table XI.

4. Range E

Failure to obtain significant results in tests of ranges A through D3 merits assignment of a tumor to RAS range E, indicating minimal antigenicity (Table X). Since statistically significant results are required for tumor assignments to all other RAS ranges, the statistical methods are important components of the assays. This represents the reason underlying inclusion of Section VII,A in the Appendix.

VI. Representative Results

A. ANTIGENICITY TESTS IN RANGES B AND C

In addition to work on long-transplanted tumors such as L1210 of DBA/2 mice, tumors newly derived in C57BL/6J mice by various methods were also tested. These included three osteogenic sarcomas induced by strontium-90, two sarcomas and two carcinomas induced by dimethylbenzanthracene (DMBA), and a spontaneous lymphoma (Table XIII).

Results for a test of relative antigenic strength in range B2 are illustrated (Table XIV). The challenge was performed with a single cell suspension of the tumor. For the challenge at 4900 cells, there is a difference in five survivors between the results obtained for the experimental group and for the control group. According to Table XXVII, Fisher's exact probability test gives $p \leq 0.01$ for such a difference when there are six animals in each of the two groups. The RAS score for this result in range B2 is 1.5 (see Table XI). Since a significant comparison between individual groups has been obtained, it is not possible to use the results for pooled groups that are listed under "corresponding totals" (Table XIV),

TABLE XIII
DETAILS OF THE INDUCTION OF TUMORS IN C57BL/6J MICE[a]

| Designation of tumor | Type of tumor | Agent used for tumor induction | | First transplant | |
		Name	Dose	Days after injection	Date
Ly-C	Lymphoma	None[b]			6/08/77
Os-B	Osteosarcoma	^{90}Sr	0.5 μCi/g	141	4/14/77
Os-E	Osteosarcoma	^{90}Sr	1.0 μCi/g	314	10/04/77
Os-G	Osteosarcoma	^{90}Sr	2.0 μCi/g	386	12/15/77
SMx-A	Sarcoma	DMBA	1.0 mg	114	2/16/78
SMx-E	Carcinoma	DMBA	1.0 mg	157	3/29/78
SMx-F	Sarcoma	DMBA	1.0 mg	169	4/11/78
SMx-G	Carcinoma	DMBA	1.0 mg	169	4/11/78

[a] Data taken in part from Argyris and Reif (1981) and Cataldo and Reif (1982).
[b] This lymphoma developed in a 224-day-old female.

even though these results also differ significantly at the 1% level of probability (see Table XXVII for a difference of eight survivors between immunized and control groups). Once a positive result has been obtained at any given range of RAS, no purpose is served in performing additional tests in lower ranges of RAS (see Table X), unless it is desired to obtain additional useful information, such as the relationship between the results of *in vivo* immunorejection assays and various *in vitro* tests.

Further illustrations of the assignment of RAS scores will be helpful. The experiment with the L1210 subline L/Ha is more extensive than required merely for determination of RAS scores in ranges B and C, since our purpose was to obtain additional information (Table V). The data relevant for the highest RAS range for which requirements are met (see Table X) are those for 6× compared to 0× immunizations. For the challenges with 500, 5000, and 50,000 cells, the numbers of survivors in the 6× groups exceed those in the 0× groups by 7, 5, and 5, respectively. These differences in survivors are all significant at the 0.01 level of probability p (see Table XXVII, and direct evaluation of Fisher's exact probability test). For each of these three dose ranges a RAS score of 1.5 is earned, for a total score of 4.5 (Table XI). Since the 2× immunization that is required for range B1 was not performed, the RAS score for tumor L1210-L/Ha lies in the range of 4.5–8.9.

For the L1210 subline L-W, immunizations performed either six times or four times yield a maximum difference of three survivors between immunized and control groups (Table VI); this difference is not statistically significant (Table XXVII). Thus, L-W fails to score in RAS range B2. The requirements for tests in the C1 range are fulfilled by the 4× immunization

TABLE XIV

TEST OF RELATIVE ANTIGENIC STRENGTH IN RANGE B2

Challenge dose of unstained SMx-F cells[a] (number)	Immunized mice[b]		Controls	
	S[c]	D	S	D
49			8	1
490			1	4
4,900	6	0	1	5
49,000	2	4	0	6
490,000	1	5	0	6
Corresponding totals[d]	9	9	1	17

[a] Challenge was performed with transplant generation 14 of the tumor 1 week after the last immunization. Challenge injections made sc on opposite side used for immunization. Numbers represent cells injected that were left unstained by vital dye.

[b] C57BL/6J females 16 weeks old at the time of challenge were immunized sc six times at weekly intervals with 25 mg irradiated tumor SMx-F.

[c] S, Survivors; D, tumor deaths.

[d] Totals for pooled groups are used for statistical comparisons only if comparisons for individual groups do not give a significant result.

with *C. parvum* (Table VI); this regimen produced differences of 9, 9, and 6 survivors, respectively, compared to the 0× control group for challenges with 3000, 30,000, or 300,000 L-W cells. All these differences are significant at the level of $p \leq 0.01$ (Table XXVII). Thus, L1210-L-W earns a score of 0.50 for the first significant result of 3000 cells, plus a "bonus" of 0.05 for significance at the 0.01 level of p at this challenge dose, plus 0.15 for each of the other two significant results, for a total RAS score of 0.85 (see Table XI).

When data for survivors/tumor deaths (Section VII,A,1) do not give significant differences between immunized and control groups, then results obtained in the same experiment for measurements of mean day of death or of tumor diameter are used to assign scores in RAS ranges C2 and C3 (Table X). The statistical analysis of the results obtained in such tests are described in the Appendix, Sections VII,A,2 and 3, respectively. Scores are assigned as listed in Table XI. An additional example illustrates not only the assignment of scores, but also the increasing level of statistical significance obtained when tumor diameters are measured more frequently.

For generation 42 of SMx-E carcinoma, antigenicity tests in range C1 proved negative with regard to data on survivors/tumor deaths (Table XV). When the mean day of death from tumor was computed for different groups and tested by the one-way analysis of variance (see Appendix,

TABLE XV

RESULTS OF CHALLENGE WITH VIABLE TUMOR: NEGATIVE RESULTS FOR
IMMUNOREJECTIVE STRENGTH TEST IN RANGE C1[a]

| | Number of weekly immunizations with 25 mg irradiated SMx-E cells | | | | | | | |
| Challenge dose of SMx-E cells (mg) | 0× | | 4× | | 4× + BCG | | 4× + C. parvum | |
	S[b]	D	S	D	S	D	S	D
2.0	2	7						
6.8	1	8	1	8	1	6	0	7
20.0	1	8	0	9	0	9	0	9

[a] Challenges were performed with transplant generation 42 of carcinoma SMx-E. The mice were DBF$_1$ females 17–18 weeks old at the time of challenge. The amount of BCG mixed with minced tumor was 1×10^6 viable organisms per mouse, and of C. parvum, 20 μg per mouse.

[b] S, Survivors; D, tumor deaths.

Section VII,A,2), no significant difference between any of the experimental groups and their corresponding control group was found. When, however, measurements of tumor diameters were tested by the proper statistical test (see Appendix, Section VII,A,3), significant reductions in tumor growth rate were detected in the two groups listed in Table XV that were immunized four times with the addition of BCG (Table XVI).

TABLE XVI

SIGNIFICANCE OF REDUCTION IN RATE OF TUMOR GROWTH: EFFECT OF FREQUENCY OF
TUMOR DIAMETER MEASUREMENTS ON STATISTICAL SIGNIFICANCE

| | Number of times tumor diameter measurements were made[b] | | |
Experimental group that is compared with its control[a]	5 (p)	8 (p)	11 (p)
4× + BCG (6.8 mg)	<0.05	<0.01	<0.01
4× + BCG (20.0 mg)	>0.05	<0.05	<0.01
All other groups	>0.05	>0.05	>0.05

[a] The experimental and control groups are those listed in Table XV. The two groups immunized 4× with addition of BCG were challenged with, respectively, 6.8 and 20.0 mg of a suspension of finely minced tumor.

[b] Measurements were performed on days 10, 14, 17, 21, 25, 28, 31, 35, 39, 42, and 45 after challenge with transplant generation 42 of tumor SMx-E (see Table XV). The 5×, 8×, and 11× measurements analyzed all began on day 10.

To determine whether the significance of differences in tumor diameter measurements between experimental and control groups is increased by more measurements, measurements were performed on 11 separate days; these began on the day palpable tumors were first observed, and continued at 3- or 4-day intervals (Table XVI). There was a progressive increase in the level of significance of the results that correlated with the larger number of instances on which tumor diameters were measured (Table XVI). The RAS score for significance ($p < 0.05$) in range C3 is 0.10 (Table XI). Since the level of significance was $p < 0.01$ for eight sets of measurements (the maximum suggested on p. 69) for group $4\times$ + BCG at a challenge dose of 6.8 mg, this earns a bonus score of 0.01. There is also a score of 0.02 for the second significant result of $p < 0.05$ for the same groups at a challenge dose of 20.0 mg. The total RAS score obtained for this data in range C3 is therefore 0.13 (see Table XI).

B. Relationship between Antigenicity and Biological Properties

The mode of induction of eight recently derived C57BL/6 tumors has already been presented (Table XIII). Within a given set of tumors, such as strontium-90-induced osteosarcomas or DMBA-induced submaxillary gland tumors, there tends to be a rough parallel between antigenic strength and the following biologic properties: doubling time, LD_{50} for the challenge of normal isogenic hosts, survival time following routine transplantation, and percentage of tumor-free survivors in the routine transplantation procedure (Table XVII). Certainly, far more extensive and convincing data than those presented here would be necessary to establish such a correlation. Perhaps future investigators will fill this informational void.

C. Advantages of Standardized Measurements of Tumor Antigenicity

There are many advantages in the use of a standardized, all-inclusive system for the measurement of the relative antigenic strength of tumors (Table XVIII). The present intent is to ask investigators to use it, so that a beginning can be made in garnering those advantages, as well as revealing its deficiencies. The system for measurement of RAS adopted by the general consensus of some future workshop in tumor immunology may bear only a scant resemblance to that suggested here. Nevertheless, it seems important that the benefits universally enjoyed by the standardization of serological reagents should also be sought and attained in the area of antigenicity.

TABLE XVII
RELATIVE ANTIGENIC STRENGTH, GROWTH AND TRANSPLANTATION CHARACTERISTICS OF RECENTLY DERIVED C57BL/6J MOUSE TUMORS

Type and name of tumor	Relative antigenic strength[a]	Doubling time (days)	LD_{50} cell dose	Transplant generation[b]	Unstained cell count[c] (%)	Data obtained from routine tumor transplantation		
						Transplant generations	Survival (mean ± SD) (days)	Survivors/ total number transplanted
Lymphoma								
Ly-C	<0.2	2.1 (1.3)[d]	2700 (140)	32	48	16–55	29.0 ± 4.6	4/180
Osteosarcoma								
Os-B	0.2	3.0	83,000	23	5	12–39	50.9 ± 17.4	4/144
Os-E	<0.2	2.2	15,000	20	10	6–35	31.4 ± 11.3	1/144
Os-G	0.25	2.2	11,000	21	3	4–45	35.9 ± 9.8	11/183
Fibrosarcoma								
SMx-A	0.5	2.3	5400	26	9	1–45	27.2 ± 13.4	2/216
SMx-F	1.5	1.9	220	19	8	1–34	35.0 ± 15.5	5/171
Carcinoma								
SMx-E	1.5	1.5	180,000	17	43	1–28	52.6 ± 26.5	5/133
SMx-G	2.0	10.0	—[e]	6	15	1–11	129.0 ± 49.8	17/70

[a] Above scoring system has been changed from its original form (Reif and Tomas, 1980; Argyris and Reif, 1981; Reif, 1981; Cataldo and Reif, 1982).

[b] The mean of the transplant generations for which the relative antigenic strengths and the LD_{50} values were determined is recorded. In all cases, the mean value is within five generations for each of the two types of determinations.

[c] Cells of a single cell suspension that do not take up vital dye.

[d] The values in parentheses refer to ip injections, while the values written above them refer to sc injections.

[e] No takes were obtained with single cell suspensions. The LD_{50} for minced tumor tissue was approximately 1 mg.

TABLE XVIII

BENEFITS OF A COMPREHENSIVE SYSTEM FOR MEASUREMENT
OF RELATIVE ANTIGENIC STRENGTH

A. For comparisons of relative antigenic strength
   1. Between early and later transplant generations of a single tumor
   2. Between different tumors of the same etiology or histologic type
   3. Between tumors of different etiology or histologic type
   4. Between tumors used by different investigators
   5. Between methods used to assess RAS for the same tumors
B. For correlation of RAS with biological properties
   1. With parameters of tumor growth
   2. With potential for metastasis
   3. With success of specific modes of therapy
   4. With other biological or immunobiological properties
C. For quantification of changes in RAS
   1. When different adjuvants are used during immunization with the tumor
   2. When immunization is done with tumor cells modified by different methods
   3. When the host is suitably conditioned prior to, at, or after tumor challenge
D. Steps required for indirect measurement of RAS for human tumors
   1. *In vitro* assay of immunogenicity and immunosensitivity of the human tumor
   2. *In vitro* assay by the same methods for several analogous animal tumors
   3. *In vivo* determination of RAS for these same animal tumors
   4. Calibration of the *in vitro* assays (step 2) in terms of the RAS scores obtained for the same animal tumors *in vivo* (step 3)
   5. Use of this calibration to interpolate the data obtained *in vitro* for human tumors (step 1) into equivalent *in vivo* RAS scores

A strong case can be made for the choice of a system that involves rejection of a tumor in its isogenic host as the basis for a comprehensive system of measurement of RAS. When clinicians involved in cancer therapy talk about the "antigenic strength" of tumors, they really mean "immunorejective strength." A tumor with a high RAS score is by definition relatively easily rejected by its host, and hence cured. Thus, accurate measurement of immunorejective strength has vital applicability to the therapy of tumors.

D. MEASUREMENT OF THE RELATIVE ANTIGENIC STRENGTH OF HUMAN TUMORS

It is possible to arrive at a very rough grading of the relative antigenic strength of human tumors on the basis of three criteria: the number of spontaneous regressions, the effectiveness of systemic chemotherapy, and laboratory data regarding antigenic cross-reactivity (Table XIX). Nevertheless, such a classification begs the important question of whether a high relative antigenic strength really ensures a good prognosis

TABLE XIX

AN APPROXIMATE RANKING OF THE ANTIGENIC STRENGTHS OF HUMAN
TUMORS BASED ON PRELIMINARY EVIDENCE[a]

Type of tumor	Substantiated cases of spontaneous regression	Effectiveness of systemic chemotherapy	Antigenic cross-reactivity for tumors of same histologic type
Hypernephroma	31	—	—
Wilms' tumor	29	High	Yes
Neuroblastoma	—	High	Yes
Rhabdomyosarcoma	Yes	High	—
Burkitt's lymphoma	—	High	Yes
Choriocarcinoma	19	Fair	Yes
Malignant melanoma	19	Fair	Yes
Acute childhood leukemia	—	Good	—
Bladder cancer	13	—	Yes
Sarcomas	19	—	Yes
Colon and rectal cancer	7	—	Yes
Ovarian cancer	7	—	Yes
Testicular cancer	7	—	—
Breast cancer	6	—	Yes

[a] Reproduced without modification from Reif (1975). Today we know that the response to high-dose multiple-agent chemotherapy tends to be very good not only for most childhood tumors, but also for selected adult tumors, many of which are included in the above list. Further, we now know that a surprisingly large number of spontaneous regressions occur in neuroblastoma of type IVS (Hann, 1981). Thus, time has served to confirm rather than confound the thrust of the above correlations.

regarding therapy when criteria such as stage of tumor and tumor burden are standardized. If this were true, then an intensive attack using the newest methods of therapy should be concentrated on the most antigenic types of tumors (Reif, 1979), since the possibiliy for gain seems greatest for such types. In fact, the random attack which is presently the rule may well serve to identify such types of tumors. These considerations are presently based largely on indirect evidence. However, they may serve as an impetus to determine the relative antigenic strength of human tumors as suggested in Table XVIII,D. Only when such determinations are made will the present uncertainty about these important issues be resolved.

VII. Appendix: Statistics and Techniques for Tumor Challenge Experiments

The most crucial part of experiments that involve a challenge with tumor—whether their purpose is to test tumor antigenicity, chemotherapy, immunotherapy, prophylaxis, or other forms of therapy—is generally the performance of the challenge. In procedures such as antigenic testing, chemotherapy, or immunotherapy, the therapeutic injections are often given several times. While this does not mean that poor technique is acceptable for such injections, the statistics of chance indicate that random errors will tend to cancel out and thereby diminish during the course of several injections. This is not the case for the challenge with tumor cells, since it is performed only once. Further, the equivalence of control and experimental groups in terms of the dose and the viability of the tumor cells injected is vital if valid results are to be obtained.

In this section, the first focus is on statistics, since the design of an experiment is greatly aided by an understanding of how many animals are needed in control and experimental groups in order to achieve statistically significant results. The section on statistics gives the information necessary for investigators to chose the right size of groups to accomplish their purpose. A prospective understanding of this matter minimizes a retrospective disappointment because of failure to obtain statistically significant results. In addition, statistical methods are described that are suitable for analysis of the type of data obtained in tests of tumor antigenicity: data on survivors/tumor deaths, on day of death from tumor, and on tumor diameter measurements. The stress is on the simplicity and ease of performance of the tests.

The second focus is on the actual performance of tumor challenge experiments. In particular, the strategies underlying the challenge injections are discussed. Because of the constraints of time imposed by the frequently experienced loss of viability of the tumor cells following their harvest, the need for careful planning and good technique is demanding.

A. Statistics for Tumor Challenge Experiments

Most investigators do not have enough time to work out complicated statistical problems. On the other hand, statistics are crucial for a determination of whether the experimental results are significant—and if this cannot be proven, all the time spent in conducting extensive laboratory work may have been wasted. Since the writer is a laboratory worker who never ceases to grudge the long hours required by attention to statistics, this appendix is written with the purpose of making the necessary statistics as easy as possible to understand and as rapid as possible to perform.

1. Data on Survivors/Tumor Deaths

By far the most important statistical test concerns the significance of data on survival as contrasted to death from tumor following challenge of an experimental and a control group with viable tumor cells. In our case, the experimental group consists of immunized animals, while the control group contains identical animals that are left uninjected or are injected with saline. Suppose we obtain 4 survivors and 6 tumor deaths in an experimental group, and 0 survivors and 10 tumor deaths in our control group: Are these results statistically significant?

The standard method for arranging such data is as a "2 × 2 table," illustrated as follows:

Group	Survivors	Tumor deaths	Totals
Experimental	A = 4	B = 6	I = 10
Control	C = 0	D = 10	H = 10
Totals	F = 4	G = 16	E = 20

There are two standard ways of treating these data statistically. The first is use of the χ^2 distribution. This has the disadvantage that it is an approximation. Further, if the value of E is under 45, then Yates' correction to the test is generally employed. Also, if any of the expected values of A, B, C, or D are under five, the χ^2 test is not valid and may not be used. The method recommended instead is Fisher's exact probability test (Fisher, 1946; Denenberg, 1976). In antigenic testing, one of the expected values of A, B, C, or D is often under five, and in any case Fisher's test gives an exact evaluation of the probability while the χ^2 test represents an approximation. Therefore, consideration is confined to the exact probability test.

  a. Fisher's Exact Probability Test. For results that can be arranged in a 2 × 2 table as illustrated above, it is remarkably simple to evaluate the precise statistical probability that mere chance (rather than an intrinsic difference between the two groups) could account for the observed difference in results. In this situation, Fisher's formula for the exact probability p is

$$p = \frac{F! \times G! \times H! \times I!}{A! \times B! \times C! \times D! \times E!}$$

Factorials are easily evaluated using a standard desk calculator. For instance, A! in our table equals $4! = 4 \times 3 \times 2 \times 1 = 24$. However, it is usually not necessary to evaluate most of the factorials, since they cancel out. For instance, for the values just presented,

$$p = \frac{4! \times 16! \times 10! \times 10!}{4! \times 6! \times 0! \times 10! \times 20!}$$

This equation can be rewritten to place factorials that can be completely or partially canceled above and below each other, with the largest values on the left:

$$p = \frac{16! \times 10! \times 10! \times 4!}{20! \times 10! \times 6! \times 4! \times 0!}$$

$$p = \frac{(10 \times 9 \times 8 \times 7)}{(20 \times 19 \times 18 \times 17) \times 1}$$

In other words, 20!/16! is represented by factorial 20 that stops at factorial 16, or $20 \times 19 \times 18 \times 17$, while 10!/6! is represented by factorial 10 that stops at factorial 6, or $10 \times 9 \times 8 \times 7$. The other two sets of factorials, 10!/10! and 4!/4!, cancel out, and the factorial of zero (0!) equals 1. The equation can be further simplified by writing $^{10}/_{20} = {}^1/_2$, and $^9/_{18} = {}^1/_2$, to become

$$p = \frac{8 \times 7}{2 \times 19 \times 2 \times 17} = \frac{56}{1292} = 0.0433$$

Unfortunately, the calculation of p using Fisher's exact probability test is more complicated when the distribution of survivors and tumor deaths is not extreme; extreme is used here in the sense that there is a zero in one of the observed values A, B, C, or D of the above example. When the distribution is nonextreme, the value of p is the sum of its value for the distribution under consideration plus the sum of the values of p for all other more extreme distributions that possess the same marginal values E, F, G, H and I. By using a sum of p values, the probability that is tested is not only whether the distribution under consideration could have arisen by chance, but also that all other distributions more extreme than this could have arisen by chance (Denenberg, 1976).

An example (Table XX) explains how p values are calculated for nonextreme distributions of survivors and tumor deaths. Suppose that our results are represented by distribution a. Then a more extreme distribution, differing by a reduction of 1 in the value of B, makes necessary the changes in the values of A, C, and D that are illustrated in distribution b, since the totals E, F, G, H, and I must all remain unchanged. The next change produces distribution c, and so on down to the extreme distribution e, which represents the end point of the chain. The true value of p, which allows us to judge whether or not any one of the distributions a, b, c, d, or e could have arisen by chance, is given not by calculating the value of p for that distribution alone, but by adding the p values for that distribution plus all more extreme ones, as shown in the right-hand column of Table XX.

TABLE XX

DERIVATION OF DISTRIBUTIONS MORE EXTREME THAN THOSE UNDER CONSIDERATION[a]

Distribution	Group	S^b	D	Totals	p value for this distribution Alone	+ more extreme ones
a	Experimental	10	*4*	14		
	Control	5	9	14		
	Totals	15	13	28	0.05352	0.06416
b	Experimental	11	*3*	14		
	Control	4	10	14		
	Totals	15	13	28	0.00973	0.01064
c	Experimental	12	*2*	14		
	Control	3	11	14		
	Totals	15	13	28	0.00088	0.00091
d	Experimental	13	*1*	14		
	Control	2	12	14		
	Totals	15	13	28	0.00003	0.00003
e	Experimental	14	*0*	14		
	Control	1	13	14		
	Totals	15	13	28	0.00000	0.00000

[a] The value of the lowest figure of the survivors/tumor deaths figures in distribution a is *4* (the number of tumor deaths in the experimental groups is shown in italics). This value is progressively reduced by 1 in distributions b, c, d, and e. Because the totals must remain unchanged, the change in this one (lowest) value determines the changes in all other figures in each distribution. Note that the increase in p values, due to inclusion of p for all distributions more extreme than that under consideration, is relatively small: it is only 20% for distribution a, and decreases progressively for the more extreme distributions b, c, d, and e.

[b] S, Survivors; D, tumor deaths.

In the case evaluated at the start of this section, the value of p is below 0.05, hence the results for the experimental group differ from the results for the control group at the 5% level of significance. The calculation is quite simple. However, if one has dozens of such calculations to perform, then one might wish to use a shortcut. I have written a program in Machine Language for the Hewlett-Packard minicomputer 9815A (Table XXI), which we utilize. This program will work with the most unsophisticated of minicomputers, since only multiplication and division are required. To run the program, the minicomputer is used in modes NORMAL and RUN. After the program is accessed, the computer's memory is cleared. Now the numbers corresponding to A, B, C, D, E, F, G, H,

TABLE XXI
Computer Program in Machine Language for Calculation of p

00 GOSUB 60	23 STOP	43 RECALL B	60 FIX 9
02 STORE A	24 GOSUB 60	44 DIVIDE	62 PRINT
03 STOP	26 STORE G	45 RECALL H	63 1
04 GOSUB 60	27 STOP	46 MULTIPLY	64 STORE J
06 STORE B	28 GOSUB 60	47 RECALL C	65 IF X $\geq$ Y
07 STOP	30 STORE H	48 DIVIDE	66 GO TO 75
08 GOSUB 60	31 STOP	49 RECALL I	68 REVERSE X & Y
10 STORE C	32 GOSUB 60	50 MULTIPLY	69 STORE $\times$ J
11 STOP	34 STORE I	51 RECALL D	70 REVERSE X & Y
12 GOSUB 60	35 STOP	52 DIVIDE	71 MINUS
14 STORE D	36 SPACE	53 RECALL E	72 1
15 STOP	37 RECALL F	54 DIVIDE	73 GO TO 65
16 GOSUB 60	38 ENTER	55 PRINT	75 RECALL J
18 STORE E	39 RECALL A	56 STORE J	76 PRINT
19 STOP	40 DIVIDE	57 STOP	77 SPACE
20 GOSUB 60	41 RECALL G	58 RECALL J	78 RETURN
22 STORE F	42 MULTIPLY	59 SPACE	79 SPACE
			80 END

and I are keyed in, being taken from a 2×2 table arranged as shown above. The RUN–STOP key is pressed after each of the numbers is entered, and again after all numbers have been entered. The program prints out each number, its factorial, and the probability p for the comparison represented by the 2×2 table. Each determination of p takes about 20 seconds. Alternatively, tables for evaluation of Fisher's exact probability test for up to 40 animals in each group (Finney et al., 1963) can be used. Values of p for more extreme distributions (see Table XX) must be added.

  b. *Evaluation of p for Data on Survivors/Tumor Deaths.* With the help of the above program, the author has evaluated commonly encountered data on survivors/tumor deaths, but only for the situation where the numbers of animals chosen for the experimental and the control groups are equal. For this particular case, Tables XXII–XXIX provide most of the required p values, so that the actual calculation of p can usually be avoided.

  The first question to be answered is, what must be the minimum number of animals in each of the two groups to ensure that the results obtained will demonstrate a statistically significant distinction between the groups? The answer depends on the degree to which the results for the two groups differ. As Table XXII shows, if the results differ by 20, 50, or 100%, a minimum of 20, 8, or 3 animals, respectively, is required in each group if such differences are to be statistically valid at the 5% level ($p \leq 0.05$). The table also gives the number of animals required to give results significant at the 1 and 0.1% level.

TABLE XXII

Probability That Stated Percentage Differences in Results Between an Experimental and a Control Group Represent True Distinctions Between the Groups and Not Random Chance under the Most Favorable Distribution of 100% Tumor Deaths in Controls or 0% in Experiments[a,b]

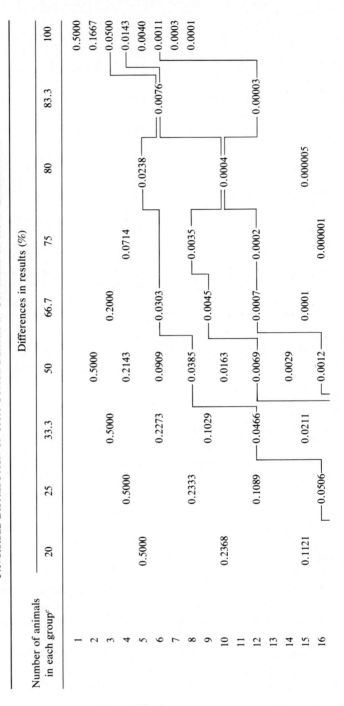

Number of animals in each group[c]	20	25	33.3	50	66.7	75	80	83.3	100
1									0.5000
2				0.5000					0.1667
3			0.5000		0.2000				0.0500
4		0.5000		0.2143		0.0714			0.0143
5	0.5000						0.0238		0.0040
6			0.2273	0.0909	0.0303			0.0076	0.0011
7									0.0003
8		0.2333		0.0385		0.0035			0.0001
9			0.1029		0.0045				
10	0.2368			0.0163			0.0004		
11									
12		0.1089	0.0466	0.0069	0.0007	0.0002		0.00003	
13									
14				0.0029					
15	0.1121		0.0211		0.0001		0.000005		
16		0.0506		0.0012		0.000001			

Differences in results (%)

58

TABLE XXII (*continued*)

Number of animals in each group[c]	Differences in results (%)								
	20	25	33.3	50	66.7	75	80	83.3	100
17									
18			0.0095	0.0005					
19									
20	0.0530	0.0236		0.0002					
21			0.0043						
22				0.0001					
23									
24		0.0110	0.0019						
25	0.0251								
27			0.0009						
28		0.0051	0.0004						
30	0.0119	0.0024							
32									
35	0.0056								
36		0.0011							
40	0.0026								
45	0.0013								

[a] For example, if there was a 50% difference in results between an experimental and a control group, and if there were eight animals in each group, then four out of eight (4/8) animals would survive in the experimental group, compared to zero out of eight (0/8) in the control group ($p = 0.0385$).

[b] Probability values calculated by Fisher's exact probability test. The solid lines join values of the probability (p) that are 0.05 or less, 0.01 or less, or 0.001 or less, computed to one significant figure.

[c] There are equal numbers of animals in the experimental group and in the control group.

Unfortunately, the value of p can vary for a given difference in results between the experimental and the control groups, depending upon how this difference is distributed. For instance, if there are 14 animals in each group, and the experimental group has 5 more survivors than the control group, the value of p varies considerably with the distribution of the difference (Table XXIII). If the control group has no survivors, or the experimental group has no tumor deaths (comparisons a and j, respectively), then the value of p is minimal, and the situation is ideal for obtaining statistically significant results. When, however, the difference between the two sets of results is distributed precisely between the extremes represented by comparisons a and j, the value of p is maximal. This is the situa-

TABLE XXIII

CHANGE OF PROBABILITY VALUES WITH CHANGE IN DISTRIBUTION OF A CONSTANT
DIFFERENCE IN RESULTS BETWEEN TWO GROUPS OF ANIMALS

Comparison	Experimental group S^b	D	Control group S	D	p value for this distribution[a] (alone + more extreme ones)
a	5	9	0	14	0.020
b	6	8	1	13	0.036 + 0.003 = 0.039
c	7	7	2	12	0.045 + 0.006 = 0.051
d	8	6	3	11	0.051 + 0.009 = 0.060
e	9	5	4	10	0.054 + 0.011 = 0.065
f	10	4	5	9	0.054 + 0.011 = 0.065
g	11	3	6	8	0.051 + 0.009 = 0.060
h	12	2	7	7	0.045 + 0.006 = 0.051
i	13	1	8	6	0.036 + 0.003 = 0.039
j	14	0	9	5	0.020

[a] Fisher's exact probability test is used to determine probability (p) values. For this situation, where the number n of animals in each group is 14 and the difference d in numbers of survivors between experimental and control groups is 5, the *least favorable distribution* of survivors occurs with either 9 or 10 survivors in the experimental group: the p value is then highest, which means that a true distinction between the two groups is least likely. For the general case where n and d may have any value, the least favorable distribution occurs when there are $(n + d)/2$ survivors in the experimental group if $(n + d)/2$ is an integer, or if it is not, when there are $(n + d)/2 \pm 0.5$ survivors in the experimental group. For the above case, with $n = 14$ and $d = 5$, this distribution occurs when the number of survivors s is either $(14 + 5)/2 + 0.5 = 10$, or else $(14 + 5)/2 - 0.5 = 9$. Once s has been determined for the experimental group, its value for the control group is $s - d$; the number of tumor deaths in each group is obtained by subtracting the number of survivors from the total number of animals n in each group.

[b] S, Survivors; D, tumor deaths.

tion for comparisons e and f, which represents the least favorable situation for obtaining a statistically significant result.

Because of the above considerations, the values of p given in Table XXII apply only to the most favorable situation, when there are either 100% tumor deaths in the controls, or 0% tumor deaths in the experimentals. The values of p for the least favorable conditions, corresponding to the situation for comparisons e and f of Table XXIII, are given in Table XXIV.

In order to give a clear overview of the results of Tables XXII and XXIV, a summary is presented in Table XXV. This table shows that the number of animals required for each of the two groups is independent of the manner in which survivors and tumor deaths are distributed when there are large differences between the results obtained for the two groups. However, when this difference falls below 75%, more animals are required to provide statistical significance when the distribution varies from the most favorable (100% tumor deaths in the controls or 0% tumor deaths in the experimentals). This tendency for divergence between the numbers of animals required for significance increases progressively as the difference between the results for the two groups becomes smaller. Table XXV shows that groups which one might think are sufficiently large if one has not gone through the present statistics (for instance, groups composed of seven experimental animals and seven controls) will not give statistically significant results, even if the true difference between the groups is as high as 50%.

Comparison between Tables XXII and XXIV, which is highlighted by the summary of Table XXV, indicates that if one wishes to achieve a statistically significant difference between the control and the experimental groups, one should arrange to obtain 100% tumor deaths in the control group, or else 0% tumor deaths in the experimental group—a condition not as easily met as the former. If it seems likely that neither of these two conditions can be met, one should use the numbers of animals evident from Table XXIV (or the numbers in brackets in Table XXV) to achieve significant results for the degrees of difference between the two groups that one expects to obtain.

Another way in which probabilities for significant differences between an experimental and a control group can be arranged is shown in Table XXVI, which is summarized in Table XXVII. To illustrate how this latter table functions, let us assume that there is a difference of 4 in the number of animals that survive in the experimental group and in the control group. If the total number of animals in each group is 4, then the experimental group must have 4 survivors/4 total animals, while the control group has 0/4; these results differ at the level of $p = 0.01$ (Table XXVII). If this dif-

TABLE XXIV

PROBABILITY THAT STATED PERCENTAGE DIFFERENCES IN RESULTS BETWEEN AN EXPERIMENTAL AND A CONTROL GROUP REPRESENT TRUE DISTINCTIONS BETWEEN THE GROUPS AND NOT RANDOM CHANCE UNDER THE LEAST FAVORABLE DISTRIBUTION OF TUMOR DEATHS WITH SOME SURVIVORS IN BOTH GROUPS[a]

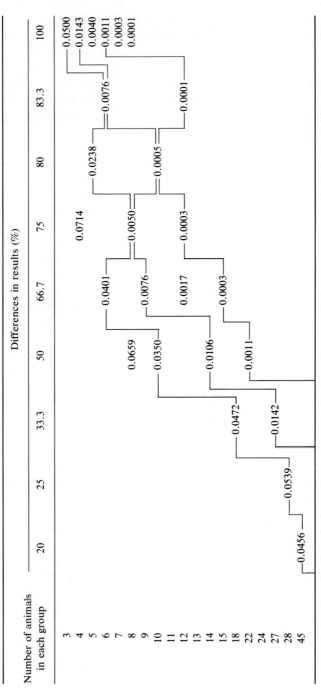

Number of animals in each group	Differences in results (%)								
	20	25	33.3	50	66.7	75	80	83.3	100
3									
4						0.0714			0.0500
5									0.0143
6								0.0076	0.0040
7							0.0238		0.0011
8				0.0659	0.0401				0.0003
9						0.0050			0.0001
10				0.0350	0.0076				
11							0.0005		
12					0.0017	0.0003			
13								0.0001	
14				0.0106					
15					0.0003				
18			0.0472						
22				0.0011					
24			0.0142						
27		0.0539							
28									
45	0.0456								

[a] See all footnotes to Table XXII regarding the explanation of this table, and the footnote to Table XXIII for derivation of the least favorable distribution of survivors in the experimental and control groups.

TABLE XXV

Minimum Numbers of Animals Required in Order for Stated Percentage Differences in Results between Experimental and Control Groups to be Statistically Significant[a]

Probability (p) of a true difference[b]	Differences in results (%)								
	20	25	33.3	50	66.7	75	80	83.3	100
0.05	20 (45)[c]	16 (28)	12 (18)	8 (10)	6 (6)	8 (8)	5 (5)	6 (6)	3 (3)
0.01	30 (>45)	24 (>28)	18 (27)	12 (14)	9 (9)	8 (8)	10 (10)	6 (6)	4 (4)
0.001	45 (>45)	36 (>36)	27 (>27)	16 (22)	12 (15)	12 (12)	10 (10)	12 (12)	6 (6)

[a] Equal numbers of animals in the experimental and the control groups.

[b] Probability values computed to one significant figure.

[c] Numbers required under the most and under the least favorable distribution of tumor deaths are represented by figures without and with parentheses, respectively (see p. 60 for explanation).

TABLE XXVI

PROBABILITY THAT STATED DIFFERENCES IN NUMBERS OF SURVIVORS BETWEEN AN EXPERIMENTAL AND A CONTROL GROUP REPRESENT TRUE DISTINCTIONS BETWEEN THE GROUPS AND NOT RANDOM CHANCE[a]

Difference in number of animals between groups	Number of animals in each group											
	1	2	3	4	5	6	7	8	9	10	14	18
A. Under ideal conditions, with tumor deaths at 100% in controls or 0% in experimentals												
1	0.500	0.500	0.500	0.500	0.500	0.500						
2		0.167	0.200	0.214	0.222	0.227						
3			0.050	0.071	0.083	0.091						
4				0.014	0.024	0.030	0.035	0.038	0.041	0.043	0.049	0.052
5					0.004	0.008	0.010	0.013	0.015	0.016	0.020	0.023
6						0.001	0.002	0.003	0.005	0.005	0.008	0.010
7							<0.001	0.001	0.001	0.002	0.003	0.004
8								<0.001	<0.001	<0.001	0.001	0.001
9									<0.001	<0.001	<0.001	<0.001
B. Under least favorable conditions, with tumor deaths and survivors in both groups												
1	0.500	0.500	0.500	0.500	0.500	0.500						
2		0.167	0.200	0.243	0.262							
3			0.050	0.071	0.103	0.121						
4				0.014	0.024	0.040	0.051	0.066				
5					0.004	0.008	0.015	0.020	0.028	0.035	0.064	0.047
6						0.001	0.002	0.005	0.008	0.012	0.029	0.022
7							<0.001	0.001	0.002	0.003	0.011	0.009
8								<0.001	<0.001	0.001	0.004	0.003
9										<0.001	0.001	0.001
10										<0.001	<0.001	0.001

[a] Equal numbers of animals used in the experimental and the control groups. Fisher's exact probability test (Fisher, 1946; Denenberg, 1976) used to determine p. As an illustration of how this table functions, here is what is implied by a *difference in number of animals between groups* of 3, and a *number of animals in each group* of 6, in terms of survivors/total number animals: (A) Under ideal conditions, the experimentals and the controls have respectively 3/6 and 0/6, or else 6/6 and 3/6 survivors/total number, and $p = 0.091$; (B) under least favorable conditions, these figures are respectively 5/6 and 2/6, or else 4/6 and 1/6, and $p = 0.121$. For an explanation how this least favorable distribution of survivors can be obtained,

TABLE XXVII

Maximum Numbers of Animals Permitted for a Stated
Difference in Numbers of Survivors between Experimental
and Control Animals to Be Statistically Significant[a]

Difference in number of animals between groups	Limits in total number of animals in each group within which the stated level of statistical significance applies
A. Statistical probability 0.05 or less	
3	3 only (3 only)[b]
4	4–18 (4–7)
5	5–>30[c] (5–12)
6	6–>50 (6–19)
B. Statistical probability 0.01 or less	
4	4 only (4 only)
5	5–8 (5–7)
6	6–>30 (6–10)
7	7–>40 (7–15)
8	8–>50 (8–21)
9	9–>60 (9–27)
10	10–>70 (10–34)

[a] Equal numbers of animals used in the experimental and the control groups. Fisher's exact probability test used to determine p to one significant figure. For an illustration of how this table functions, see text.

[b] Numbers required under the most and least favorable distribution of tumor deaths are represented by figures without and with parentheses, respectively.

[c] Here, ">" denotes that the given probability applies somewhat beyond the stated number of animals.

ference of 4 occurs when the total number of animals in each group is either 5, 6, or 7, the results for the experimental and control groups differ at the level of $p = 0.05$, irrespective of the distribution of survivors in the two groups. For instance, when the total of animals in each group is 7, the results for the number of survivors/total number in the experimental group and in the control group, respectively, could be either $4/7$ and $0/7$ (most favorable distribution), $5/7$ and $1/7$, $6/7$ and $2/7$, or $7/7$ and $3/7$ (also a most favorable distribution); for all these distributions of survivors, the comparison between the two groups is still statistically significant at the 0.05 level of probability. If, however, the same difference of 4 survivors between the two groups occurred when the total number of animals in each group was 18, this result would only be significant if the distribution of survivors in the two groups was, respectively, $4/18$ and $0/18$, or $18/18$ and

$^{12}/_{18}$ (both are most favorable distributions), but *not* if it was $^{5}/_{18}$ and $^{1}/_{18}$, $^{6}/_{18}$ and $^{2}/_{18}$, or $^{7}/_{18}$ and $^{3}/_{18}$, etc. If the actual distribution of survivors lies between the most favorable distribution and the least favorable distribution of $(18 + 4)/2$ or 11 survivors/18 total for experimentals and $^{7}/_{18}$ for controls (see footnote to Table XXIII for calculation of this least favorable distribution), then one has to evaluate p by setting up a 2×2 table, as illustrated at the beginning of this section. Table XXVII will not give the answer for intermediate distributions of survivors, since it lists results only for the most and for the least favorable distributions.

The above discussion has been confined to the case where the numbers of animals in the experimental and control groups are equal. Is this the most efficient assignment of a given number of animals, or are there distributions more likely to give statistically significant results for a certain minimum difference between the two groups? This question is addressed in Table XXVIII. It is seen that if we impose the condition that the difference between the experimental and the control groups, in terms *both* of the number of survivors *and* of the number of tumor deaths, must be as small as possible and yet result in the highest possible level of statistical significance for this difference, then the most economical use of a given number of animals is indeed to assign equal numbers to the experimental group and to the control group. However, when more than one experimental group is compared to a single control group, the best strategy probably consists of assigning more animals to the control group than to each of the experimental groups. (Regarding reduction of animals in groups, see Note Added in Proof, p. 84.)

2. Data on Day of Death from Tumor

One-way analysis of variance is superior to use of the t test in situations where data are available from groups of animals additional to the two groups which are to be compared. However, the additional groups must comprise part of the same experiment and be of comparable nature. Use of the data from these additional groups increases the precision of the statistical analysis.

Textbooks on statistics give detailed instructions for performance of AOV. Better yet, most computer facilities associated with universities or medical schools have the capability to run an AOV program on behalf of an investigator. For those who have access to a minicomputer such as the Hewlett-Packard model 9815A in their own laboratories, software that includes AOV is generally available. Use of such a program for the statistical analysis of data on the day of death following challenge with tumor is both rapid and simple. Here, use of such a program is illustrated for data obtained for the challenge of five groups of mice with 30,000 viable cells of the ascites tumor L1210-L-W (Table XXIX).

The total numbers of mice in the latter experiment were actually 9, 7, 9,

TABLE XXVIII

EFFECT OF UNEQUAL NUMBERS OF ANIMALS IN THE CONTROL AND EXPERIMENTAL
GROUPS ON THE STATISTICAL SIGNIFICANCE OF A GIVEN DIFFERENCE
IN RESULTS BETWEEN THE GROUPS

Comparison	Number of animals		Difference between experimentals and controls		Experimentals		Controls		Probability[a]
	Experimentals	Controls	S[b]	D	S	D	S	D	(p)
A. Most favorable conditions: 100% tumor deaths in controls, 0% in experimentals									
a	14	14	5	5	5	9	0	14	0.020
b	15	13	5	3	5	10	0	13	0.031
c	15	13	6	4	6	9	0	13	*0.013*
d	13	15	5	7	5	8	0	15	*0.013*
e	13	15	4	6	4	9	0	15	0.035
B. Least favorable conditions: symmetrical distribution of survivors and deaths									
f	14	14	5	5	10	4	5	9	0.065
g	15	13	5	3	10	5	5	8	0.133
h	15	13	6	4	11	4	5	8	0.072
i	13	15	5	7	10	3	5	10	*0.026*
j	13	15	4	6	9	4	5	10	*0.064*

[a] The total number of animals for the experimental and control groups combined is constant at a figure of 28. Values of p are italic when they are lower than those obtained for comparisons a and f, for which the number of animals in the two groups is equal.

[b] S, Survivors; D, tumor deaths.

9, and 9, respectively. Since none of the mice in group 5 died of tumor, this group is not shown in Table IX. Even if one mouse had died of tumor, its day of death could not be used in AOV, since one cannot obtain a standard deviation for a single value. In group 4, only $2/9$ mice died from tumor, but the days of death of these mice can be used in AOV, as long as the conclusions drawn from AOV take into account the data on survivors/tumor deaths, which do not enter directly into AOV computations.

Data for the days of death of animals that died with tumor in groups 1–4 are entered into the computer program. The computer then prints out the following statistics: mean, variance, and standard deviation for each group (which have been entered into Table XXIX), and an AOV table that lists the total degrees of freedom (df) calculated as (total number of values in all groups − 1), in our case (9 + 7 + 9 + 2 − 1), or 26, which is the value of the parameter n_2 in a table of F that can be found in most text-

TABLE XXIX

ILLUSTRATION OF ANALYSIS OF VARIANCE FOR DATA ON DAY OF DEATH FROM TUMOR[a]

Group	Number of mice	Days on which mice died following challenge with viable tumor cells									Mean	Variance	Standard deviation
1	9	11	11	11	11	11	11	11	13	13	11.4	0.8	0.9
2	7	12	18	24	24	26	29	36			24.1	58.8	7.7
3	9	9	11	11	12	13	14	16	22	24	14.7	26.5	5.1
4	2	16	22								19.0	18.0	4.2

[a] Challenge performed with 30,000 viable cells of the ascites tumor L1210-L-W.

books on statistics. Also printed are the df for the treatments, calculated as (number of treatment groups − 1), in our case (4 − 1), or 3, which represents the parameter n_1 in a table of F. Finally, an F value is printed out, in our case 8.86. When this value is entered in a table of F, with $n_2 = 26$ and $n_1 = 3$, we find that it represents $p < 0.01$. This p value expresses the probability that the subsequent comparisons between sets of two groups may give rise to a false claim that results for two groups are significantly different, when in fact they are not different. As long as this probability is less than 0.05, the subsequent comparisons between sets of two groups are valid. We may therefore proceed with these comparisons.

The computer program permits us to contrast the data obtained for one group with that obtained for another. On the Hewlett-Packard program for AOV, the only complication lies in entering into the contrast program those two groups that one wishes to compare. If one wishes to compare groups 1 and 2, one must enter first the number of animals in the second group, then the negative number of animals in the first group, followed by zero for each of the other groups not involved in the comparison. In the case where the numbers of animals are equal in the two groups that are to be compared, one can enter 1 and − 1 instead of the actual number of animals in these two groups. The computer prints out an F ratio, the df numerator n_1 (number of treatment groups − 1)—in our case (2 − 1) or 1, and the df denominator n_2 (total number of observations in the two groups being compared − 2)—in our case (16 − 2), or 14. In our case, the F ratio for comparison of groups 1 and 2 is 24.8, which is found to correspond to a value of $p < 0.01$ when entered into an F table for $n_1 = 1$ and $n_2 = 14$. This indicates that groups 1 and 2 of Table XXVII differ below the 1% level of statistical significance.

Most computer programs for AOV follow the determination of treatment contrasts with a second test that examines whether or not the use of AOV for the data under consideration is valid. This is Bartlett's test, which examines the variances of the different treatment groups to determine whether they are close to each other within acceptable limits, such as a range of 3:1 for the highest:lowest variance. The results of Bartlett's test printed by the computer for the present data (Table XXIX) give $\chi^2 =$ 20.0, with a df value evaluated as (number of treatment groups $-$ 1), in our case $(4 - 1)$ or 3. The corresponding value of p read from a standard table of χ^2 is under 0.01, which indicates that there is a highly significant difference in the variance of the various groups. This difference is easily observed from the listing of variances in Table XXIX; it is commonly seen in therapy experiments, where the control group (in our case, group 1) consists of animals that die in closely homogeneous fashion relatively early after injection of the challenge dose of tumor cells. In contrast, the other groups contain animals that have reacted in widely differing manners to the therapy treatments they have received, as evidenced by non-uniform prolongation of survival time prior to death from tumor. However, Norton's work (see Lindquist, 1956) suggests that the robustness of AOV analysis is sufficient enough that Bartlett's test need not be used to invalidate an AOV analysis. This would be the function of Bartlett's test in the present case, where its results are highly significant. Snedecor's (1946) treatment of Bartlett's test in reference to AOV also makes it clear that a highly significant result need not invalidate the AOV analysis if the reasons for large differences in variances between groups are understood and taken into account in evaluating the results of the AOV analysis. Also available are nonparametric procedures such as the Kruskal–Wallis test.

3. Data on Tumor Diameter Measurements

In most previous studies, the size of tumors in different groups of animals was measured on one day only, and either the t test or the analysis of variance were used for analysis of the data. A far better opportunity to obtain statistically significant differences between experimental and control groups is achieved if tumor sizes are measured on several days; the data obtained in this way are then subjected to analysis of variance for independent groups with repeated measures (Kirk, 1968). The considerations that led to the choice of this approach are outlined below.

Measurements of tumor lengths and breadths are begun when tumors are first discovered using mice anesthetized with ether. Caliper readings to the nearest millimeter are made on each tumor in two directions (length and breadth) at right angles to each other. Depending upon the rate of tumor growth, measurements are performed every 3 or 4 days, or else every 7 days, for a total of 5 to 8 times.

In the experiment illustrated here (Table XXX), measurements were ended before any mouse had died from tumor. Alternatively, measurements can be continued beyond the death of one or more mice, and the data for subsequent days of measurements are simply reduced in size by the absence of dead mice. This poses no problem for the type of AOV analysis found ideally suited to the present data (see p. 72). If alternative statistical methods are used that cannot accommodate a reduction in the numbers of animals, it is possible to restitute mice that have died from tumor by a convention: the largest tumor dimensions measured in the relevant group immediately prior to the death of the mouse are carried forward to subsequent days of measurement. In any case, if a mouse is inadvertently killed with anesthetic or lost for reasons unconnected with the experiment, it is eliminated from all tumor measurement data; but if it had already developed a tumor by the time it died or was lost, it may be retained in the data reported for survivors/tumor deaths.

Before statistical tests are applied to raw data on size measurements such as those in Table XXX, it is essential that each length and breadth measurement be converted to a single number representative of tumor diameter. Otherwise, the number of measurements equals twice the number of tumors measured, and this leads to serious difficulties in the correct application of the concept of degrees of freedom when the results of statistical tests are evaluated. Ideally, a single number representative of tumor diameter would be the cube root of tumor (length) × (breadth) × (width). If one is unable to perform easily three such measurements at right angles to each other, the next best representation of tumor diameter would be the square root of tumor (length) × (breadth), measured in two directions at right angles. The author has performed many statistical tests in which tumor diameters were calculated by this formula. In no instance was a different statistical result obtained when tumor diameters were calculated by the mathematically less satisfactory formula (length + breadth)/2. Therefore, investigators are advised to use the simplest possible statistic, namely, the latter, the mean of length and breadth, as representative of tumor diameter.

The simplest and most straightforward method by which the difference between experimental and control group measurements can be tested for statistical significance is Student's t test (Fisher, 1946). When this test is applied to the data in Table XXX (once these have been converted to tumor diameters as suggested above) values of t 1.80, 0.85, 1.53, 1.72, and 1.58 are obtained for the data gathered on days 7, 10, 14, 17, and 25, respectively. The corresponding values of the probability p were < 0.1, < 0.5, < 0.2, < 0.2, and < 0.2, indicating that there were no statistically significant differences between groups on any of the days on which measurements were made.

A slightly more sophisticated approach is to subject the data (for instance the results in Table XXX converted to tumor diameters) to analysis

TABLE XXX

Tumor Diameter Measurements for an Experimental and a Control Group[a]

| Group | Day after challenge with viable tumor cells | | | | | | | | | |
| | 7 | | 10 | | 14 | | 17 | | 25 | |
	L[b]	B	L	B	L	B	L	B	L	B
Experimentals	0	0	0	0	9	9	17	8	23	15
	0	0	0	0	10	8	19	13	8	7
	0	0	0	0	7	7	14	8	24	15
	0	0	0	0	7	5	13	12	10	8
	7	5	10	7	12	7	9	6	19	7
	0	0	9	7	6	4	9	9	10	7
	0	0	8	7	8	6	11	6	17	12
Mean	0.9		3.4		7.5		11.0		13.0	
Controls	0	0	0	0	11	7	16	14	21	16
	0	0	7	6	13	12	22	15	27	19
	8	7	10	9	14	13	9	7	10	9
	5	3	7	7	14	12	16	15	22	16
	10	7	8	7	12	12	13	9	23	19
	0	0	8	5	14	13	16	10	14	12
	9	7	0	0	0	0	19	16	21	10
Mean	4.0		5.3		10.5		14.1		17.1	

[a] The experimental group consisted of seven C57BL/6J females immunized six times at weekly intervals with approximately 25 mg of irradiated tumor Os-B, an isogenic strontium-90-induced osteogenic sarcoma. The seven control mice were left uninjected. One week after the last immunization, both groups were challenged subcutaneously with a predetermined dose of a suspension of minced viable Os-B tumor in transplant generation 24.
[b] L, Length; B, breadth, in millimeters.

of variance. This method is described in virtually every modern textbook on statistics, and is available in the statistical programs of the Hewlett-Packard 9815A minicomputer, as well as in the software library of virtually every modern university-based computer facility. First the data obtained on all 5 days of measurement are entered, then the measurements obtained for the two groups on one particular day of measurement are compared. When this analsis was applied to the above data for measurements performed on days 7, 10, 14, 17, and 25, the values of F obtained were, respectively, 2.32, 0.81, 2.11, 2.21, and 3.89. All of these values of F correspond to values of p that are statistically insignificant.

Both of the above tests compare the results of the measurements made on the experimental and the control group *only a single day at a time.* In contrast, the analysis of variance for independent groups with repeated measures (called "split-plot repeated measures design SPF-2.3" by Kirk, 1968) compares the data obtained on all days of measurements for the two groups in a single statistical test. To avoid the laborious calculations required for performance of this statistical test, use of the program for it available at most research computing facilities is suggested. When the data of Table XXX (reduced to tumor diameters) were entered into such a computer program, a value of $F = 14.93$ was obtained. Using 1 degree of freedom for groups (2 groups $- 1 = 1$) and 12 degrees of freedom for repeated measures (2 groups $\times$ 7 animals in each group $- 2$), the corresponding value of the probability p is < 0.01, indicating a significant difference in the measurement data for the experimental as compared to the control group. The program at the Boston University facility available to us had the capability of converting our data into logarithms, and of substituting a value of 2 mm for all values of 0 mm obtained for tumor diameters; this substitution is justified on the basis that the smallest tumor diameter that could be measured by us was occasionally 4 mm and more usually 5 mm, so that absence of a palpable tumor could actually imply the presence of a tumor in the range 0–4 (mean $= 2$) mm. Analyses performed with logarithmic conversion of the data, and with substitution of "2" every time "0" appeared in the data plus logarithmic conversion, gave values of p of, respectively, < 0.05 and < 0.05. Hence, these transformations were not useful for analysis of the present data (Table XXX).

4. Correction for Repeated Tests of Statistical Significance

One caution must be included regarding the use of any of the tests described in Sections VII,A,1,2, or 3, in which results obtained for a single control group are compared with the results obtained for several experimental groups. If we compare a particular set of results obtained for a control group with just one set of results obtained for an experimental group, we correctly set our limits for a statistically significant difference between these two sets of results as $p \leq 0.05$. This means that 19 times out of 20, the results observed will indicate a true difference between the two groups, while 1 time in 20 the discordance of the results is a chance event caused by sampling error. On the other hand, if we compare 5 sets of experimental results (obtained for 5 different experimental groups) with a single set of results obtained for a control group, the chance that a value of $p < 0.05$ represents a chance event due to sampling error is still only $1:20$ for any one experimental group. But looked at together, values of $p \leq 0.05$ obtained for comparisons of each of the 5 experimental groups with the control group means that now there are 1×5 chances out of 20 that *one* of the experimental groups would achieve a value of $p \leq 0.05$! To compensate for this inequity, Bonferroni (see Glantz, 1981) has suggested that if more than one comparison (for instance, n comparisons) between experimental and control groups is made, the value of p for statistical significance should be taken to be not 0.05, but instead $0.05/n$. In our case, this value of p would be $\leq 0.05/5$ or $p \leq 0.01$.

Another way in which the above correction can be made for any situation in which the t distribution is used is to construct a new table for evaluation of the probability p that takes into account Bonferroni's considerations regarding multiple comparisons that involve repeated use of a single set of data. Such a table has been published by Dunnett (1955). However, there continues to be a controversy about the application of Bonferroni's and Dunnett's corrections, since in many cases these are not linear, as assumed by the authors. The problem posed by such corrections can be circumvented by the restriction of comparisons to the fewest possible number.

B. PERFORMANCE OF TUMOR CHALLENGE INJECTIONS

As in most laboratory operations, success in performance of challenges with viable tumor cells depends both on the availability of good equipment and supplies, and on manipulative skill. These aspects are discussed below under separate headings.

1. Equipment and Supplies

The most important piece of equipment for animal injections is a hood with a strong exhaust fan (Fig. 1). Plexiglas carrying-tops and carrying-trays for rack cages with wire-mesh floors are valuable time-savers (Fig. 1). They make it unnecessary to transfer animals from rack-type cages into totally enclosed carrying cages, which is the practice in many laboratories. Perhaps least important is the Micromedic Automatic Pipet, which is used to deliver 0.1 ml of 95% ethanol when a foot pedal is pressed. While this frees the hands, use of a plastic squeeze bottle to apply ethanol to the animal skin in the area intended for injections is not very much more cumbersome. To prevent ether from wetting the animal skin, the floor of the 4000-ml beaker that serves as anesthesia chamber is raised about 2 cm by insertion of a circular stainless-steel screen, with ends turned downward to provide this elevation. To minimize the inhalation of ether by the person who performs the injections, three steps are taken: the sliding door of the hood is kept as low as is convenient for free access to the anesthesia chamber, this vessel is pushed to the rear of the hood as far as is possible, and, most important, the working surface of the hood

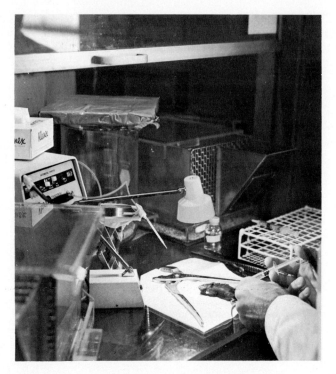

FIG. 1. Equipment for tumor challenge injections. From left to right, cage with plastic carrying-top and carrying-bottom for mice to be injected, Micromedic Automatic Pipet model 25004 for delivery of 0.1 ml 95% ethanol through a catheter (shown held in place above injection area) and activated by foot pedal (not shown), high-intensity lamp (Tensor), anesthesia chamber (4000-ml Kimax beaker no. 14005) and cover, cage for receipt of injected mice with plastic carrying-top and carrying-bottom, sterile bottle containing tumor cell suspension, and sterile syringe and needle. Injections are performed with the mouse resting on disposable tissue, prevented from flapping in the draft caused by the hood exhaust by weighting down with a heavy object. To reduce the operator's exposure to the ether used for anesthesia, the hood's sliding door is kept as low as is practical. Further, a 9.5-mm-thick sheet of Plexiglas has been placed over the entire floor of the hood extending 23 cm out beyond the floor of the hood so that all injections can be performed where exposure to ether is minimal.

is extended into the room by insertion of a heavy sheet of Perspex (Fig. 1).

With regard to supplies, presterilized physiological saline, antibiotics, and culture media can all be purchased. In addition, Wheaton serum bottles (Fisher No. 06-406-F) with sleeve-type rubber stoppers (Fisher No. 06-406-10B), which need to be sterilized in one's own laboratory, are very useful for the preparation of standardized cell suspensions and for storage of the laboratory's own solutions and media that are intended for animal injection.

2. Design and Performance of Challenge Injections

a. Preliminary Experiments. Before a definitive challenge of control and immunized animals is attempted, the following information vital to the success of the challenge experiments should be determined in preliminary experiments: the LD_{10} (lethal dose of tumor cells for 10% of the mice), LD_{50}, and LD_{90} for the tumor cells in question when tested in the inbred strain in which the tumor originated, or (not quite as desirable) in an F_1 hybrid of which one parent represents the isogenic strain. In addition, it is very helpful to repeat this determination 120 minutes after the first series of challenge injections, to test the decrease in tumor cell viability with time of storage during the challenge procedure, and on another day, to test the reproducibility of the results when the same or the next transplant generation of the tumor is used.

Perhaps the most important decision in the design of challenge experiments is the time permitted between harvest of the tumor to be used for challenge and injection of the last animal that is challenged in the experiment. Ascites tumors yield a single cell suspension that can generally be stored for 2 to 3 hours without serious loss in viability, especially when tissue culture media are employed. In contrast, mincing or enzymatic degradation of solid tumors yields cell suspensions that tend to be more fragile. It is therefore important to perform preliminary experiments to determine the conditions under which the tumor cell suspension deteriorates least rapidly, and to use these standarized conditions for all challenges.

Cell viability is often equated with the ability of the cells to prevent permeation by vital dyes, such as eosin or trypan blue, when the cells are placed in a dilute solution containing 0.15% eosin plus 0.05% trypan blue for 1 to 3 minutes at room temperature. While exclusion of vital dyes is useful for rough assessment of cell viability, transplantation tests indicate that the true viability can be far lower than indicated by dye exclusion, especially when the percentage of cells able to exclude dye drops below 50% (Reif and Norris, 1960). For this reason, it would be wrong to conclude that because the degree of vital staining has dropped only slightly during the time interval required for challenge injections, the transplantation viability has not dropped radically. Therefore, it is wise to perform transplantation tests, rather than merely vital staining, to test the decline of cell viability during the time required for challenge injections.

b. Planning and Preparation. Loss of tumor cell viability is more readily apparent when a small rather than a large inoculum of tumor cells is used. Therefore, injections should begin at the lowest dose and end at the highest dose. If the highest dose chosen requires use of cell suspensions more concentrated than about 1×10^7 cells/ml, clumping may occur if the cells are permitted to stand for more than 30 to 60 minutes. In that case, clumping can be avoided by the addition of 100 units of heparin/ml; or better, by using a suspension medium free of Ca^{2+} and Mg^{2+} ions to which 10% EDTA has been added (Lawler et al., 1981). Alternatively, challenges performed at any other cell dose can be preceded by challenges at the highest dose. If many different groups of mice require injection and loss of tumor cell viability represents a problem, it is often essential to perform the experiment in two portions, each with newly prepared cell suspensions. However, the injections at any given cell concentration are performed all together, with a minimum of time lag between injection of the first and the last group.

If cell viability drops significantly during the time required to challenge several groups of mice with a given number of tumor cells, then it can happen that the later a group is injected, the more numerous the survivors in that group. For this reason, the group expected to yield the highest number of survivors is challenged first, and the control group is challenged last. In this way, prejudice that might lead to a false-positive result for the experimental group is avoided. If the control group is challenged last, it may develop more survivors than some of the experimental groups (see challenge at 5.0 mg tumor, Table XXXI; however, the increase in survivors was not statistically significant in this example).

In order to evaluate adequately the results of challenge experiments, one needs to determine the LD_{50} for the cells used in the actual challenge experiment; this permits expression of the various challenge doses in terms of multiples of LD_{50}. For this reason, control groups challenged with progressively fewer tumor cells are included in the challenge experiment, since evaluation of LD_{50} requires data both from a control group in which there are more than 50% survivors, and from a control group with fewer survivors. The number or weight of tumor cells used for the challenge is plotted logarithmically along the x axis of semilogarithmic paper, while the percentage of tumor deaths that result from the challenge is plotted arithmetically along the y axis. The LD_{50} cell dose is read off at 50% tumor deaths.

Preparation and labeling of animal groups and cages prior to the challenge experiment reduces the time required for it. Cages are arranged in the order of the injections. Each mouse is routinely earmarked with the group's number prior to the challenge. The Jackson Laboratory's system for numbering ears with a small punch (Fisher No. 01-337B) is best modified by omission of the numbers 5, 7, and 8, which are easily confused.

TABLE XXXI

RESULTS OF CHALLENGE WITH VIABLE TUMOR: TEST OF IMMUNOREJECTIVE
STRENGTH WHEN CELL VIABILITY DECLINES RAPIDLY DURING THE ASSAY[a,b]

Challenge dose[c] of SMx-E tumor (mg)	Number of weekly immunizations with 25 mg irradiated SMx-E tumor mince									
	6×		4×		3×		2×		0×	
	S[d]	D	S	D	S	D	S	D	S	D
0.8									8	1
2.0									0	9
5.0	7	2	0	9	1	8	2	7	3	6
12	1	8	1	8	0	9	3	6	2	7
30	0	9	0	9	0	9	0	9	0	9
75	0	8	0	9	0	8	0	9	0	9

[a] Trial of transplant generation 39 of carcinoma SMx-E of C57BL/6J mice in DBF$_1$ hybrid females 16 weeks old at the time of challenge with tumor.

[b] The experiment was performed in two portions, using freshly harvested tumor in each case. In the morning, groups of mice immunized 6×, 4×, 3×, 2×, and 0× (controls) were challenged in that order with 12, 30, and 75 mg of viable tumor per mouse. In the afternoon, two control groups were challenged with 0.8 and 2.0 mg, then groups 6×, 4×, 3×, 2×, and 0× were challenged in that order with 5.0 mg of viable tumor.

[c] Challenge doses specify the wet weight of tumor tissue injected sc through an 18-gauge needle in finely minced form.

[d] S, Survivors; D, tumor deaths.

Sufficient numbers remain to number a plethora of groups. With this modification, looking down on the back of a mouse, earmarks are coded as follows. On the periphery of the right earlobe: 1, 2, and 3, one mark each on top, middle, and bottom, respectively; 4 and 6, two marks each on top and bottom, respectively; 9, one mark both on top and on bottom. On the periphery of the left ear lobe: to denote the double digits 10, 20, and 30; 40 and 60; and 90, the same code is used as for single digits on the right ear. Near the center of the right ear lobe: for 100, 200, and 300, one, two, and three punches, respectively. Near the center of the left ear lobe: for 1000, 2000, and 3000, one, two, and three punches, respectively. With the convention that 0 is represented by the absence of a mark, this system permits the numbering of $(7 \times 7 \times 4 \times 4 - 1)$, or 783 different groups.

c. Standardization of Cell Suspensions and Animal Injections. Single cell suspensions of tumor cells are standardized either by hemacytometer count or by use of the Coulter counter. Having decided what numbers of cells should be injected during the challenge experiment, it is usually convenient to prepare a cell suspension that contains the highest number of cells one intends to inject in a convenient volume such as 0.5 ml. If one wished to inject 1×10^6 cells into each mouse, then one would prepare a cell suspension containing 2×10^6 cells/ml and inject 0.5 ml into each mouse.

Depending upon the circumstances, each one of three different methods for changing the concentration of a standardized cell suspension has particular usefulness.

1. Rapid method.

> Where i = initial cell concentration
> and f = final cell concentration desired (where $i > f$)

Now measure out f ml of the suspension of initial concentration i, add an amount $(i - f)$ ml of buffer, and mix. The cell concentration is now f. Instead of using f ml of the suspension of concentration i, one can use rf ml. Then one should add $r(i - f)$ ml of buffer, and mix, to attain a cell concentration of f. Here, r = a constant that can have any desired value.

2. Initial volume of suspension fixed. If i and f have the above meaning, and i is greater than f, then if

> U ml = initial volume of cell suspension (at concentration i)
> and V ml = final volume of cell suspension (at concentration f),

then the final volume is

$$V \text{ ml} = U(i/f) \text{ ml}$$

and the amount of buffer to add in order to attain volume V is

$$W \text{ ml} = V - U \text{ ml} = U(i - f)/f \text{ ml}$$

3. Buffer volume is fixed. Suppose we have a certain fixed volume of

$$W \text{ ml} = \text{volume of buffer}$$

and it is this buffer to which we would like to add

> X ml = volume of suspension (at concentration i),
> where f = final cell concentration desired (and $i > f$)
> then $X = Wf/(i - f)$ ml

While method (*1*) is very simple, it wastes some of the cell suspension, whereas method (*2*) does not waste a drop. Method (*3*) is useful when a large volume of dilute suspension must be prepared from a small volume of concentrated suspension.

As an example, suppose i = 9000 cells/ml, f = 6000 cells/ml, U = 10 ml, and W = 5 ml. Then for (*1*), one measures out rf = 6 ml of suspension i, and adds $r(i - f) = (9 - 6) = 3$ ml buffer. While one need not evaluate r to use this method, its value here is 0.001. For (*2*), to

$U = 10$ ml of suspension i one adds $W = 10(9 - 6)/6 = 5$ ml of buffer. For (3), to $W = 5$ ml of buffer one adds $X = 5 \times 6000/(9000 - 6000) = 10$ ml suspension i.

To ensure that there is a sufficient amount of material for injections, 10% more than one desires to inject should be prepared. In addition, the quantities required for serial dilutions should be provided for.

To prevent the settling out of suspensions of single cells or of tumor mince, we have devised a "stirrer" method to load syringes with uniform amounts for use in injections. The cell suspension is placed in a disposable sterile plastic flask and stirred magnetically at a rate just sufficient to maintain a uniform suspension. The plastic-coated stirrer bar is previously sterilized by dipping in 95% ethanol, burning this off by passing it rapidly through a Bunsen burner flame, and then letting it cool. While stirring is in progress, all the syringes needed to inject animals at a single cell concentration are then filled with suspension and stored in the refrigerator at 5°C.

After each syringe is filled, a bubble of air approximately 0.15 ml in volume is drawn into the syringe, and then the needle attached to the syringe is once again filled with suspension. The bubble is used to mix the contents of the syringe by repeated inversion of the syringe immediately prior to its use for injections. In addition, once the needle has penetrated to the site where the inoculum is to be injected into the animal, the syringe is rotated 360° about its axis immediately prior to the actual injection. In this way, a close correspondence between the number of tumor cells injected into each animal is maintained. This is vital in order to avoid inequity in the injection of different animals and different groups.

In order to inject mice rapidly, one should work only with one group at a time, but introduce between three and nine mice into the ether chamber at one time, as long as there is an appropriate time interval between the introduction of each mouse. After practice, one can arrange to have the next mouse enter an appropriate stage of anesthesia just when the previous mouse has been injected. In this way, an experienced worker can inject 50 to 60 mice per hour during challenges by routes such as ip, sc, im, or id. In contrast, iv injections are far more time consuming.

ACKNOWLEDGMENTS

Thanks are due to the following research assistants for their excellent work: Cynthia Robinson, Dovile Eiva Cooper, Ann T. Fidler, Francesca Holinko, Clara Tomas, Chantal I. Charles, Walter Gonzalez, and Samuel Bechar. Thanks are also due to R. Ernest Clark, Ph.D., Professor and Head, Division of Biostatistics, Tufts University School of Dental Medicine, and to Herbert Kayne, Ph.D., Chief, Biostatistics Laboratory, Boston University School of Medicine, for their help with and review of the section on statistics in the Appendix.

REFERENCES

Abelev, G. I., Engelhardt, N. V., and Elgort, D. A. (1979). *Methods Cancer Res.* **18**, 1–37.

Alaba, O., and Law, L. W. (1978). *J. Exp. Med.* **148**, 1435–1439.

Andersen, V., Bjerrum, O., Bendixen, G., Schiødt, T., and Dissing, I. (1970). *Int. J. Cancer* **5**, 357–363.

Argyris, B. F., and Reif, A. E. (1981). *Cancer Res.* **41**, 839–844.

Bach, M. L., Bach, F. H., and Joo, P. (1969). *Science* **166**, 1520–1522.

Barth, R. F., Gillespie, G. Y. III, and Gobuty, A. (1972). *Natl. Cancer Inst. Monogr.* **35**, 39–47.

Bartlett, G. L. (1972a). *J. Natl. Cancer Inst.* **49**, 493–504.

Bartlett, G. L. (1972b). *Natl. Cancer Inst. Mongr.* **35**, 27–35.

Bartlett, G. L., Katsilas, D. C., Kreider, J. W., and Purnell, D. M. (1977). *Cancer Immunol. Immunother.* **2**, 127–133.

Basombrio, M. A., and Prehn, R. T. (1972). *Cancer Res.* **32**, 2545–2550.

Bauma, R., and Marks, A. (1981). *Cancer Res.* **41**, 2598–2604.

Black, M. M., Moore, D. H., Shore, B., Zachrau, R. E., and Leis, H. P. (1974). *Cancer Res.* **34**, 1054–1060.

Bloom, B. R. (1980). *J. Immunol.* **124**, 2527–2528.

Broder, S., and Waldmann, T. A. (1978a). *N. Engl. J. Med.* **299**, 1281–1284.

Broder, S., and Waldmann, T. A. (1978b). *N. Engl. J. Med.* **299**, 1335–1341.

Brunner, K. T., Mavel, J., Cerottini, J.-C., and Chapuis, B. (1968). *Immunology* **5**, 181–196.

Cantrell, J. L., Killion, J. J., and Kollmorgen, G. M. (1976). *Cancer Res.* **36**, 3051–3057.

Cataldo, E., and Reif, A. E. (1982). *Cancer*, in press.

Churchill, W. H., Jr., Rapp, H. J., Kronman, B. S., and Borsos, T. (1968). *J. Natl. Cancer Inst.* **41**, 13–29.

Crane, J. L., Jr., Glasgow, L. A., Kern, E. R., and Younger, J. S. (1978). *J. Natl. Cancer Inst.* **61**, 871–874.

Crispen, R. G., ed. (1976). "Neoplasm Immunity: Mechanisms." ITR, Chicago.

Davis, M.-T. B., and Preston, J. F. (1981). *Science* **213**, 1385–1388.

Denenberg, V. H. (1976). "Statistics and Experimental Design for Behavioral and Biological Researchers. An Introduction," p. 269. Wiley, New York.

Dunnett, C. W. (1955). *J. Am. Stat. Assoc.* **50**, 1096–1121.

Eilber, F. R., and Morton, D. L. (1970). *J. Natl. Cancer Inst.* **44**, 651–657.

Fidler, I. J. (1978). *Methods Cancer Res.* **15**, 399–439.

Finney, D. J., Latscha, R., Bennett, E. M., and Hsu, P. (1963). "Tables for Testing Significance in a 2 × 2 Contingency Table." Cambridge Univ. Press, London and New York.

Fisher, B. (1975). *In* "Immunity and Cancer in Man: An Introduction" (A. E. Reif, ed.), pp. 81–90. Dekker, New York.

Fisher, R. A. (1946). "Statistical Methods for Research Workers," 10th Ed., p. 96. Oliver & Boyd, Edinburgh.

Forni, G., Giovarelli, M., Varesio, L, and Landolfo, S. (1979). *In* "Current Trends in Tumor Immunology" (S. Ferrone, S. Gorini, R. B. Herberman, and R. A. Reisfeld, eds.), pp. 73–84. Garland STPM, New York.

Gibson, T. G., and Martin, W. J. (1978). *Cancer Immunol. Immunother.* **3**, 201–205.

Gilbert, J. R., ed. (1972). *Natl. Cancer Inst. Monogr.* **35**, 1–477.

Glantz, S. A. (1981). "Primer of Biostatistics," p. 88. McGraw-Hill, New York.

Gold, P., Shuster, J., and Freedman, S. O. (1978). *Cancer* **42**, 1399–1405.

Goldenberg, D. M., ed. (1980). *Cancer Res.* **40**, 2953–3087.

Golub, S. H. (1975). *In* "Cancer. A Comprehensive Treatise" (F. F. Becker, ed.), Vol. 4, pp. 259–300. Plenum, New York.

Gorer, P. A., and Amos, D. B. (1956). *Cancer Res.* **16**, 338–343.
Green, I., Cohen, S., and McCluskey, R. T. (1977). "Mechanisms of Tumor Immunity." Wiley, New York.
Greenberg, P. D., Cheever, M. A., and Fefer, A. (1981). *J. Immunol.* **126**, 200–203.
Gross, L. (1943). *Cancer Res.* **3**, 326–333.
Gunby, P. (1981). *J. Am. Med. Assoc.* **246**, 205.
Hager, J. C., and Heppner, G. H. (1978). *Handb. Cancer Immunol.* **4**, 195–218.
Halliday, W. J., and Miller, S. (1972). *Int. J. Cancer* **9**, 477–483.
Hann, H.-W. L., Evans, A. E., Cohen, I. J., and Leitmeyer, J. E. (1981). *N. Engl. J. Med.* **305**, 425–429:
Harris, J. E., and Sinkovics, J. G. (1976). "The Immunology of Malignant Disease." Mosby, St. Louis, Missouri.
Hattler, B., and Amos, B. (1966). *Monogr. Surg. Sci.* **3**, 1–34.
Hellström, K. E., and Hellström, I. (1971). *In* "Immunobiology" (R. A. Good and D. W. Fisher, eds.), pp. 209–218. Sinauer, Stamford.
Hellström, K. E., and Möller, G. (1965). *Prog. Allergy* **9**, 158–245.
Hersh, E. M., and Sinkovics, J. G., eds. (1978). "Immunotherapy of Human Cancer." Raven, New York.
Humphrey, J. H., and White, R. G. (1970). "Immunology for Students of Medicine," 3rd Ed. Davis, Philadelphia, Pennsylvania.
Humphrey, L. J., Estes, N. C., Morse, P. A., Jewel, W. A., Boudet, R. A., and Hudson, M. J. K. (1974). *Cancer* **34**, 1516–1520.
Jamasbi, R. J., and Nettesheim, P. (1977). *Int. J. Cancer* **20**, 817–823.
Jamasbi, R. J., and Nettesheim, P. (1979). *Cancer Res.* **39**, 2466–2470.
Jamasbi, R. J., Nettesheim, P., and Kennel, S. J. (1978). *Cancer Res.* **38**, 261–267.
Jami, J., Rubio, N., and Ritz, E. (1976). *Eur. J. Cancer* **12**, 13–18.
Jones, F. R., Yoshida, L. H., Ladiges, W. C., and Kenny, M. A. (1980). *Cancer* **46**, 675–684.
Kahan, B. D. (1972). *In* "Transplantation Antigens" (B. D. Kahan and R. A. Reisfeld, eds.), pp. 311–338. Academic Press, New York.
Kaiser, C. W., and Reif, A. E. (1975). *In* "Immunity and Cancer in Man: An Introduction" (A. E. Reif, ed.), pp. 19–46. Dekker, New York.
Kirk, R. E. (1968). "Experimental Design: Procedures for the Behavioral Sciences," pp. 246–255. Brooks-Cole, Belmont, California.
Klein, E., and Klein, G. (1964). *J. Natl. Cancer Inst.* **32**, 547–568.
Klein, G. (1968). *Cancer Res.* **28**, 625–634.
Klein, G. (1969). *Fed. Proc. Fed. Am. Soc. Exp. Biol.* **28**, 1739–1753.
Klein, G. (1975). *Harvey Lect.* **69**, 71–102.
Klein, J. (1975). "Biology of the Mouse Histocompatibility-2 Complex," p. 517. Springer-Verlag, Berlin and New York.
Kobayashi, H. (1981). *In* "Immunological Aspects of Cancer Therapeutics" (E. Mihich, ed.), in press.
Kobayashi, H., Kodama, T., and Gotohda, E. (1977). *Hokkaido Univ. Med. Libr. Ser.* **9**, 1–124.
Kobayashi, H., Takeichi, N., and Kuzumaki, N. (1978). *Hokkaido Univ. Med. Libr. Ser.* **10**, 1–174.
Kripke, M. L. (1980). *Cancer Biology Rev.* **1**, 221–250.
Kronman, B. S., Rapp, H. J., and Borsos, T. (1969a). *J. Natl. Cancer Inst.* **43**, 869–875.
Kronman, B. S., Wepsic, H. T., Churchill, W. H., Jr., Zbar, B., Borsos, T., and Rapp, H. J. (1969b). *Science* **165**, 296–297.
Lavrovsky, V. A., and Viksler, V. K. (1980). *Cancer Res.* **40**, 3252–3258.

Law, L. W. (1969). *Cancer Res.* **29**, 1–21.
Law, L. W., Rogers, M. J., and Appella, E. (1980). *Adv. Cancer Res.* **32**, 201–235.
Lawler, E. M., Outzen, H. C., and Prehn, R. T. (1981). *Cancer Immunol. Immunother.* **11**, 87–91.
LeGrue, S. J., Kahan, B. D., and Pellis, N. R. (1980). *J. Natl. Cancer Inst.* **65**, 191–196.
Leibo, S. P. (1978). *Cancer Immunol. Immunother.* **3**, 211–213.
Lindquist, E. F. (1956). "Design and Analysis of Experiments in Psychology and Education," pp. 78–86. Houghton, Boston, Massachusetts.
McCollester, D. L. (1980). *Cancer Immunol. Immunother.* **8**, 249–256.
Mathé, G. (1978). *Cancer Immunol. Immunother.* **5**, 149–152.
Mazuran, R., Majugic, H., Malenica, B., and Silobrevic, V. (1976). *Int. J. Cancer* **17**, 14–20.
Middle, J. G., and Embleton, M. J. (1981). *J. Natl. Cancer Inst.* **67**, 637–643.
Mizushima, Y., Sendo, F., Miyake, T., and Kobayashi, H. (1981) *J. Natl. Cancer Inst.* **66**, 659–665.
Möller, G. (1961). *J. Exp. Med.* **114**, 415–434.
Mousawy, K. M., Rees, R. C., and Potter, C. W. (1980). *Cancer Immunol. Immunother.* **8**, 119–126.
Müller, D., and Sorg, C. (1975). *Eur. J. Immunol.* **5**, 175–178.
Murphy, S. G., Laufman, H., and LoBuglio, A. F. (1977). *J. Natl. Cancer Inst.* **58**, 1815–1818.
Murthy, M. S., Belehradek, J., Jr., and Barski, G. (1976). *Eur. J. Cancer* **12**, 33–39.
Nadler, L. M., Stashenko, P., Hardy, R., Kaplan, W. D., Button, L. N., Kufe, D. W., Antman, K. H., and Schlossman, S. F. (1980). *Cancer Res.* **40**, 3147–3154.
Nelson, R. A., Jr. (1953). *Science* **118**, 733–737.
Old, L. J. (1981). *Cancer Res.* **41**, 361–375.
Old, L. J., and Boyse, E. A. (1964). *Annu. Rev. Med.* **15**, 167–186.
Oldham, R. K., Ortaldo, J. R., Holden, H. T., and Herberman, R. B. (1977). *J. Natl. Cancer. Inst.* **58**, 1061–1067.
Order, S. E. (1975). *In* "Immunity and Cancer in Man: An Introduction" (A. E. Reif, ed.), pp. 91–102. Dekker, New York.
Osband, M. E., Shen, Y.-J., Shlesinger, M., Brown, A., Hamilton, D., Cohen, E., Lavin, P. and McCaffrey, R. (1981). *Lancet* **1**, 636–638.
Pellis, N. R., and Kahan, B. D. (1976). *Methods Cancer Res.* **13**, 291–330.
Perlmann, P., and Perlmann, H. (1970). *Cell. Immunol.* **1**, 300–315.
Peters, L. C., Brandhorst, J. S., and Hanna, M. G., Jr. (1979). *Cancer Res.* **39**, 1353–1360.
Pimm, M. V., and Baldwin, R. W. (1977). *Int. J. Cancer* **20**, 923–932.
Phillips, J. H., Babcock, G. G., and Nishioka, K. (1981). *J. Immunol.* **126**, 915–921.
Pinkel, D. (1976). *J. Am. Med. Assoc.* **235**, 1049–1050.
Prager, M. D. (1975). *In* "Cellular Membranes and Tumor Cell Behavior," pp. 523–540. Williams & Wilkins, Baltimore, Maryland.
Prager, M. D., and Baechtel, F. S. (1973). *Methods Cancer Res.* **9**, 339–400.
Price, M. R., Preston, V. E., Robins, R. A., Zöller, M., and Baldwin, R. W. (1978). *Cancer Immunol. Immunother.* **3**, 247–252.
Rapp, H. J. (1979). *Natl. Cancer Inst. Monogr.* **52**, 457–460.
Reif, A. E. (1975). *In* "Immunity and Cancer in Man: An Introduction" (A. E. Reif, ed.), pp. 1–18. Dekker, New York.
Reif, A. E. (1978). *Handb. Cancer Immunol.* **1**, 173–240.
Reif, A. E. (1979). *Cancer Immunol. Immunother.* **7**, 141–142.

Reif, A. E. (1981). *Fed. Proc. Fed. Am. Soc. Exp. Biol.* **40**, 984.
Reif, A. E., and Kim, C.-A. H. (1971). *Immunology* **20**, 1087–1097.
Reif, A. E., and Norris, H. J. (1960). *Cancer Res.* **20**, 1235–1245.
Reif, A. E., and Tomas, C. (1980). *Proc. Am. Assoc. Cancer Res* **21**, 251.
Reif, A. E., Curtis, L. E., Duffield, R., and Shauffer, I. A. (1974). *J. Surg. Oncol.* **6**, 133–150.
Rivera, E. S., Hersh, E. M., Bowen, J. M., Barnett, J. W., Wharton, T., and Murphy, S. G. (1979). *Cancer* **43**, 2297–2305.
Rosenberg, S. A., and Terry, W. D. (1977). *Adv. Cancer Res.* **25**, 323–388.
Ruppert, B., Wei, W., Medina, D., and Heppner, G. H. (1978). *J. Natl. Cancer Inst.* **61**, 1165–1169.
Schmidt, M., Fruchter, G., Stergiopoulous, G., and Babott, D. (1981). *Cancer Immunol. Immunother.* **10**, 167–168.
Shields, R. (1975). *Nature (London)* **256**, 537–538.
Shiku, H., Takahashi, T., Oettgen, H. F., and Old, L. J. (1976). *J. Exp. Med.* **144**, 873–881.
Snedecor, G. W. (1946). "Statistical Methods," 4th Ed., pp. 249–252. Iowa State Univ. Press, Ames.
Snell, G. D. (1963). In "Conceptual Advances in Immunology and Oncology," p. 323–353. M. D. Anderson Hospital Symposium, Houston, Texas.
Southam, C. M., and Friedman, H., eds. (1976). *Ann. N. Y. Acad. Sci.* **277**, 1–741.
Southam, C. M., Brunswig, A., Levin, A. G., and Dizon, Q. S. (1966). *Cancer* **19**, 1743–1753.
Suit, H. D., Sedlacek, R. S., and Wiggins, S. (1977). *Cancer Res.* **37**, 3836–3837.
Sulitzeanu, D., and Weiss, D. W. (1981). *Cancer Immunol. Immunother.* **11**, 291–292.
Takasugi, M., and Klein, E. (1970). *Transplantation* **9**, 219–227.
Talmadge, J. E., Key, M., and Fidler, I. J. (1981). *J. Immunol.* **126**, 2245–2248.
Task Force on Immunology and Disease (1977). "Immunology. Its Role in Disease and Health." DHEW Publ. No. 77-940. National Institutes of Health, Bethesda.
Terman, D. S., Young, J. B., Shearer, W. T., Ayus, C., Lehane, D., Mattioli, C., Espada, R., Howell, J. F., Yamamoto, T., Zaleski, H. I., Miller, L., Frommer, P., Feldman, L., Henry, J. F., Tillquist, R., Cook, G., and Daskal, Y. (1981). *N. Engl. J. Med.* **305**, 1195–1200.
Terry, W. D., and Windhorst, D. (1978). "Immunotherapy of Cancer: Present Status of Trials in Man." Raven, New York.
Thaler, M. S., Klausner, R. D., and Cohen, H. J. (1977). "Medical Immunology." Lippincott, Philadelphia, Pennsylvania.
Urist, M. M., Boddie, A. W., Holmes, E. C., and Morton, D. L. (1976). *Int. J. Cancer* **17**, 338–341.
Vaage, J. (1973). *Methods Cancer Res.* **8**, 33–58.
Vaage, J. (1978). *Cancer Res.* **38**, 331–338.
Vaage, J. (1979). *Cancer Immunol. Immunother.* **6**, 185–189.
Vaage, J. (1980). *Cancer Res.* **40**, 3495–3501.
Vaage, J., and Agarwal, S. (1978). *Methods Cancer Res.* **14**, 1–27.
Vaage, J., and Medina, D. (1978). *Cancer Res.* **38**, 2443–2447.
Voller, A., and Bidwell, D. E. (1980). *Clin. Immunol. Newsletter.* **1**, 5–7.
Wagner, H., and Rollinghoff, M. (1973). *J. Exp. Med.* **138**, 1–15.
Weiss, D. W. (1980). "Tumor Antigenicity and Approaches to Tumor Immunotherapy—An Outline." Springer-Verlag, Berlin and New York.
Winn, H. J. (1961). *J. Immunol.* **86**, 228–239.

Witz, I. P., and Hanna, M. J., Jr., eds. (1980). *Contemp. Top. Immunobiol.* **10,** 1–348.

Wood, G. W., and Gellespie, G. Y. (1975). *Int. J. Cancer* **16,** 1022–1029.

Woodruff, M. F. A. (1980). "The Interaction of Cancer and the Host." Grune & Stratton, New York.

Yefenof, E., Tchakirov, R., and Kedar, E. (1980). *Cancer Immunol. Immunother.* **8,** 171–178.

Zichelboim, J., Bonavida, B., and Fahey, J. L. (1973). *J. Immunol.* **111,** 1737–1742.

NOTE ADDED IN PROOF: ATTEMPT TO REDUCE NUMBER OF ANIMALS PER GROUP. When assay conditions can be arranged to assure tumor deaths of 100% in the controls and of 0% in the experimentals, then three animals per group suffice to give statistical significance (see result of 2× immunization at a challenge dose of 1.5 million Lk-B cells, Table XXXII). In contrast, results of 1× immunization were not significant, even though there was a 66.7% difference in survivors compared to controls; this difference would have been significant if six or more animals had been used instead of only three (see Table XXV).

TABLE XXXII

RESULTS OF CHALLENGE WITH VIABLE TUMOR: RELATIVE ANTIGENIC STRENGTH ASSAY IN RANGE B1: EFFECT OF REDUCTION IN THE NUMBER OF MICE ASSIGNED TO GROUPS[a]

Challenge dose of Lk-B cells[b] (millions)	Number of weekly immunizations with 25 mg irradiated tumor					
	0×		1×		2×	
	S[c]	D	S	D	S	D
0.08	2	1				
1.5	0	3	1	2	3[d]	0
4.5	0	6	1	2	2	1
12.1	0	6	0	3	2	4
38.0	0	6	0	3	0	6

[a] Results added *in proof* on day 43 after challenge with tumor.

[b] Lk-B is a lymphoma induced in our laboratory by injection of MuLV into newborn C57BL/6J mice. The original transplant was made 86 days after injection of the virus, and tumor from transplant generation 4 was used for challenge.

[c] S, Survivors; D, tumor deaths.

[d] Results significant at the 5% level (see Table XXVII). This result merits award of a RAS score of 5.0 in range B1 (see Table XI). If, however, 8 animals had been used in each group as suggested in Table IV (line 3), then the result at a challenge dose of 4.5 million cells might have been significant and the RAS score higher.

CHAPTER II

ALLOGENEIC CELL IMMUNITY*

M. HOSOKAWA AND H. KOBAYASHI

I. Introduction

In connection with the findings of alien histocompatibility antigens on tumor cells (Invernizzi and Parmiani, 1975; Martin *et al.*, 1976; Wrathmell *et al.*, 1976; Bonavida *et al.*, 1980), it has been of interest to note that immunization with allogeneic, neoplastic, or normal cells produces transplantation resistance against syngeneic tumors. Since immune responses to allogeneic cells have been extensively investigated for years in conjunction with concepts for the rejection mechanism in syngeneic tumor

* This work was in part supported by Grant-in-Aid for Cancer Research from the Ministry of Education, Science, and Culture, Japan.

cells, these findings of alien histocompatibility antigens on tumor cells as tumor-associated transplantation antigens (TATA) are attractive. With regard to the immunizing effects of allogeneic tumor cells, there is the further consideration that allogeneic tumor cells share cross-reactive tumor-specific transplantation antigens (TSTA) with syngeneic tumor cells.

However, such cross-reactive antigens are not always responsible for the immunizing effects of allogeneic cells. The authors have previously observed that antigenically unrelated allogeneic cells produce strong transplantation resistance to various lines of syngeneic tumors in rats (Kobayashi et al., 1974; Hosokawa et al., 1976). The phenomenon referred to as "allogeneic cell immunity" has been thought to be due to nonspecific stimulation of host resistance to tumors, and not to cross-reactive antigens between immunizing allogeneic cells and challenging syngeneic tumor cells. Similar nonspecific immune resistance to leukemic cells can be obtained by the "allogeneic effect," first proposed by Katz et al. (1971a), which is evoked by the transient graft-versus-host (GVH) reaction following transfer of allogeneic immunocompetent cells (Katz et al., 1971a,b; 1972; Osborne and Katz, 1977a,b). The GVH reaction, however, is not necessary for the production of allogeneic cell immunity, since allogeneic tumor cells and skin grafts could produce the immunizing effects in our system. It has been reported that the responsiveness in vitro of spleen cells to syngeneic tumor cells in mice was augmented by priming in vivo with allogeneic cells (Dennert, 1975; Bach et al., 1980). At present, the authors are unable to propose a conclusive explanation for the mechanism of allogeneic cell immunity. However, investigation of these phenomena may be an efficient way to discover the means by which stimulation of the host's immunological resistance against tumors is achieved.

II. Inhibition of Tumor Growth in Syngeneic Rats Immunized with Allogeneic Cells

A. IMMUNIZING EFFECTS OF ALLOGENEIC TUMOR CELLS

During attempts in this laboratory to induce specific antitumor resistance in syngeneic rats by immunization with murine leukemia virus-infected viable tumor cells (Kobayashi et al., 1969, 1970a, 1977), it was accidentally noticed that the growth of a transplanted tumor was also inhibited in syngeneic rats after immunization with viable allogeneic tumor cells which had been used as control, antigenically unrelated immunizing tumor cells. This growth inhibition of transplanted tumor after immunization with allogeneic tumor cells was studied extensively. Vari-

TABLE I

INHIBITION OF KMT-17 TUMOR GROWTH IN SYNGENEIC WKA
RATS IMMUNIZED WITH VARIOUS ALLOGENEIC
TUMOR LINES FROM DONRYU RATS

Immunized with		Growth of KMT-17	
Tumor	Type	Died/used	(Temporary)[a]
None	—	32/32	(32/32)
AH-66	Liver cancer	1/106	(3/106)
AH-66F	Liver cancer	0/4	(1/4)
AH-60C	Liver cancer	0/4	(1/4)
AH-272	Liver cancer	0/4	(1/4)
DLT	Lung cancer	0/4	(1/4)
AS-D653	Fibrosarcoma	0/7	(0/7)
DBLA-6	Leukemia	0/4	(4/4)
DBLA-10	Leukemia	4/8	(8/8)

[a] Growth of tumor more than 10 mm in diameter.

ous types of allogeneic tumor cells from Donryu strain rats induced a strong transplantation resistance to KMT-17 tumor—a methylcholanthrene-induced fibrosarcoma in Wistar King Aptekman (WKA)/Hok rats (Table I). Moreover, immunization with AH-66 tumor cells, which were used mainly for analysis of this phenomenon, effectively inhibited the growth of several lines of syngeneic tumors in WKA rats (Table II), as reported by Kobayashi *et al.* (1974, 1980). From these results the authors postulate that a cross antigen between allogeneic and syngeneic tumor

TABLE II

INHIBITION OF GROWTH OF VARIOUS LINES OF SYNGENEIC TUMORS IN WKA RATS
IMMUNIZED WITH ALLOGENEIC AH-66 TUMOR CELLS FROM DONRYU RATS

Challenge with[a]			Growth of tumor (died/used)	
Tumor	Type	Number of cells	In immune rats	In normal rats
KMT-50	Fibrosarcoma	16^6	0/8	8/8
KST-1	Hemangiosarcoma	10^6	0/5	5/5
NRT	Neurosarcoma	Trocal	0/4	4/4
KBT-10	Breast cancer	Trocal	0/7	4/4
KDH-8	Liver cancer	10^6	0/8	11/11

[a] Syngeneic tumor cells were challenged 1 week after the last immunization with 10^7 AH-66 cells.

cells is not responsible for the immunizing effects of allogeneic cells because it is unlikely that such a number of tumor lines should have cross-reactive antigens as tumor-specific transplantation antigens. In fact, AH-66 tumor cells were antigenically different from KMT-17 tumor cells, as described in Section V,A.

B. Immunizing Effects of Allogeneic Skin Grafts

Since the immunizing effects of allogeneic tumor cells seemed to be unrelated to TSTA, it was important to clarify whether strong inhibition could be induced not only by allogeneic tumor cells, but also by allogeneic normal cells. Although the immunizing effects of normal allogeneic cells were comparatively weak when the immunization was performed with suspended cells from various tissues, skin grafting from Donryu strain rats completely inhibited the growth of KMT-17 tumors (Table III). This inhibition by immunization with skin grafts was as strong as by immunization with tumor cells (Hosokawa et al., 1976). The authors observed, thereafter, that allogeneic kidney and urinary bladder tissues, as well as skin grafts, from Donryu strain rats induced a complete resistance to tumor when they were patched to the skin graft bed of the recipients (Table IV). These organ tissues induced weaker resistance if they were inserted subcutaneously (sc) for immunization. These results indicated that immunizing effects were dependent on the site in the recipient rats

TABLE III

Inhibition of KMT-17 Growth in Syngeneic WKA Rats
Immunized with Various Types of Allogeneic
Normal Cells from Donryu Rats

| | Growth of KMT-17 | |
Immunized with	Died/used	(Temporary)[a]
None	32/32	(32/32)
Liver cells	2/4	(4/4)
Spleen cells	1/7	(4/7)
Kidney cells	1/4	(2/4)
Embryo cells	1/5	(2/5)
Whole blood	2/9	(3/9)
White blood cells	10/24	(14/24)
Red blood cells	1/4	(4/4)
Platelets	3/4	(4/4)
Skin grafts	0/34	(0/34)

[a] Growth of tumor more than 10 mm in diameter.

TABLE IV

INHIBITION OF KMT-17 GROWTH IN WKA RATS IMMUNIZED WITH
ALLOGENEIC EPITHELIAL TISSUES FROM DONRYU RATS

Immunization[a]		Lethal growth of KMT-17		
Tissue	Route	Died/used	(%)	MSD ± SD[b]
None		0/9	(100)	18 ± 3
Skin	Grafted to skin	0/13	(0)	—
Skin	Inserted sc	5/11	(46)	27 ± 12
Kidney	Patched to skin	0/10	(0)	—
Kidney	Inserted sc	4/10	(40)	25 ± 8
Urinary bladder	Patched to skin	0/10	(0)	—
Urinary bladder	Inserted sc	2/5	(40)	24 ± 7

[a] One million cells of KMT-17 were sc inoculated 10 days after the immunization with allogeneic tissues.
[b] MSD ±SD, Mean survival days ± standard deviation.

where the reaction to allogeneic cells occurred rather than on the kinds of donor cells used. In the experiments in which the immunizing effects of spleen cells introduced by various routes were compared, intradermal (id) immunization was the most efficient means of inhibiting the growth of tumors (Table V). The reaction to allogeneic cells in the skin of recipients was effective for induction of allogeneic cell immunity just as cellular response was effectively stimulated by the intradermal immunization.

TABLE V

INHIBITION OF KMT-17 GROWTH IN WKA RATS IMMUNIZED WITH
ALLOGENEIC SPLEEN CELLS FROM DONRYU
RATS BY DIFFERENT ROUTES

Route of immunization[a]	Lethal growth of KMT-17 (died/used) Number of cells challenged			LTD$_{50}$[b]
	10^5	10^6	10^7	
Not immunized	9/9	4/4	4/4	<3 × 10^4
id	0/4	1/4	1/4	>1470 × 10^4
sc	1/9	3/10	4/4	164 × 10^4
ip	1/5	5/5	5/5	24 × 10^4

[a] Fifty million (5 × 10^7) allogeneic spleen cells were inoculated 10 days before challenge of KMT-17 tumor cells as the immunization.
[b] LTD$_{50}$, 50% lethal tumor dose.

C. Necessity of Immunization with Viable Allogeneic Cells

Studies on nonspecific antitumor resistance induced by bacteria indicate that administration of living materials favors tumor inhibition (Woodruff and Boak, 1966; Zbar et al., 1971; Zbar, 1972). In allogeneic cell immunity, it was seen that immunization with viable allogeneic cells is necessary to elicit immunizing effects. Viable AH-66 cells and fresh skin grafts induced complete resistance to syngeneic tumors. However, immunization with freeze-thawed cells showed no effect and treatments which attenuate the viability of allogeneic cells reduced their immunizing effects (Table VI). It should be pointed out that allogeneic tumor cells or skin grafts were able to survive in the recipients for several days before rejection. This suggests that the reaction to viable allogeneic cells might stimulate nonspecifically an immunity in the host resulting in resistance to syngeneic tumor cells. It was observed that alloreactive lymphocytes, but not lymphocytes reacting to syngeneic tumor cells, could be induced even if immunization was performed with freeze-thawed allogeneic cells (Section V,B).

D. Abrogation of Immunizing Effects by Low-Dose Whole-Body Irradiation

In the investigation to clarify whether the resistance is due to an immunological mechanism, recipients were given whole-body irradiation 24 hours before the tumor challenge. The immunizing effects of allogeneic tumor cells and skin grafts were abrogated by irradiation in both groups (Table VII). These results indicated that the inhibition of syngeneic tumor growth by allogeneic cells was due to an immunological mechanism. Moreover, it was observed that the immunizing effects of allogeneic cells were easily abrogated by low-dose irradiation (250 or 350 rad), which ought to abrogate only nonspecific resistance against tumors, as described by Klein and Klein (1962).

E. Strength of Antitumor Transplantation Resistance

It should be emphasized that antitumor resistance was very strong after immunization with allogeneic cells. That is the reason why the authors have paid special attention to this phenomenon. For example, the KMT-17 tumor—a fibrosarcoma in WKA rats—is a very fast growing tumor and grew lethally in 50% of the nonimmunized syngeneic rats when it was transplanted subcutaneously with a dose of less than 10^4 cells [50% lethal

TABLE VI

INHIBITION OF KMT-17 TUMOR IN SYNGENEIC WKA RATS IMMUNIZED WITH
INACTIVATED ALLOGENEIC CELLS FROM DONRYU RATS

Experiment	Immunized with	Growth of KMT-17		
		Died/used	(%)	MSD[a]
I	None	8/8	(100)	17.5
	Viable AH-66 cells	0/9	(0)	—
	Mitomycin C-treated AH-66 cells	5/9	(56)	25.0
	Formaldehyde-treated AH-66 cells	8/8	(100)	23.0
	Glutaraldehyde-treated AH-66 cells	9/9	(100)	24.2
	Freeze-thawed AH-66 cells	13/13	(100)	19.8
II	None	5/5	(100)	13.0
	Fresh skin graft	0/7	(0)	—
	Skin graft stored for 1 day at 4°C	1/8	(13)	28.0
	Skin graft stored for 7 days at 4°C	4/8	(50)	15.3
	Freeze-thawed skin graft	8/8	(100)	18.4

[a] MSD, Mean survival days.

tumor dose (LTD_{50}) is less than 10^4 cells in normal rats]. One million cells of KMT-17 tumor failed to grow at all in rats after a single immunization with 10^7 allogeneic tumor cells. Further immunization with allogeneic tumor cells produced even stronger effects, resulting in 5×10^7 cells of the tumor being completely inhibited after three immunizations (Table VIII). The strong immunizing effect was also observed after allogeneic skin grafting. The LTD_{50} of KMT-17 cells increased 7500 times when the

TABLE VII

ABROGATION OF IMMUNIZING EFFECTS OF ALLOGENEIC
CELLS BY IRRADIATION

Immunization with[a]	Irradiation with[b] (rad)	Growth of KMT-17 (died/used)
None	None	10/0
AH-66 cells	None	0/6
AH-66 cells	250	7/9
AH-66 cells	600	6/6
Skin graft from Donryu rat	None	0/3
Skin graft from Donryu rat	350	4/5

[a] Immunization was performed 10 days before challenge of 10^6 KMT-17 tumor cells.

[b] Recipient rats received whole-body irradiation 24 hours before tumor challenge.

TABLE VIII

STRENGTH OF ANTITUMOR RESISTANCE AGAINST KMT-17 TUMOR IN WKA
RATS IMMUNIZED WITH ALLOGENEIC AH-66 CELLS

Immunization[a]		Growth of tumor[b] [died/used (%)]			
		Number of cells challenged			
Number of cells	Number of times	1×10^6	5×10^6	1×10^7	5×10^7
None	—	30/30 (100)	4/4 (100)	20/20 (100)	14/14 (100)
1×10^7	1	0/30 (0)	—	0/25 (0)	1/4 (25)
1×10^6	3	0/13 (0)	0/4 (0)	—	—
5×10^6	3	0/4 (0)	—	0/4 (0)	—
1×10^7	3	0/10 (0)	0/4 (0)	—	0/8 (0)

[a] Immunization was performed by sc inoculation of AH-66 cells at 1-week intervals.
[b] KMT-17 cells were challenged sc 10 days after the first immunization and 7 days after the last.

tumor cells were challenged subcutaneously in rats immunized by alloge-neic skin grafting, and increases in LTD_{50} were by 4500 and 600 times in cases of intraperitoneal (ip) and intravenous (iv) challenging, respectively (Table IX). There has previously been no report indicating such a strong resistance to syngeneic tumors. The authors have not been able to offer any exact explanation of the strong resistance in allogeneic cell immunity, but it is postulated that viable allogeneic cells may efficiently elicit the host immunity to tumor as described previously.

TABLE IX

INCREASE OF LTD_{50} IN WKA RATS IMMUNIZED WITH
ALLOGENEIC SKIN GRAFTS AND CHALLENGED
WITH KMT-17 BY DIFFERENT ROUTES

Route of challenge	$LTD_{50}{}^a$ of KMT-17		
	In immune rats[b]	In nonimmune rats	Increase of $LTD_{50}{}^c$
sc	$22,400 \times 10^3$	$<3 \times 10^3$	$7500\times$
ip	$>150,000$	<32	$4700\times$
iv	$>2400 \times 10^4$	$<4 \times 10^4$	$600\times$

[a] LTD_{50}, 50% lethal tumor dose.
[b] Rats were immunized with allogeneic skin grafts from Donryu rats 10 days before challenged with KMT-17.
[c] Increase of LTD_{50} is LTD_{50} in immune rats/LTD_{50} in non-immune rats.

III. Exception of Leukemia and Lymphoma Cells in Allogeneic Cell Immunity

Various types of tumor were involved in this matter of the induction of resistance and inhibition of tumor growth in allogeneic cell immunity. However, the authors observed some exceptional tumors which were not inhibited in rats immunized with allogeneic cells. These exceptions were leukemias and lymphomas. The characteristics of leukemic tumors in allogeneic cell immunity may relate to the nature of the immunostimulation of allogeneic cells (Hosokawa *et al.*, 1978).

A. Lack of Inhibition of Growth of Leukemias and Lymphomas

Although six lines of nonleukemic tumor were rejected in syngeneic rats by immunization with allogeneic cells (Table II), the growth of two lines of leukemias (KNL-1 and KNL-6) and two lines of lymphomas (WRT-1N and WFT-2N) was not inhibited at all in similarly immunized rats. In addition, immunization with allogeneic leukemic cells (DBLA-6 and DBLA-10) from Donryu strain rats was not effective in inhibiting the growth of the leukemic tumors either (Table X).

TABLE X

LACK OF INHIBITION OF LEUKEMIA AND LYMPHOMA GROWTH IN SYNGENEIC
RATS IMMUNIZED WITH ALLOGENEIC TUMOR CELLS

Immunized with tumor[a] (type)	Challenged with tumor[b] (type)	Growth of tumor (died/used)	MSD[c]
None	KNL-1 (leukemia)	10/10	23 ± 4
AH-66 (liver cancer)	KNL-1 (leukemia)	12/12	21 ± 2
DBLA-6 (leukemia)	KNL-1 (leukemia)	4/4	21 ± 6
DBLA-10 (leukemia)	KNL-1 (leukemia)	4/4	21 ± 2
None	KNL-6 (leukemia)	2/2	59 ± 4
AH-66	KNL-6 (leukemia)	2/2	68 ± 6
None	WRT-1N (lymphoma)	6/6	39 ± 5
AH-66	WRT-1N (lymphoma)	6/6	43 ± 3
None	WFT-2N (lymphoma)	6/6	28 ± 1
AH-66	WFT-2N (lymphoma)	6/6	30 ± 2

[a] Immunization was performed subcutaneously with allogeneic tumor cells three times at 1-week intervals.

[b] Tumor cells were challenged subcutaneously 7 days after the last immunization.

[c] MSD, Mean survival days.

To substantiate the above findings, additional experiments were carried out. Lethally growing syngeneic tumor cells and temporarily growing allogeneic tumor cells were mixed and inoculated subcutaneously. This was to test the hypothesis that nonspecific cellular immunity evoked by temporarily growing allogeneic tumor cells at the site of inoculation might inhibit the growth of syngeneic tumor. The growth of a fibrosarcoma (KMT-17) after mixing with allogeneic AH-66 and AH-272 cells was strongly inhibited, but the growth of a leukemia (KNL-1) mixed with allogeneic AH-66 cells was not inhibited (Hosokawa et al., 1978). These results correlated well with preimmunization experiments.

B. CHARACTERISTICS OF LEUKEMIAS AND LYMPHOMAS IN ALLOGENEIC CELL IMMUNITY

There are several possible explanations for these results. First, if these leukemic tumors were of extremely low antigenicity, their growth could not be affected by host immunity. However, it was noted that one of these lymphomas which was not inhibited by allogeneic cell immunity was antigenic in WKA rats (Kobayashi et al., 1970b; Hosokawa et al., 1978). Second, if the immunizing effect was due to certain organ-specific antigens, this could explain why leukemia and lymphoma could not be inhibited even after immunization with nonleukemic tumors. This explanation is unlikely because the leukemic tumors were not inhibited even in rats immunized with allogeneic leukemia or normal lymphoid cells, while the nonleukemic tumors were inhibited. Third, it is well known that better resistance to tumors is acquired by stimulation of cell-mediated rather than humoral immunity. In fact, spleen cells from rats immunized with allogeneic tumors have inhibited syngeneic fibrosarcoma cells in certain circumstances (Sendo et al., 1976; Nakayama et al., 1977). However, it is difficult to find any evidence that humoral response was stimulated in rats immunized with allogeneic cells. It has been speculated that the balance between cellular and humoral immunity is important as a means to inhibit nonleukemic tumor growth in allogeneic cell immunity.

There are several reports that immunization with allogeneic cells inhibits growth of leukemic tumor cells. Wrathmell et al. (1976) mentioned that immunization with allogeneic cells induced resistance to transplantable leukemia in rats. They showed definite cross-antigenicity between allogeneic cells and leukemic cells using the immunofluorescence test with humoral antibody. Truitt et al. (1980) have reported that transferred immunocompetent cells from CBA mice immunized with individual or pooled lymphoid cells from various allogeneic strains resulted in the elimination

of leukemic cells in AKR mice. They offered the possibility that alloimmunization induced a population of cells in donor CBA mice which was
considered to be T cells and which helped antigen-specific or nonspecific
reactions to the leukemia cells. We are unable to draw conclusions as to
whether their observations are relevant to our allogeneic cell immunity.
However, they did mention an observation similar to an aspect of our system: namely, that the transfer of alloimmunized lymphoid cells was effective only in recipients treated with antitumor drugs and irradiation (Gotohda et al., 1976; Nakayama et al., 1977). A syngeneic leukemia in
guinea pigs and a murine plasmacytoma were inhibited in the F_1 hybrid
hosts after the transfer of parental spleen cells (Katz et al., 1972; Osborne
and Katz, 1977a,b). The inhibition of leukemic tumor growth was based
on the phenomenon referred to as the allogeneic effect, in which the host
immune response was stimulated after induction of a transient GVH reaction (Katz et al., 1971a). A major difference between allogeneic cell immunity and the allogeneic effect is that allogeneic cell immunity can be
induced by nonimmunocompetent cells, such as tumor cells and skin
grafts, without induction of GVH reactions, whereas the latter is induced
only by transfer of immunocompetent cells and is able to stimulate humoral responses (Katz et al., 1971b). In allogeneic cell immunity, transfer
of mitomycin C-treated allogeneic lymphoid cells induced resistance to
syngeneic tumor as well as did live allogeneic lymphoid cells (Oikawa et
al., 1977). It has been considered from the comparison of the above two
phenomena that the balance between cellular and humoral immune responses might be an important means of inhibiting leukemic or nonleukemic tumor growth after nonspecific immunostimulation. Allogeneic leukemic cells were somewhat weaker as a means of inhibiting syngeneic tumor
(Table I). The findings were further confirmed by the experiment of a
transplantation of a mixture of syngeneic tumor and allogeneic leukemic
cells (Hosokawa et al., 1978).

IV. Strain Difference of Donors for Allogeneic Cell Immunity

Allogeneic cell immunity by which the growth of syngeneic tumor is inhibited was first observed in WKA/Hok rats ($RT1^k$) immunized with allogeneic tumor cells from Donryu strain rats. This inhibition was not, however, restrictively observed in the relationship of the above host and
donor rats (Kobayashi et al., 1974). It was noted that the strain difference
between the tumor host and the donor of the allogeneic cells might be important in determining allogeneic cell immunity.

A. Immunizing Effects of Allogeneic Skin Grafts from Various Strains of Rats

A syngeneic tumor was inhibited in WKA rats immunized by allogeneic skin grafts not only from Donryu rats but also from several other strains of rats. Table XI indicates that the degree of inhibition of KMT-17 tumor growth differed among the donor strains of skin grafts used for immunization. Some strains showed a strong resistance, while other strains did not. Strains of Donryu, Kyoto, SHR, LEJ, LEW, ACI, and BUF were able to produce a strong resistance to the challenge of syngeneic tumors, but strains of SD, F344, Tokyo, ALB, WKS, NIG$_{III}$, and W/Hok were not. Skin grafts from Donryu and Kyoto strain rats were most effective in the

TABLE XI

INHIBITION OF KMT-17 GROWTH IN WKA RATS (RT1^k)
IMMUNIZED WITH ALLOGENEIC SKIN GRAFTS
OBTAINED FROM VARIOUS RAT STRAINS

Immunized with skin from			Growth of KMT-17[a]		
Strain of rat	RT1[b]	Cross antigen[c] with RT1^k	Died/used	(%)	Inhibition
Donryu	ND[d]	+	0/25	(0)	+++
Kyoto	ND	+	0/15	(0)	+++
SHR	k	+	2/8	(25)	++
LEJ	u	−	1/11	(9)	+++
LEW	l	−	1/4	(25)	++
ACI	a	−	5/14	(36)	++
BUF	b	−	2/5	(40)	++
SD	u	−	3/6	(50)	+
F344	l	−	6/10	(60)	+
Tokyo	t	−	7/10	(70)	+
ALB	b	−	4/5	(80)	±
WKS	ND	−	4/5	(80)	±
NIG$_{III}$	ND	−	15/18	(83)	±
W/Hok	k	+	4/4	(100)	−
WKA	k	+	17/17	(100)	−
None			32/32	(100)	−

[a] One million cells of KMT-17 were challenged sc 10 days after the immunization with allogeneic skin grafts.

[b] RT1 is rat major histocompatibility antigen; see report of the first international workshop on the alloantigenic system in the rat (Gill *et al.*, 1978).

[c] Cross-reactivity of MHC in each strain was examined by the dextran hemagglutination test with anti-RT1^k.

[d] ND, Not determined.

TABLE XII
INHIBITION OF KMT-17 GROWTH IN WKA RATS (RT1^k)
IMMUNIZED WITH ALLOGENEIC FIBROSARCOMAS
FROM VARIOUS RAT STRAINS

Immunized with			Growth of KMT-17[a]		
Tumor line[b]	Strain	RT1	Died/used	(%)	Inhibition
AS-D653	Donryu	ND[c]	0/7	(0)	+++
AMC-60	ACI/N	a	0/13	(0)	+++
FMT-2	F344	l	2/5	(40)	+
BMT-4	BUF	b	4/5	(80)	±
NMT-2	NIG$_{III}$	ND	4/5	(80)	±
None			5/5	(100)	−

[a] One million cells of KMT-17 were challenged 10 days after the immunization with allogeneic tumor cells.

[b] All tumors were fibrosarcomas induced by methylcholanthrene in each rat strain.

[c] ND, Not determined.

production of resistance. Regarding the strain difference of the immunizing effects, similar results were obtained in the experiments using allogeneic blood transfusions (Oikawa et al., 1977). Some allogeneic fibrosarcomas induced by methylcholanthrene in Donryu, ACI, F344, BUF, and NIG$_{III}$ rat strains also showed different degrees of immunizing effects. The immunizing effect of each allogeneic fibrosarcoma was approximately parallel to that of the skin grafts from the respective rat strains (Table XII). This result suggests that the immunizing effect of allogeneic tumors does not depend on tumor-associated or tissue-specific antigens, but on histocompatibility antigens.

B. ROLE OF MAJOR HISTOCOMPATIBILITY ANTIGENS OF DONOR CELLS

The recipient rats which the authors used were mainly inbred Wistar King Aptekman/Hok strain rats maintained by sister–brother breedings for more than 200 generations at the Department of Science of Hokkaido University.

The major histocompatibility antigen of the WKA rats is designated RT1^k (Gill et al., 1978) and those in the donor rat strains are indicated in Table XI. Unfortunately, the major histocompatibility antigens of the Donryu, Kyoto, and NIG$_{III}$ rats, which were the most important strains as donors of allogeneic cells, have not yet been determined. However, Donryu and Kyoto strains which induced the strongest resistance to syngeneic tumor in WKA rats share the cross antigens with $RT1^k$ in recipient WKA rats. This was investigated by the dextran hemagglutination test with LEJ anti-WKA antiserum (anti-$RT1^k$ typing serum). NIG_{III}, whose skin grafts showed weak immunizing effects, does not share the $RT1^k$ antigen. Preliminary experiments indicated that the immunizing effects of allogeneic cells from (Donryu × NIG)F_2 and (Donryu × NIG_{III}) × NIG_{III} backcrossed rats were not segregated by the RT1 antigen (unpublished data). Moreover, allogeneic cells from strains which share the RT1 antigen with the host WKA rats (except W/Hok) seemed to induce a stronger resistance than those from other rat strains which do not share RT1 with the host WKA rats. These results indicate that not RT1 itself but non-RT1 alloantigen is responsible for the stimulation of the host immune resistance to tumors.

The question of the relationship between the host WKA rats and the donor rats for allogeneic cell immunity will remain unanswered until analysis of the rats' major histocompatibility complexes has been completed. The authors described allogeneic skin graft rejections in WKA with their immunizing effects (Kobayashi and Hosokawa, 1981). No correlation of mean days for the rejection of skin grafts and the degree of the immunizing effects was observed, while W/Hok skin grafts were accepted for more than 100 days and an immunizing effect of W/Hok was not observed at all. For example, the skin grafts from Donryu rats were rejected after 7.9 days and gave strong resistance, and those from F344 rats were also rejected after 8.0 days and gave weaker resistance. Although the SHR rat has $RT1^k$, as well as the same RT1 as the host WKA rat, the skin graft was rejected after 8.1 days and gave strong resistance. The second-set rejection of Donryu skin graft was accelerated in the host preimmunized with Donryu skin graft. However, syngeneic skin grafts were never rejected in those hosts preimmunized with allogeneic cells. It was seen that immunostimulation with alloantigens was effective as a means of rejecting syngeneic tumors but not syngeneic normal cells.

Regarding MHC in the host, it was observed that WKA and W/Hok rats with $RT1^k$ were the rat strains in which the antitumor resistance was produced after immunization with allogeneic cells. The resistance to a methylcholanthrene-induced fibrosarcoma (SMT-2 tumor) was observed in SHR rats ($RT1^k$) after immunization with allogeneic Donryu cells in the earlier experiments (Kobayashi and Hosokawa, 1981); however, the result was not reproducible in repeated experiments. In ACI ($RT1^a$), BUF ($RT1^b$), and F344 ($RT1^l$) rats, no resistance to respective syngeneic tumors was observed after immunization with allogeneic cells from Donryu, WKA ($RT1^k$), LEW ($RT1^l$), or ALB ($RT1^b$) rats (Kobayashi and

Hosokawa, 1981). At present, the phenomenon seems to be restricted to the host with RT1^k. The question whether the restriction of this phenomenon is due to the different immune responses to allogeneic cells or to the susceptibility of respective syngeneic tumors to such a nonspecific immunostimulation induced by allogeneic cell immunity should be resolved in further experiments.

V. Mechanisms of Allogeneic Cell Immunity

It is obvious that the inhibition of syngeneic tumors by allogeneic cell immunity is due to immunological mechanisms, since the inhibiting effect was easily abrogated by whole-body irradiation or administration of anti-lymphocyte serum into immunized rats prior to the challenging of tumor cells (Kobayashi *et al.*, 1974). Other characteristics of the inhibition are thought to be as follows. (1) The immunizing effects develop a short time after the immunization and disappear in shorter periods (within 2 months) as compared with the specific antitumor resistance produced by xenogenized tumor cells (Kobayashi *et al.*, 1970a) that lasts for more than 5 months. (2) The immunizing effects are abrogated by low-dose irradiation (250–350 rad) which does not affect specific immunity (Kobayashi *et al.*, 1974). (3) The strong resistance is produced by immunization with viable allogeneic cells only and not with inactivated cells. (4) The resistance cannot to be transferred to normal syngeneic recipients by means of spleen cells except for conditioning of the recipients with irradiation (Nakayama *et al.*, 1977). These characteristics indicate that the immunizing effects might be due to nonspecific stimulation of host immunity to syngeneic tumor cells.

A. Lack of Cross-Reactive Antigens between Challenging Syngeneic Tumor Cells and Immunizing Allogeneic Cells

There have been several reports that inhibition of primary or syngeneic tumor growth can be observed after immunization with allogeneic cells (Sjögren and Ankerst, 1969; Oth and Liegey, 1975; Invernizzi and Parmiani, 1975; Martin *et al.*, 1976; Usubuchi *et al.*, 1972; Wrathmell *et al.*, 1976; Bear *et al.*, 1980). It is reasonable to suspect some cross antigen between the immunizing allogeneic cells and the challenging syngeneic tumor cells. In fact, it has been reported that a chemically induced tumor in BALB/c mice possesses antigens which cross-react with normal histocompatibility antigens of allogeneic mice (Invernizzi and Parmiani, 1975). The alien histocompatibility antigens in some syngeneic tumors in mice have been revealed by other investigators (Gipson *et al.*, 1978; Bonavida *et al.*, 1980). In rat tumors, myelogenous leukemia cells in August rats showed cross antigen to alloantigen found in both normal and malignant cells derived from Hooded rats (Wrathmell *et al.*, 1976). It has also been suspected that virus-associated antigens caused by viral oncogenes are responsible for resistance induced by immunization with allogeneic tumor cells (Huebner *et al.*, 1976). The present authors have also suspected cross antigens between syngeneic tumor cells and allogeneic cells in allogeneic cell immunity. However, in our system there has been no evidence to show cross-antigenicity between them. First, the immunizing effects with allogeneic cells were easily abrogated by low-dose irradiation on the immunized host and lasted for a short period of time after the immunization (Kobayashi, 1974; Hosokawa, 1976). If specific immunity had been established after immunization with allogeneic cells, it is curious that the resistance could be abrogated with such a low dose of irradiation. In fact, the immunizing effects in rats immunized specifically with xenogenized identical tumor cells remained after the irradiation with 250 rad, and were only abrogated by 600-rad irradiation. Second, sera from WKA rats immunized with allogeneic AH-66 cells from Donryu rats showed a positive reaction to AH-66 cells as well as other tumor cells from Donryu rats, and this could not be absorbed with syngeneic tumor cells. Anti-KMT-17 tumor antibody in WKA rats could not be absorbed by any allogeneic tumor cells from Donryu rats (Sendo *et al.*, 1976). Third, spleen cells from WKA rats immunized with allogeneic cells killed allogeneic cells but not syngeneic tumor cells (Table XIII). These results of humoral and cellular

TABLE XIII

CYTOTOXIC ACTIVITY OF SPLEEN CELLS OBTAINED FROM WKA
RATS IMMUNIZED WITH ALLOGENEIC CELLS AGAINST
ALLOGENEIC AND SYNGENEIC TUMOR CELLS

Spleen cells from rats immunized with	Specific percentage cytolysis[a]		
	Donryu spleen cells	AH-66 cells	KMT-17 cells
Spleen cells from Donryu rats	42.1 ± 3.0	NT[b]	0.4 ± 0.8
AH-66 cells from Donryu rats	NT	26.2 ± 2.0	5.1 ± 0.2
KMT-17 cells from WKA rats	3.0 ± 2.1	0.5 ± 0.6	23.6 ± 10.1

[a] Specific percentage cytolysis: percentage cytolysis with normal spleen cells was subtracted from percentage cytolysis with tested spleen cells. Percentage cytolysis was calculated from the following formula: (release with spleen cells − spontaneous release)/(maximum release − spontaneous release by 12-hour chromium release test at 1/100 of target/effector ratio).

[b] NT, Not tested.

TABLE XIV

NEUTRALIZING ACTIVITY OF SPLEEN CELLS OBTAINED FROM
WKA RATS IMMUNIZED WITH LIVE OR FREEZE-THAWED
AH-66 CELLS AGAINST SYNGENEIC AND
ALLOGENEIC TUMOR CELLS

Spleen cells from rat immunized with[a]	Neutralizing activity against[b]	
	KMT-17 cells	AH-66 cells
None	−	−
Viable AH-66 cells	+ + +	+ + +
Freeze-thawed AH-66 cells	−	+ +

[a] Spleen cells were harvested from three rats in each group 1 week after the last immunization.

[b] A mixture of 10^5 tumor cells and 10^7 spleen cells was inoculated into five WKA rats irradiated (600 rad) and rescued with 10^6 syngeneic bone marrow cells; and the growth inhibition of tumor cells was observed.

immune responses indicate that there is no cross antigen between alloge-neic cells and syngeneic tumor cells in our system. The indications are also supported by the evidence that alloreactive lymphocytes differed from lymphocytes which are effective in inhibiting syngeneic tumor cells in the *in vitro–in vivo* neutralization test (Winn assay) (Nakayama *et al.*, 1977). It has also been observed that spleen cells from WKA rats immu-nized with freeze-thawed AH-66 cells had a strong inhibiting activity on AH-66 tumor cells, but they were unable to inhibit syngeneic KMT-17 tumor cells in Winn's assay. On the other hand, immunization with viable AH-66 cells had a neutralizing activity on both AH-66 and KMT-17 cells (Table XIV). These results indicate that freeze-thawed allogeneic cells could induce alloreactive lymphocytes but not effective lymphocytes to inhibit syngeneic tumor growth, so that lymphocytes effective in inhib-iting syngeneic tumor cells differ from alloreactive lymphocytes. Al-though it is still difficult to exclude completely the possibility of some un-known cross antigen, the above evidence supports the suggestion that there is no cross-reactive antigen between the immunizing allogeneic cells and challenging syngeneic tumor cells in our system.

B. ENHANCEMENT OF THE HOST IMMUNE RESPONSE TO TUMOR CELLS BY IMMUNIZATION WITH ALLOGENEIC CELLS

The inhibition of syngeneic tumor in allogeneic cell immunity is consid-ered to be due to nonspecific immunity, since no cross antigen was de-tected between immunizing cells and challenging tumor cells. Analysis of the effector mechanism to inhibit syngeneic tumor *in vivo* has been carried out by our colleagues (Sendo *et al.*, 1976). They clearly demonstrated that spleen cells obtained from WKA rats immunized with allogeneic AH-66 cells inhibited *in vivo* growth of admixed syngeneic tumor cells when the immune spleen cells were stimulated by inactivated AH-66 cells. They indicated that AH-66 immune spleen cells produce a soluble factor which activates polymorphonuclear (PMN) leukocytes or macrophages to inhibit syngeneic tumor cells in the diffusion chamber and in the thymidine uptake inhibition test with cultured tumor cells (Nakayama *et al.*, 1978; Sendo *et al.*, 1980). The activated PMN or macrophage inhibited not only syngeneic tumor cells but also Meth-A cells in BALB/c mice in culture system, so that the killing activity of activated cells is considered nonspecific. Although there is no direct evidence that the same effector mechanisms play any role in *in vivo* resistance to syngeneic tumors, they may possibly be mechanisms that are involved in allogeneic cell immunity. As described earlier, syngeneic tumor growth was completely inhibited after being mixed with allogeneic tumor cells which can produce antitumor resistance through preimmunization (Section III,A). One explanation for the inhibition of antigenically unrelated tumors is that antigen-stimulated immune lymphocytes kill the syngeneic tumor cells directly or through activation of macrophages; this was proposed by Zbar *et al.* (1970) as a two-step mechanism of *in vivo* tumor rejection.

Another possibility is that immune reactions to allogeneic cells activate the specific immune reactions to tumor-specific antigens on the challenged tumor cells. Spleen cells from WKA rats immunized with allogeneic AH-66 tumor cells showed no cytotoxic activity to syngeneic KMT-17 tumor cells. These immune spleen cells showed a higher cytotoxic activity to KMT-17 tumor cells after *in vitro* sensitization with inactivated KMT-17 tumor cells than did normal spleen cells. When the immune spleen cells were sensitized with AH-66 cells, they showed cytotoxicity only to AH-66 cells (unpublished data). Although further experiments will be required for an interpretation of these results, it seems that alloimmunization activates the generation of cytotoxic cells to syngeneic tumor cells. Dennert (1975) reported that spleen cells of mice immunized with allogeneic or xenogeneic tumor cells showed an enhanced capacity to generate cytotoxic cells in *in vitro* sensitization. Two subpopulations of T lymphocytes were thought to develop after priming with allogeneic or xenogeneic tumor cells. The precursors of cytotoxic T cells were found in both normal and primed spleen cells, whereas the stimulating T cells were found only in primed spleen cells. Dennert (1975) proposed that the stimulating T cells were not descendants of cytotoxic T cells but helped a development of cytotoxic T cells in *in vitro* sensitization with tumor cells. We do not know whether alloimmunization expands the precursors of cytotoxic T cells or induces the stimulating cells that help the generation of cytotoxic cells to syngeneic tumor cells in our rat system.

There have been reports indicating that immunization with pooled allogeneic cells induces antitumor resistance in mice (Oth and Liegey, 1975; Bear et al., 1980). The phenomenon may involve two different effector mechanisms: the induction of specific cytotoxic cells based on alien histocompatibility antigens in syngeneic tumor cells, and a nonspecific immunostimulation of the host defense mechanism against tumor as we propose in allogeneic cell immunity. It was reported that stimulation in vitro with an allogeneic mixture of pooled spleen cells from several strains of mice resulted not only in the generation of cytotoxic T lymphocytes, but also in the activation of cells cytotoxic for syngeneic solid tumor cells that were resistant to treatment with anti-Thy 1 serum and maybe activated natural killer (NK) cells as well (Paciucci et al., 1980; Bach et al., 1980). However, the NK cell activity of spleen cells in WKA rats immunized with AH-66 cells was not enhanced when compared with those of normal spleen cells in our system as far as we investigated by means of the short-time chromium release assay (unpublished data). The question whether natural cytotoxicity to syngeneic tumor cells is enhanced in alloimmunized rats still remains, since natural cytotoxicity to solid tumor cells requires a long-term cytotoxicity assay. However, the cytotoxicity assay may involve the generation of specific cytotoxic cells during incubation for long periods such as 48 or 72 hours.

With regard to nonspecific stimulation of host immunity, protective effects against the infection of Listeria monocytogens were investigated. However, no protective effect against Listeria monocytogens was observed in WKA rats immunized with allogeneic AH-66 cells (Kobayashi and Hosokawa, 1981). It was therefore concluded that allogeneic cell immunity was restricted to the syngeneic tumor challenge.

VI. Conclusions

The induction of resistance to syngeneic tumors in WKA rats following immunization with allogeneic cells is believed to be due to nonspecific stimulation of host immunity against tumor cells. The phenomenon termed allogeneic cell immunity is one of the most powerful means of inducing resistance to tumor challenges. The feasibility of allogeneic cell immunity in experimental immunotherapy on transplanted tumor in syngeneic rats has been reported elsewhere (Gotohda et al., 1976, 1980; Yamada et al., 1980).

With regard to the generality of allogeneic cell immunity, strong transplantation resistance to syngeneic tumors was observed only in rats strains with MHC of RT1ᵏ as far as we investigated using mice and other rat strains as tumor hosts. However, similar immunizing effects on the growth of tumor in mice were reported by others (Sjögren and Ankerst, 1969; Usubuchi *et al.*, 1972; Oth and Liegey, 1975; Bear *et al.*, 1980). Although they did not completely exclude the possibility of cross-reactive antigens, the question of responsibility for nonspecific stimulation of host immunity still remains for their system. Allogeneic cell immunity, therefore, may not be restricted to our rat system.

In consideration of the immunogenetic relationship of the host and the donor of allogeneic cells, immunostimulation seems to be produced by the non-MHC antigen (Section IV,B). Regardless of the identification of alloantigens which may stimulate the host resistance to tumor cells, we would like to stress that immunization with viable cells is advantageous for the production of an *in vivo* resistance to tumors. It has also been observed that immunization with viable tumor cells infected with foreign antigenic viruses (xenogenized tumor cells) produces a strong resistance to original noninfected tumor cells (Kobayashi *et al.*, 1969, 1970a, 1977). At present, a conclusive explanation cannot be offered to show why these viable cells are able to produce such strong antitumor resistance in either specific or nonspecific immunization. It might be due not only to an increase of immunizing cells prior to their being rejected but also to qualitatively different responses of the host to living materials. From the standpoint of cancer immunotherapy, the means to produce a stronger resistance are required. The immunological role of viable-cell immunization needs, therefore, to be resolved in future studies.

ACKNOWLEDGMENT

We would like to thank Miss J. Yamamoto for her secretarial assistance in the preparation of this manuscript.

REFERENCES

Bach, F. H., Paciucci, P. A., Macphail, S., Sondel, P. M., Alter, B. J., and Zarling, J. M. (1980). *Transplant. Proc.* **12**, 2–7.
Bear, R. H., Roholt, O. A., and Pressman, D. (1980). *Transplant. Proc.* **12**, 150–151.
Bonavida, B., Roman, J. M., and Hutchinson, I. V. (1980). *Transplant. Proc.* **12**, 59–64.
Dennert, G. (1975). *J. Immunol.* **114**, 1570–1573.
Gill, T. J., III, Kunz, H. W., Cramer, D. V., and Stark, O. (1978). *Transplant. Proc.* **10**, 271–284.
Gipson, T. G., Imamura, M., Conliffe, M. A., and Martin, W. J. (1978). *J. Exp. Med.* **147**, 1363–1373.

Gotohda, E., Kawamura, T., Sendo, F., Nakayama, M., Akiyama, J., Oikawa, T., Hoso-kawa, M., Kodama, T., and Kobayashi, H. (1976). *Cancer Res.* **36**, 2119–2123.

Gotohda, E., Kawamura, T., Yamada, Y., Hosokawa, M., Kodoma, T., and Kobayashi, H. (1980). *Transplant. Proc.* **12**, 147–149.

Hosokawa, M., Imamura, M., Oikawa, T., Nakayama, M., Gotohda, E., Sendo, F., Ko-dama, T., and Kobayashi, H. (1976). *Int. J. Cancer* **18**, 369–374.

Hosokawa, M., Yamashita, T., Gotohda, E., Takaichi, N., Kodama, T., and Kobayashi, H. (1978). *Int. J. Cancer* **22**, 91–97.

Huebner, R. J., Gilden, R. V., Lane, W. T., Toni, R., Trimmer, R. W., and Hill, P. R. (1976). *Proc. Natl. Acad. Sci. U.S.A.* **73**, 620–624.

Invernizzi, G., and Parmiani, G. (1975). *Nature (London)* **254**, 713–714.

Katz, D. H., Paul, W. E., Goidl, E. A., and Benacerraf, B. (1971a). *J. Exp. Med.* **133**, 169–186.

Katz, D. H., Paul, W. E., and Benacerraf, B. (1971b). *J. Immunol.* **107**, 1319–1328.

Katz, D. H., Ellmann, L., Paul, W. E., Green, I., and Benacerraf, B. (1972). *Cancer Res.* **32**, 133–140.

Klein, G., and Klein, E. (1962). *Cold Spring Harbor Symp. Quant. Biol.* **27**, 463–470.

Kobayashi, H., and Hosokawa, M. (1981). *Transplant. Proc.* **13**, 1922–1926.

Kobayashi, H., Hosokawa, M., and Oikawa, T. (1980). *Transplant. Proc.* **12**, 156–159.

Kobayashi, H., Kodama, T., Shirai, T., Kaji, H., Hosokawa, M., Sendo, F., Saito, T., and Takeichi, N. (1969). *Hokkaido J. Med. Sci.* **44**, 133–134.

Kobayashi, H., Sendo, F., Kaji, H., Shirai, T., Saito, H., Takeichi, N., Hosokawa, M., and Kodama, T. (1970a). *J. Natl. Cancer Inst.* **44**, 11–19.

Kobayashi, H., Shirai, T., Takeichi, N., Hosokawa, M., Saito, H., Sendo, F., and Kodama, T. (1970b). *Eur. J. Clin. Biol. Res.* **15**, 426–428.

Kobayashi, H., Gotohda, E., Kuzumaki, N., Takeichi, N., Hosokawa, M., and Kodama, T. (1974). *Int. J. Cancer* **13**, 522–529.

Kobayashi, H., Kodama, T., and Gotohda, E. (1977). *Hokkaido Univ. Med. Libr. Ser.* **9**, 43–121.

Matin, W. J., Gipson, T. G., Martin, S. E., and Rice, J. M. (1976). *Science* **26**, 532–533.

Nakayama, M., Sendo, F., Gotohda, E., and Kobayashi, H. (1977). *Gann* **68**, 509–512.

Nakayama, M., Sendo, F., Miyakae, T., Fuyama, S., Arai, S., and Kobayashi, H. (1978). *J. Immunol.* **120**, 619–623.

Oikawa, T., Hosokawa, M., Imamura, M., Sendo, F., Nakayama, M., Gotohda, E., Ko-dama, T., and Kobayashi, H. (1977). *Clin. Exp. Immunol.* **27**, 549–554.

Osborne, D. P., and Katz, D. H. (1977a). *J. Immunol.* **118**, 1441–1448.

Osborne, D. P., and Katz, D. H. (1977b). *J. Immunol.* **118**, 1449–1455.

Oth, D., and Liegey, A. (1975). *Biomedicine* **23**, 17–19.

Paciucci, P. A., Macphail, S., Zahling, J. M., and Bach, F. H. (1980). *J. Immunol.* **124**, 370–375.

Sendo, F., Nakayama, M., Gotohda, E., and Kobayashi, H. (1976). *J. Immunol.* **117**, 1340–1345.

Sendo, F., Seiji, K., Watanabe, S., Fuyama, S., and Arai, S. (1980). *Transplant. Proc.* **12**, 160–163.

Sjögren, H. O., and Ankerst, J. (1969). *Nature (London)* **221**, 863–864.

Truitt, R. L., Bortin, M. M., and Rimm, A. A. (1980). *Transplant. Proc.* **12**, 143–146.

Usubuchi, I., Sobajima, Y., Kudo, H., Kano, M., and Sato, T. (1972). *Tohoku J. Exp. Med.* **107**, 253–262.

Woodruff, M. F. A., and Boak, J. L. (1966). *Br. J. Cancer* **20**, 345–355.

Wrathmell, A. B., Gauci, C. L., and Alexander, P. (1976). *Br. J. Cancer* **33**, 187–194.

Yamada, Y., Kawamura, T., Gotohda, E., Akiyama, J., Hosokawa, M., Kodama, T., and Kobayashi, H. (1980). *Cancer Res.* **40,** 954–958.
Zbar, B. H. (1972). *Natl. Cancer Inst. Monogr.* **35,** 341–344.
Zbar, B. H., Wepsic, T., Borsos, T., and Rapp, H. J. (1970). *J. Natl. Cancer Inst.* **44,** 473–481.
Zbar, B. H., Bernstein, I. D., and Rapp, H. J. (1971). *J. Natl. Cancer Inst.* **46,** 831–839.

CHAPTER III

LYMPHOCYTE-MEDIATED TUMOR CYTOLYSIS AFTER TREATMENT WITH IMMUNE RNA

GLENN STEELE, JR., BOSCO S. WANG, AND JOHN A. MANNICK

I. Background

The potential infectivity of viral ribonucleic acid for tissue-cultured mammalian cells was demonstrated as early as 1956 (Alexander *et al.*, 1958; Ellem and Colter, 1960; Gierer and Schramm, 1956). Niu *et al.* (1961) attempted to show cytoplasmic incorporation of ^{14}C-labeled immune RNA (I-RNA) after *in vivo* injection by autoradiography of single cells in an ascites tumor model. In 1962, several investigators postulated that RNA extracted from normal tissues might inhibit tumor isograft growth in rats (Aksenova *et al.*, 1962) and that RNA extracted from normal human bone marrow cells might "redifferentiate" exposed human leukemic cells (DeCarvalho, 1963).

The first unequivocal demonstration, however, of what seemed to be transfer of immunologic information affecting humoral immune response was reported in 1961 by Fishman. After incubation of macrophages with bacteriophage T2, a lysate was prepared, filtered, and added to a culture of lymph node cells. Antibody directed against T2 was generated by the lysate-exposed lymph node cells. In 1964, Fishman and Adler demonstrated that RNA seemed to be the most likely active component in this macrophage extract. Mannick and Egdahl (1964) were the first investigators to report that immune responsiveness could be amplified by RNA extracted from lymphoid tissues of specifically immunized animals. They demonstrated that autologous lymphocytes incubated with specific immune RNA *in vitro* could, upon reinfusion, cause second-set rejection of skin allografts in rabbits. Adoptive transfer of *in vivo* skin allograft immunity was donor specific. Third-party grafts did not undergo second-set rejection. Furthermore, in the *in vivo* models of Mannick (1964), second-set allograft immunity could not be adoptively transferred by direct intravenous (iv) injection of immune RNA. This work was subsequently confirmed by Sabbadini and Sehon (1967) and later by Ramming and Pilch (1968).

The passive transfer of antibody production *in vitro* by an RNA-like substance extracted in the manner of Fishman and Adler has been reported to have a high degree of specificity. By using antiallotypic sera, Bell and Dray (1970, 1972, 1973) reported their ability to transfer immune RNA donor allotype (not present in the cells of the recipient) on anti-SRBC-directed IgM and IgG after exposure of recipient lymphoid cells to immune RNA from SRBC-immunized rabbits. Host and donor immunoglobulin allotypes on the induced anti-SRBC antibody were claimed to be present up to 37 days after immune RNA treatment. These investigators speculated that the RNA had either an informational role and functioned as a template for protein synthesis via an RNA-dependent DNA polymerase, or modified specific regulatory genes in the host lymphoid tissues.

Although these allotype transfer experiments have been criticized (Sell, 1976), they have at least been reproducible by Adler, Fishman, and Dray (Adler, 1976) who have continued to focus their *in vitro* studies on the ability of immune RNA to induce specific antibody formation and have defined the RNase sensitivity of the phenomenon, its Pronase and DNase resistance, the size of the active RNA species involved (16–28 S), and the lack of cell proliferation involved in their *in vitro* information transfer models (Adler and Fishman, 1975; Meiss and Fishman, 1972; Schaefer *et al.*, 1974).

The production of cytotoxic antibodies with specificity to a benzopyrene-induced sarcoma by treatment of naive mice with xenogeneic antitumor immune RNA was first reported by Pilch and co-workers in 1976 (Fritze *et al.*, 1976). Antitumor antibody synthesis induced *in vitro* in mouse spleen cells after xenogeneic immune RNA exposure was reported by this same group in 1978 (Kern and Pilch), and human lymphoblastoid B-cell lines were shown to be immunizable to tumor cell specificities by *in vitro* incubation using immune RNA from specifically immunized sheep. Purportedly, the information transferred to the exposed cell line was shown to be replicated in tissue culture for at least 10 weeks (Viza *et al.*, 1978).

The initial observation by Mannick and Egdahl that immune RNA could augment specific cell-mediated immune responses was expanded by numerous other investigators in both *in vitro* and *in vivo* models. Paque, Dray, and associates repeatedly demonstrated the ability to transfer cellular immune responses to defined delayed-type hypersensitivity antigens [such as keyhole limpet hemocyanin (KLH), purified protein derivative (PPD), or coccidiodin (COCCI)] by *in vitro* incubation of naive lymphocytes with xenogeneic immune RNA obtained from specifically sensitized donors (Paque and Dray, 1972; Paque *et al.*, 1973; Paque and Dray, 1974). Recipient lymphocytes included human white cells, and the initial *in vitro* assay used was inhibition of macrophage migration. White cells exposed to immune RNA harvested from specifically immunized donors were challenged *in vitro* with KLH, PPD, or COCCI and compared for migration inhibition response with white cells incubated with RNA extracted from the lymphoid tissues of nonsensitized xenogeneic donors. Using similar *in vitro* assays for migration inhibition, Paque *et al.* (1975) reported that specific immune RNA exposure could "restore" delayed-type hypersensitivity responses to the peritoneal exudate cells obtained from strain 13 guinea pigs. Braun and Dray (1977) reported that tumor-specific immune RNA could reestablish the *in vitro* migration inhibition response to peritoneal exudate cells obtained during the unresponsive phase 10–14 days after plasmacytoma growth in MOPC-315 bearing hosts.

The ability to transer *in vitro* proliferative responses to xenogeneic lymphocytes challenged with specific antigen was demonstrated using immune RNA harvested from lymphoid cells of bacillus Calmette-Guérin (BCG)-immunized cattle (Wang *et al.*, 1974) and using a tumor-antigen-immunized sheep RNA (Coates and Pilch, 1977). In both the tumor and the nontumor system, blastogenesis of antigen-challenged lymphocytes was compared to nonspecific proliferation after *in vitro* challenge of the treated lymphocytes with histoplasm versus PPD. Specificity of the proliferative response was found.

The most frequently exploited *in vitro* parameter of cell-mediated immune function affected by immune RNA has been the lymphocyte-mediated cytotoxic, cytolytic, or antiadherent effect. Bondevick and Mannick (1968) reported that immune RNA-exposed lymphocytes could be induced to "attack" allogeneic target tissue *in vitro* with specificity determined by the skin allograft-sensitized RNA donor. The initial assay used in these experiments was a 48-hour microcytotoxicity test with trypan blue defining residual viable target cells after effector cell exposure. By using an *in vitro* adherent assay modified from Cohen *et al.* (1971), Pilch and co-workers demonstrated that lymphocytes from nonimmune Fisher rats could be made cytotoxic to methylcholanthrene-induced tumor cells after *in vitro* incubation using immune RNA harvested from spleens of Fisher rats hyperimmunized with methylcholanthrene sarcoma isografts. The concentration of immune RNA effecting this cell-mediated immune transfer was 100 μg/ml. Immune RNA was RNase sensitive, but DNase and Pronase resistant. The level of cytotoxic effect after *in vitro* immune

RNA exposure of nonsensitized syngeneic lymphocytes was purported to be similar to lymphocytes harvested from hyperimmunized animals and tested for cytotoxicity directly on the methylcholanthrene sarcoma targets (Kern *et al.*, 1974). These workers reported similar findings using naive spleen cells obtained from murine donors exposed to immune RNA harvested from methylcholanthrene sarcoma-hyperimmunized rats (Kern and Pilch, 1974). Identical experimental conditions were shown to successfully mediate tumor-specific cytotoxic immune responses after exposure of naive human peripheral blood lymphocytes to xenogeneic RNA directed at human tumor targets. The initial xenogeneic donors used were sheep or guinea pigs. Pilch *et al.* (1974) showed not only increased tumor-specific lymphocyte-mediated cytotoxicity (LMC) (as monitored by the Cohen assay) on human tumor targets, but a lack of effect when these same lymphocytes were incubated on normal human fibroblast target controls (Kern *et al.*, 1976a; Pilch *et al.*, 1974; Veltman *et al.*, 1974). In addition, human lymphocytes exposed to tumor-specific allogeneic or xenogeneic RNA demonstrated cell-mediated immunity not only against the specific tumor target used to sensitize the immune RNA donor, but also against other human tumor targets of the same histologic type (Kern *et al.*, 1976b).

These findings were confirmed by others (Singh *et al.*, 1977) and extended by Mannick, Wang, and Deckers to models of concomitant tumor immunity. Thus, lymphocyte-mediated cytotoxicity against tumor targets could be augmented by *in vitro* immune RNA incubation even though the exposed lymphocytes were harvested from animals already bearing tumor (Deckers *et al.*, 1975). Augmentation of the cellular immune response after immune RNA exposure of lymph node cells or peripheral blood lymphocytes harvested from animals and humans bearing tumor could be shown *in vitro* by either the [125I]iododeoxyuridine (IUdR) cytotoxicity assay or by proliferation assays monitoring tritiated thymidine uptake after specific antigen exposure of test lymphocytes (Wang and Deckers, 1976).

In addition to the early experiments of Mannick and Egdahl using skin allograft models, the possibility of immunologic information transfer by immune RNA has focused on the sensitization of monocytes in *in vivo* protection models using experimental Salmonellosis. Immune RNA-treated monocytes were said to demonstrate marked inhibition of intracytoplasmic bacterial replication (Mitsuhashi *et al.*, 1967; Saito and Mitsuhashi, 1965; Tohoku, 1966). Other *in vivo* models of resistance to various parasite infections were also postulated to be due to specific immune RNA activation of macrophages in treated recipients (Araujo and Remington, 1974; Barr *et al.*, 1977). The first direct *in vivo* evidence of adoptive transfer of cell-mediated immunity in humans by immune RNA was claimed in a brief report by Han *et al.* (1975) and concerned the transfer of PPD skin test response from a PPD-positive to a PPD-negative individual by intradermal (id) injection of immune RNA extracted from the peripheral blood lymphocytes of the tuberculin-sensitive human donor.

II. Mechanism of Action/Optimization of Technique

Discussion continues concerning antigen or antigen fragments in association with RNA in contrast to information transfer by an intact immune RNA molecule without associated antigen. The existence of antigen–immune RNA complexes has been reported in numerous cell-free systems (Fishman and Adler, 1972; Herscowitz and Stelos, 1970b), in numerous *in vitro* cellular systems (Garvey *et al.*, 1972; Herscowitz and Stelos, 1970a; Nakamura, 1976; Williams and Wu, 1971), and in various *in vivo* immune RNA transfer models (Reilly and Garvey, 1978; White and Johnson, 1976; Yaun and Campbell, 1972). An equal number of investigators have maintained that immune RNA functions to provide specific information exchange in the absence of associated antigen (Gottlieb *et al.*, 1972; Juras and Abramoff, 1970; Roelants *et al.*, 1971; Schlager *et al.*, 1974).

Evidence has accumulated that immune RNA has messenger RNA capability (Bilello *et al.*, 1976; Greenup *et al.*, 1978; Honjo *et al.*, 1976; Mikami *et al.*, 1971; Paque and Nealon, 1977; Paque and Nealon, 1979; Wang and Mannick, 1978). Identification of particular molecular moieties capable of transferring tumor-specific cellular cytotoxicity and the identification of the cell types involved have recently been published in a number of laboratories. Wang and Mannick (1978) fractionated and purified immune RNA with subsequent *in vitro* microcytotoxicity testing in a murine fibrosarcoma system. They showed that xenogeneic immune RNA extracted from the spleens and lymph nodes of guinea pigs previously immunized with murine fibrosarcoma could convert normal mouse lymphocytes to effector cells specifically cytolytic to the same murine tumor *in vitro*. The effect of this immune RNA was dose dependent and destroyed by treatment with RNase but not with DNase or Pronase (Fig. 1). After ultracentrifugation on a 5–20% sucrose density gradient, the RNA fraction capable of transferring cell-mediated cytotoxicity (CMC) sedimented at 8–16 S (Fig. 2). Immune RNA was also fractionated by these investigators using an oligo(dT)-cellulose affinity chromatography technique and the active fraction was found to possess polyadenylic acid [poly(A)] sequences resembling messenger RNA (Fig. 3). The immunologic activity of the poly(A)-containing RNA fraction was tumor specific and RNase sensi-

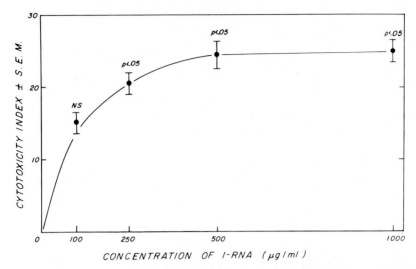

FIG. 1. Dose–response curve of I-RNA. Normal mouse lymphocytes were incubated with various concentrations of I-RNA and then tested against [^{125}I]IUdR-labeled, specific tumor cells *in vitro* at a lymphocyte:target cell (L:T) ratio of 500:1.

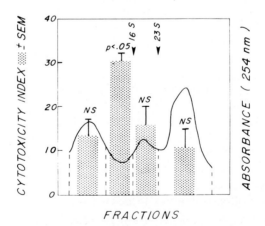

FIG. 2. Cell-mediated cytotoxicity mediated with RNA fractions. Immune RNA fractionated by 5–20% sucrose density gradient ultracentrifugation was optically analyzed at 254 nm. Three peaks were formed at 4 S, 18 S, and 28 S from left to right. Four fractions, sedimenting at 0–8 S, 8–16 S, 16–23 S, and 23–30 S were collected and their activities in transferring CMC were tested individually against specific tumor cells at an L:T ratio of 500:1. Arrows indicate the sedimentation coefficients of *Escherichia coli* ribosomal RNA used as a marker.

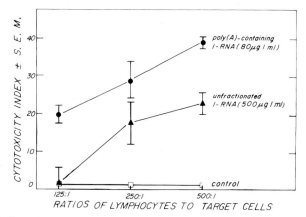

FIG. 3. Effect of I-RNA-incubated lymphocytes at various L:T ratios. Normal mouse lymphocytes incubated with 500 μg/ml of unfractionated I-RNA or 80 μg/ml of poly(A)-containing I-RNA were tested against specific tumor cells *in vitro* at L:T ratios of 125:1, 250:1, and 500:1. Normal lymphocytes incubated with no RNA were also tested at the same L:T ratios and served as controls.

tive. In subsequent experiments, immune RNA fractionated by sucrose density gradient ultracentrifugation was also chromatographed on an oligo(dT)-cellulose column. Cell-mediated cytotoxicity could be transferred only by the fractions sedimenting at 8–16 S and also containing poly(A) (Table I).

TABLE I

CELL-MEDIATED CYTOTOXICITY MEDIATED WITH RNA FRACTIONS OBTAINED FROM THE
COMBINATION OF SUCROSE DENSITY GRADIENT CENTRIFUGATION
AND OLIGO(dT)-CELLULOSE AFFINITY CROMATOGRAPHY

Normal mouse lymphocytes incubated with I-RNA fractionated with				
Sucrose density gradient centrifugation	Oligo(dT)-cellulose chromatography	Concentration of I-RNA (μg/ml)	Cytotoxic index (mean ± SEM)	p^a
8–16 S	Poly(A) containing	20	32.3 ± 6.3	<0.01
8–16 S	Poly(A) lacking	100	−0.5 ± 12.4	NS^b
0–8 S + 16–30 S	Poly(A) containing	20	3.5 ± 8.5	NS
0–8 S + 16–30 S	Poly(A) lacking	100	5.0 ± 6.4	NS
Unfractionated I-RNA		500	24.7 ± 7.4	<0.01

[a] p indicates significance of differences from effect of control lymphocytes.
[b] NS, Not significant.

Other investigators using specific antigens such as ARSNAT or KLH (Paque and Nealon, 1979) have confirmed the work of Wang and Mannick by showing that *in vitro* immune responses can be transferred by oligo(dT)-binding fractions obtained from sucrose density gradients (5–16 S) of whole donor lymphocyte RNA. Purification procedures have been demonstrated to increase the specific activity of immune RNA (Mikami *et al.*, 1971) and similar to the experiment of Mannick, the purified fractions remain RNase sensitive, but Pronase and DNase resistant (Paque, 1976).

The particular cell type or types which are the source of immune RNA capable of transferring tumor-specific cell-mediated cytotoxicity have been examined. Wang *et al.* (1978b) immunized Hartley guinea pigs with syngeneic murine fibrosarcomas BP-10 or BP-11 induced by 3,4-benzopyrene in C3H/HeJ mice. The immune RNA was extracted individually from the spleens, lymph nodes, and peritoneal exudate cells of the immunized guinea pigs. All three immune RNA preparations were shown to convert normal C3H/HeJ mouse lymphocytes to effector cells significantly cytolytic to the specific syngeneic mouse tumor *in vitro*. The $[^{125}I]IUdR$ assay was used to monitor the lymphocyte-mediated cytolytic effect. Lymphocytes and macrophages were purified from the spleens, lymph nodes, and peritoneal exudate cells from the tumor-immunized guinea pigs. Immune RNA was extracted from these purified cell populations by the conventional hot phenol technique and also from pooled guinea pig lymphoid tissues. Normal C3H/HeJ lymphocytes were incubated with each type of immune RNA and tested *in vitro* for cell-mediated cytolysis against the specific tumor targets. A significant cell-mediated cytolytic effect against BP-10 targets was observed with mouse lymphocytes incubated with immune RNA extracted from pooled lymphoid tissues of BP-10 tumor-immunized guinea pigs. There was a reduced but still significant cytotoxic effect when mouse lymphocytes were incubated with immune RNA extracted from purified guinea pig lymphocytes, but there was a markedly increased cytotoxic effect when the immune RNA was extracted from purified guinea pig macrophages (Table II).

As indicated by sucrose density gradient analysis, the less effective lymphocyte immune RNA was not due to RNA degradation resulting from lymphocyte purification or extraction techniques. Treatment of immune RNA with RNase abrogated the transfer of CMC, but treatment of immune RNA with DNase or Pronase did not. Tumor specificity of the immunity transfer by the macrophage immune RNA was also demonstrated (Table III). These results suggested that macrophages were the principal source of immune RNA capable of transferring tumor-specific cell-mediated cytotoxicity in this system.

TABLE II

TRANSFER OF CMC WITH I-RNA EXTRACTED FROM VARIOUS LYMPHOID CELL TYPES

Experiment	Treatment of normal mouse lymphocytes	Cytotoxic index (mean ± SEM)	p
A	None	0	
	Pooled lymphoid I-RNA	47.9 ± 4.1	<0.001
	Lymphocyte I-RNA	25.5 ± 5.6	<0.05
	Macrophage I-RNA	73.4 ± 1.9	<0.001
	Pooled lymphoid CFA-RNA[a]	12.6 ± 3.9	NS[b]
B	None	0	
	Pooled lymphoid I-RNA	32.3 ± 5.3	<0.001
	Lymphocyte I-RNA	14.9 ± 3.3	<0.05
	Macrophage I-RNA	51.5 ± 4.7	<0.001
	Macrophage I-RNA + RNase[c]	12.5 ± 3.0	NS
	Macrophage I-RNA + DNase[d]	58.3 ± 1.9	<0.001
	Macrophage I-RNA + Pronase[e]	45.7 ± 4.6	<0.001

[a] Complete Freund's adjuvant RNA was extracted from guinea pigs immunized with CFA without murine tumor.
[b] NS, Not significant.
[c] Immune RNA was treated with 50 μg/ml of pancreatic RNase A.
[d] Immune RNA was treated with 50 μg/ml of pancreatic DNase.
[e] Immune RNA was treated with 50 μg/ml of Pronase.

Wang *et al.* (1978a) have also recently described some details of the kinetics of transfer of tumor-specific cytotoxicity with immune RNA. In the murine fibrosarcoma C3H/HeJ model, unsensitized mouse lymphocytes were converted to effector cells specifically cytolytic to syngeneic tumor cells by incubation with immune RNA extracted from the lymphoid tissues of guinea pigs immunized with the murine tumor being tested. Using the modified Cohen [125I]IUdR release microcytotoxicity assay, these investigators examined the optimal time of immunization of the guinea pig immune RNA donors. They found that the most effective immune RNA was harvested from guinea pigs 14 days after immunization with the murine tumor. Maximum cytolytic activity was observed with mouse lymphocytes that had been incubated with immune RNA at a concentration of 500 μg/ml at 37°C for 30 minutes. Significant tumor cell destruction did not occur until 48 hours after the addition of RNA-incubated lymphocytes to target cells. Significant cell-mediated cytotoxicity was seen at a broad range of lymphocyte-to-target cell ratios in this assay system (100/1–1000/1) (Figs. 4–7). Lymphoid cells obtained from spleen, bone marrow, thymus, and lymph node were converted by immune RNA incubation to become effector cells. The treatment of lymphocytes with anti-θ

TABLE III
SPECIFICITY OF CMC TRANSFERRED WITH I-RNA

Treatment of normal mouse lymphocytes	BP-10 target cells		BP-11 target cells	
	Cytotoxic index (mean ± SEM)	p	Cytotoxic index (mean ± SEM)	p
None	0		0	
BP-10 pooled lymphoid I-RNA	68.7 ± 4.1	<0.001	10.1 ± 6.2	NS[a]
BP-10 lymphocyte I-RNA	34.1 ± 9.1	<0.05	8.9 ± 4.4	NS
BP-10 macrophage I-RNA	73.5 ± 1.9	<0.001	8.3 ± 6.4	NS
BP-11 pooled lymphoid I-RNA	12.9 ± 7.2	NS	46.1 ± 11.4	<0.01
BP-11 lymphocyte I-RNA	12.2 ± 6.1	NS	20.8 ± 5.6	<0.05
BP-11 macrophage I-RNA	12.8 ± 5.8	NS	68.4 ± 4.1	<0.001
BP-11 pooled lymphoid I-RNA + RNase[b]	ND[c]		9.1 ± 3.2	NS
BP-11 lymphocyte I-RNA + RNase	ND		3.3 ± 1.0	NS
BP-11 macrophage I-RNA + RNase	ND		2.4 ± 1.5	NS

[a] NS, Not significant.
[b] RNA was treated with 50 μg/ml of pancreatic RNase A.
[c] ND, Not done.

serum and complement prior to incubation with immune RNA abolished the ability to transfer cell-mediated cytotoxicity.

The mechanisms involved in the conversion of normal lymphocytes to cytolytic cells by immune RNA remain unclear. Treatment with immune RNA may influence a sizable number of lymphocytes to become tumor-specific killer cells. Alternatively, only a few genetically preprogrammed lymphocytes may be triggered by immune RNA and the large number of effector cells may be generated after one or more proliferative steps. Wang and Mannick (1979) have recently investigated the relationship between antigen-specific blastogenesis and cytotoxicity mediated by RNA treatment in an attempt to determine whether both phenomena were manifested by the same or by different subsets of treated lymphocytes. After confirming the murine sarcoma immune RNA cell-mediated cytotoxicity transfer system with the expected tumor specificity, Wang and Mannick demonstrated that treatment of lymphocytes after immune RNA incubation with mitomycin C completely inhibited lymphocyte proliferation in mixed lymphocyte tumor culture, but left the cell-mediated cytotoxicity response intact, suggesting that a proliferative step was not necessary for immune RNA-incubated lymphocytes to manifest tumor-specific cell-mediated cytotoxicity (Fig. 8; Table IV).

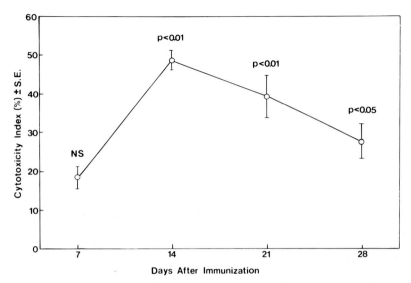

FIG. 4.   Optimal time of immunization of RNA donor guinea pigs. Guinea pigs immunized with murine tumor were killed at days 7, 14, 21, and 28 after immunization. Immune
RNA was extracted from their lymphoid tissues. Unsensitized lymphocytes were incubated
with these RNAs and tested in the microcytotoxicity assay.

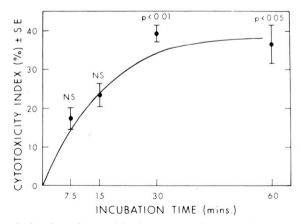

FIG. 5.   Incubation time of unsensitized mouse lymphocytes with I-RNA. Incubation of
unsensitized mouse lymphocytes with BP-8 I-RNA was performed at 37°C for various periods of time. These RNA-incubated lymphocytes were then tested for cytotoxicity against
BP-8 target cells.

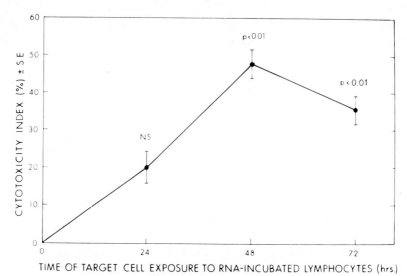

FIG. 6. Time required for RNA-incubated lymphocytes to manifest cytotoxicity. RNA-incubated lymphocytes were added to BP-8 tumor cells and incubated for 24, 48, and 72 hours.

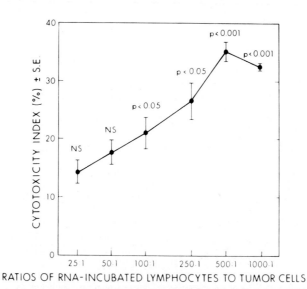

FIG. 7. Optimal ratios of RNA-incubated lymphocytes to target cells. Unsensitized mouse lymphocytes incubated with I-RNA were tested at various L:T ratios from 25:1 to 1000:1.

TABLE IV
EFFECT OF MITOMYCIN C ON THE DEGREE AND SPECIFICITY OF
TUMOR IMMUNITY TRANSFERRED BY I-RNA

| | BP-10 targets | | | BP-11 targets | |
| | Cytotoxic index | | | Cytotoxic index | |
Lymphocyte treatment	(mean ± SEM)	p^a		(mean ± SEM)	p
BP-10 I-RNA	25.6 ± 6.5	0.01		13.0 ± 5.4	NS[b]
BP-10 I-RNA + mitomycin C[c]	28.3 ± 5.5	0.01		11.0 ± 8.4	NS
BP-11 I-RNA	14.5 ± 8.7	NS		36.4 ± 7.0	<0.05
BP-11 I-RNA + mitomycin C	−5.1 ± 13.2	NS		35.8 ± 10.4	<0.05

[a] p values were determined by comparing the cytotoxic effect of I-RNA-incubated lymphocytes with that of control lymphocytes incubated with no RNA.
[b] NS, Not significant.
[c] Normal mouse lymphocytes were incubated with I-RNA and subsequently treated with mitomycin C before exposure to target cells.

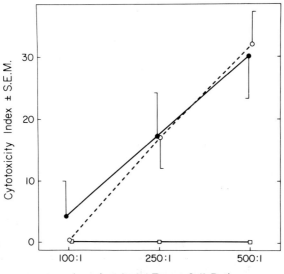

Lymphocyte to Target Cell Ratio

FIG. 8. Normal mouse lymphocytes were incubated with I-RNA and then tested against [^{125}I]IUdR-labeled BP-10 tumor cells at L:T ratios of 100:1, 250:1, and 500:1 (●——●). Some lymphocytes were treated with mitomycin C after I-RNA incubation and then similarly tested (○——○). Normal lymphocytes incubated with no RNA were also treated as controls (□——□).

Thus, immune RNA appeared to convert a sizable fraction of normal mouse lymphocytes to cells capable of tumor-specific cytolysis rather than to trigger the proliferation of a few specifically programmed cells. It appeared, however, that the cell-mediated cytotoxicity in the [^{125}I]IUdR assay system required more than 24 hours of exposure of the specific targets to the immune RNA-treated lymphocytes to produce lysis of the tumor cells. Thus, a differentiation step not involving proliferation could take place during this time. Such differentiation did not appear to take place without exposure to specific tumor antigens since there was no significant difference in the time necessary to manifest cytotoxicity by immune RNA-incubated lymphocytes that had been cultured for various periods of time before being added to the target cells (Table V; Fig. 9).

The results thus indicate that once immune RNA-treated lymphocytes have been committed to become killer cells, cellular proliferation is un-

TABLE V

CYTOTOXIC EFFECTS OF I-RNA-INCUBATED LYMPHOCYTES
CULTURED *in Vitro* FOR VARIOUS PERIODS BEFORE
EXPOSURE TO TARGET CELLS

Experiment	Time in culture of I-RNA-treated lymphocytes[a] (hours)	Cytotoxic index (mean ± SEM)	p[b]
A	0	29.1 ± 5.4	<0.05
	24	31.5 ± 2.3	<0.05
	48	32.0 ± 3.0	<0.001
	72	23.3 ± 6.4	<0.05
B	0	46.8 ± 2.6	<0.001
	24	48.4 ± 3.6	<0.01
	48	39.1 ± 3.4	<0.001
	72	39.5 ± 4.3	<0.001
C	0	28.7 ± 9.3	<0.05
	24	35.4 ± 3.9	<0.001
	48	26.5 ± 2.5	<0.01
	72	31.3 ± 3.9	<0.001

[a] After I-RNA incubation, normal mouse lymphocytes were cultured for various periods of time (0 to 72 hours) before exposure to target cells.

[b] Probability value (p) was determined by comparing the CMC of I-RNA-incubated lymphocytes with that of control lymphocytes which had been incubated with no RNA and cultured for the same period of time.

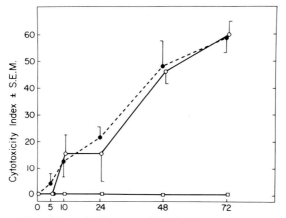

Time of Target Cell Exposure to I-RNA-incubated Lymphocytes (hours)

FIG. 9. Normal mouse lymphocytes incubated with I-RNA were either immediately tested for their cytolytic activity [group A lymphocytes (○———○)] or cultured for 48 hours before testing [group B lymphocytes (●———●)]. Cytolytic reactions were terminated at 0, 5, 10, 24, 48, and 72 hours after the addition of effector lymphocytes to target cells. Normal lymphocytes incubated with no RNA were similarly tested and served as controls (□———□).

necessary. The results also suggest that immune RNA acts upon at least two different subsets of lymphocytes: one manifesting cell-mediated cytotoxicity and the other undergoing antigen-specific proliferation (Table VI). Although not directly proving the absence of tumor antigen in these immune RNA preparations, the failure of mitomycin C to inhibit induction of cell-mediated cytotoxicity by immune RNA increases the likelihood that the transfer of tumor-specific cell-mediated cytotoxicity was not simply due to an *in vitro* sensitization of normal lymphocytes with tumor antigen present in the immune RNA preparations, since several other investigations have reported that cellular proliferation is absolutely essential for the *in vitro* induction of cytotoxic lymphocytes exposed to antigen (Bernstein, 1977; Nedrud *et al.*, 1975; Sondel *et al.*, 1976).

III. Application to Animal Tumor Models

The first application of tumor-specific xenogeneic immune RNA to the *in vivo* therapy of tumors was reported by Pilch and co-workers in 1969 and 1971 (Deckers and Pilch, 1971). These investigators showed that murine isograft challenge resistance could be altered by foot-pad injections of tumor-specific xenogeneic immune RNA. Direct injection of immune RNA without an RNase inhibitor (sodium dextran sulfate) did not

TABLE VI

CYTOTOXIC AND PROLIFERATIVE RESPONSES OF NORMAL MOUSE
LYMPHOCYTES AFTER I-RNA TREATMENT

Lymphocyte treatment	Cytotoxic index (mean ± SEM)	p^a	Stimulation index (mean ± SEM)	p^b
None	0		0.7 ± 6.8	NS[c]
I-RNA	27.9 ± 2.7	<0.01	76.5 ± 8.4	<0.01
I-RNA + RNase[d]	12.0 ± 3.2	NS	1.4 ± 2.3	NS
I-RNA + DNase[d]	23.2 ± 5.3	0.05	ND[e]	
I-RNA + Pronase[d]	24.9 ± 5.0	0.05	ND	
I-RNA + mitomycin C[f]	35.9 ± 2.6	0.001	−4.6 ± 19.2	NS
CFA-RNA[g]	12.0 ± 2.0	NS	9.4 ± 3.5	NS

[a] Probability values (p) were determined by comparing the cytotoxic effect of I-RNA-incubated lymphocytes with that of control lymphocytes not incubated with I-RNA.

[b] Probability values (p) were determined by comparing the proliferative effect of lymphocytes cocultured with tumor cells with that of the same treated lymphocytes cultured without tumor cells.

[c] NS, Not significant.

[d] Immune RNA was treated with 50 μg/ml of RNase, DNase, or Pronase before incubation with normal mouse lymphocytes.

[e] ND, Not done.

[f] Normal mouse lymphocytes were incubated with I-RNA and subsequently treated with mitomycin C before exposure to target cells.

[g] Complete Freund's adjuvant RNA was extracted from the lymphoid tissues of guinea pigs that had been immunized with CFA without tumor.

provide *in vivo* isograft challenge resistance. In 1975, Schlager and Dray reported the successful therapy of an already-established strain 2 guinea pig hepatoma by injection of either syngeneic or xenogeneic tumor-specific immune RNA plus naive syngenetic lymphocytes plus a tumor-specific antigen vaccine. Regression was obtained not only in the primary injected tumors but also at secondary noninjected sites. Survival was prolonged in animals in which tumor regression was obtained.

In 1976, Deckers *et al.* attempted to establish the therapeutic effect on murine sarcoma isograft outgrowth of xenogeneic tumor-specific immune RNA treatment. Although these investigators showed a temporary and significant delay in isograft outgrowth among animals treated with tumor-specific xenogeneic immune RNA, isograft growth in treated animals soon caught up with non-tumor-specific-treated controls. There was, however, a reportedly specific *in vitro* augmentation of splenocyte-mediated antitumor effect in the tumor-bearing animals treated with immune RNA. A major difference in the protocol of Mannick and associates as compared to that of Pilch and colleagues was the *in vitro* incubation of syngeneic splenocytes with xenogeneic tumor-specific immune RNA prior to the injection of effector cells into the mice bearing sarcoma isografts. This was thought to obviate the need for RNase inhibitors, since Mannick and co-workers (unpublished) had earlier found that direct injection of immune RNA was ineffective.

The minimal effect of immune RNA in preventing isograft outgrowth was disappointing; however, it was felt to be a consequence of the particular tumor model chosen and the extremely rapid tumor isograft outgrowth. A more suitable model with at least a superficial analogy to the human "minimal residual disease" situation was first reported by Pilch *et al.* (1976b). Using a metastasizing rat mammary carcinoma, Pilch reported that tumor-specific immune RNA in combination with an RNase inhibitor could prevent development of metastases after primary isograft excision. Animals protected against metastases were long-term survivors. Although this immunotherapy protocol included animals treated with RNase-neutralized immune RNA and RNA harvested from nonimmunized donors, tumor specificity controls were not presented.

Since immune RNA (for that matter, any immunotherapy) might be more applicable to patients or animals at risk for recurrence after all primary tumor has been surgically excised, Wang, Mannick, Steele, and their associates reported tumor-specific immune RNA therapy in a different minimal residual disease model (Wang *et al.*, 1978c, 1979). These investigators reported a consistent reduction in death from pulmonary metastases in C57BL/6J mice by immune RNA treatment after excision of primary B16 melanoma isografts. Furthermore, lymphocytes from these immune RNA-treated animals were examined in numerous *in vitro* assays for cytolytic activity against B16 melanomas in order to correlate the *in vivo* and *in vitro* effects of immune RNA therapy. The overall experimental design in the *in vivo* part of this animal study is illustrated in Fig. 10. A group of C57BL/6J mice was injected with 2×10^3 B16 tumor cells in their hind limbs. Approximately 2.5 weeks later, tumor isografts became palpable and the limbs were amputated. At days 2, 4, 6, 8, and 10 after tumor excision, each animal received 75×10^6 syngeneic normal lymphocytes or lymphocytes that had been incubated *in vitro* with RNA that was tumor specific or RNase protected. 3LL (Lewis lung carcinoma) was used as a control for tumor specificity. The survival rate of each group was recorded until 100 days after the excision of the primary B16 isografts. Selected survivors were killed and autopsied to prove absence of metastases. The significance of the difference in survival between the various groups was analyzed by Fischer's exact χ^2 test.

Control animals that received untreated lymphocytes or lymphocytes treated with RNase began to die of pulmonary metastases within 24 days

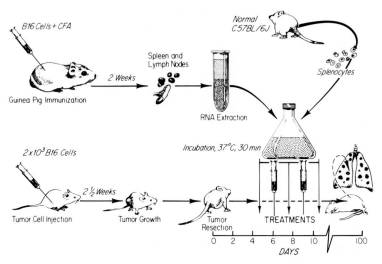

Fig. 10. Experimental design of *in vivo* study. Guinea pigs were immunized with B16 murine melanoma and complete Freud's adjuvant. Two weeks later spleens and lymph nodes were removed from these immunized animals and I-RNA was extracted from these lymphoid tissues. A group of C57BL/6J mice was injected with 2×10^6 B16 cells into their hind limbs. Approximately 2.5 weeks later the limbs were amputated after B16 isografts became palpable. Each animal then received five treatments, administered at 2-day intervals, with normal syngeneic splenocytes that had been incubated with I-RNA *in vitro*. Control animals received untreated splenocytes or splenocytes incubated with various control RNAs. The survival rate of each group was recorded until 100 days after the primary isograft excision. Dead animals were autopsied to prove presence of metastases. Selected mice surviving 100 days after amputation were killed and also autopsied to prove absence of metastases.

after the primary B16 isografts were excised. However, this survival rate was significantly improved by injection of normal mouse lymphocytes previously incubated *in vitro* with B16 specific immune RNA (Table VII). Only 2 out of 24 control mice receiving untreated lymphocytes survived until 100 days after excision of the primary B16 isografts. Treatment of mice with immune RNA-incubated lymphocytes that were tumor-specific significantly increased the survival rate: 11 out of 21 mice were still alive at 100 days ($p < 0.001$). Degradation of immune RNA with RNase prior to incubation with lymphocytes destroyed the therapeutic effect: only 2 out of 22 mice survived. RNA prepared from guinea pigs injected with complete Freund's adjuvant (CFA) without tumor was ineffective: 1 out of 7 animals survived. RNA prepared from guinea pigs that had been immunized against 3LL murine tumor, which is antigenically distinct from B16, did not prevent deaths from B16 metastases: all 13 mice died. Con-

TABLE VII
IMMUNOTHERAPY OF B16 MELANOMA WITH I-RNA

Lymphocyte treatment[a]	Animal survival after excision of the primary B16 isografts at days						
	20	25	30	35	40	45	100
None	23/24[b]	22/24	19/24	13/24	6/24	2/24	2/24
B16 I-RNA	21/21	21/21	20/21	17/21	13/21	12/21	11/21
B16 I-RNA + RNase	22/22	20/22	17/22	12/22	4/22	2/22	2/22
CFA-RNA	7/7	7/7	5/7	3/7	3/7	2/7	1/7
3LL I-RNA	13/13	12/13	9/13	7/13	1/13	1/13	0/13
B16 I-RNA (in animals with 3LL isografts)	4/10	4/10	4/10	1/10	1/10	1/10	1/10

[a] After excision of B16 isografts, C57BL/6J mice were injected with untreated lymphocytes or lymphocytes that had been treated with various RNAs in vitro.

[b] Survivors/total animals in group.

versely, B16 immune RNA had no effect on animals that had had 3LL isografts amputated: 1 out of 10 mice survived, indicating the "crisscross" in vivo specificity of tumor immunity transferred by immune RNA in this minimal residual disease protocol.

In a parallel study, animals that had been treated with either normal syngeneic lymphocytes, immune RNA-incubated lymphocytes, RNase-degraded immune RNA-incubated lymphocytes, or lymphocytes preincubated with 3LL immune RNA were killed at 7-day intervals starting 10 days after excision of the primary B16 isografts. Lymphocytes were obtained from the spleens and lymph nodes of these mice and examined for their cytolytic activity in vitro against B16 tumor cells using three different in vitro assay techniques (Wang et al., 1979). In the modified Cohen assay with prelabeled [^{125}I]IUdR B16 tumor cells, lymphocytes obtained from mice receiving untreated lymphocytes served as controls. As indicated in Table VIII, significant cytotoxicity was demonstrated only with lymphocytes harvested from mice that had received B16 immune RNA therapy. Lymphocytes from mice treated with immune RNA previously degraded by RNase had no killing effect on B16 targets, nor did lymphocytes obtained from mice that were treated with nonspecific 3LL immune RNA.

Clear-cut and significant increases in lymphocyte-mediated cytolysis specific to the B16 targets was also demonstrated in microcytotoxicity and chromium release assays using splenocytes harvested from animals 24 days after primary isograft rejection and 14 days after completing im-

TABLE VIII

In Vitro CYTOTOXICITY OF LYMPHOCYTES HARVESTED
FROM I-RNA-TREATED ANIMALS

Experimental treatment[a]	Cytotoxic index after excision of the primary B16 isografts at days[b]				
	10	17	24	31	38
None (control)	0	0	0	0	0
B16 I-RNA	18.1	24.7	40.2	16.0	44.9
B16 I-RNA + RNase	0	0	ND[c]	0	0
3LL I-RNA	ND	0	10.0	1.5	0

[a] After excision of primary B16 isografts, C57BL/6J mice were injected with untreated lymphocytes (control) or lymphocytes that had been incubated with B16 I-RNA, RNase-degraded B16 I-RNA, or 3LL I-RNA.

[b] At 7-day intervals as indicated, lymphocytes were harvested from mice of each group and then tested for cytotoxicity against B16 tumor cells *in vitro* at a lymphocyte-to-target cell ratio of 500:1.

[c] ND, Not done.

munotherapy, as shown in Tables IX and X. Serial *in vitro* cell-mediated cytotoxicity data documented that *in vivo* xenogeneic immune RNA treatment was capable of modifying a specific host immune response measurable *in vitro*. Three different cytotoxicity techniques demonstrated a similar specific *in vitro* cytotoxicity of splenocytes from immune RNA-treated animals. This significant cytotoxicity was found only in the group of animals whose survival was improved by specific immune RNA therapy. These results suggested that the combination of surgery and immunotherapy with immune RNA might be useful in preventing tumor recurrence in certain patients with cancer.

IV. Human Studies

deKernion *et al.* (1975) published the first anecdotal reports of xenogeneic immune RNA therapy in humans with a variety of malignant lesions. These investigators updated their human-treatment immune RNA protocols in 1976 and again in 1977 (Pilch *et al.*, 1976a,b, 1977; Ramming and deKernion, 1977). Despite earlier animal experience demonstrating the ineffectiveness of direct immune RNA injection without RNase inhibitors, their protocols for immunotherapy in man consisted of direct intravenous xenogeneic immune RNA injection. Immune RNA was harvested

TABLE IX

In Vitro CYTOTOXICITY OF SPLENOCYTES HARVESTED FROM I-RNA-TREATED
AND CONTROL MICE ON B16 MELANOMA TARGETS[a]

Comparisons of effects of splenocytes from animals receiving	Effector:target ratio	Differences in effects of splenocytes by	
		^{51}Cr released	^{51}Cr retained
Tumor-specific B16 I-RNA 1	100:1	17[b]	10.5[b]
versus 3LL I-RNA	30:1	8.4[c]	1.8[d]
	10:1	8.3[c]	1[d]
Tumor-specific B16 I-RNA 2	100:1	8.5[b]	5[c]
versus 3LL I-RNA	30:1	8.7[b]	3[b]
	10:1	−2[d]	−2[d]
RNase-pretreated B16 I-RNA	100:1	10.1[b]	5.6[b]
versus 3LL I-RNA	30:1	−2.1[d]	−1[d]
	10:1	−1[d]	−1[d]

[a] Long-term ^{51}Cr assay was performed at day 24 after isograft excision. Difference in effects assayed by ^{51}Cr released is calculated as the difference between mean percentage of ^{51}Cr released after exposure to test splenocytes minus mean percentage of ^{51}Cr released after exposure to 3LL splenocytes. Difference in effects assayed by ^{51}Cr retained is defined as the difference between mean percentage of ^{51}Cr retained in targets after exposure to 3LL splenocytes minus mean percentage of ^{51}Cr retained after exposure to test splenocytes. Differences were analyzed for statistical significance by Student's *t* test.

[b] $p < 0.05$.
[c] $p < 0.01$.
[d] Not significant.

from sheep or guinea pigs immunized with the patient's own tumor or with "tissue-type-specific" human tumor. Treated patients had a variety of cancer diagnoses, including melanoma, renal cell carcinoma, sarcoma, and gastric and breast carcinoma, and no uniform conclusions concerning tumor response or effect on survival could be made. On the other hand, there was no toxicity from the immunotherapy regimen and no evidence that tumor course was exacerbated. Most of these studies also included *in vitro* tests of lymphocyte-mediated cytotoxicity (as monitored by the Cohen assay using autologous or allogeneic tissue-type-specific target cells). In general, host cell-mediated cytotoxicity seemed to have been stimulated immediately after immune RNA treatment, but strict relationships between *in vitro* parameters and *in vivo* response were not obtained, and *in vitro* specificity controls were not always possible.

Because of the repeated success in preventing pulmonary metastases by adjuvant immune RNA treatment in the B16 melanoma animal model,

TABLE X

In Vitro Cytotoxicity of Splenocytes Harvested from I-RNA-Treated and
Control Mice on B16 Melanoma Targets[a]

Splenocytes harvested from animals receiving	Effector:target ratio	Surviving B16 target cells	Percentage of cytotoxicity
3LL non-tumor-specific I-RNA	3000:1	275 ± 18[b]	
	2000:1	230 ± 13	
	1000:1	150 ± 13	
Tumor-specific B16 I-RNA 1	3000:1	127 ± 7	54[c]
	2000:1	123 ± 7	47[c]
	1000:1	139 ± 7	7[d]
Tumor-specific B16 I-RNA 2	3000:1	110 ± 10	56[c]
	2000:1	149 ± 5	35[c]
	1000:1	141 ± 7	6[d]
RNase-pretreated B16 I-RNA	3000:1	246 ± 23	11[d]
	2000:1	283 ± 21	0
	1000:1	224 ± 11	0

[a] Microcytotoxicity assay with visual counting of remaining target cells was performed at day 24 after isograft excision. Percentage of cytotoxicity is expressed as the percentage of reduction in surviving cells after exposure to test splenocytes compared to 3LL splenocytes.
[b] Mean ± SEM.
[c] $p < 0.001$.
[d] Not significant.

a human immune RNA trial was proposed by Wang *et al.* (1979). However, before application to a randomized, prospective study in patients with minimal tumor burden, the potential toxicity of the treatment protocol and the predicted effect on specific *in vitro* parameters of host antitumor immunity were examined in patients with metastatic renal cell cancer or widespread melanoma. These patients were chosen since no conventional therapy has been shown to be beneficial to them. (Steele *et al.*, 1980, 1981). The seven patients included in this initial phase I clinical trial of xenogeneic immune RNA are summarized in Table XI. The clinical protocol designed adhered as closely as possible to the previous animal treatment protocol. After excision of primary or recurrent tumor, each patient's tumor tissue was used for immunization of guinea pigs in the usual manner. After recovery from surgery, patients had Scribner arteriovenous shunts placed in their left forearms. These shunts were used for serial leukapheresis to obtain autologous lymphocytes for *in vitro* immune RNA incubation and to reinfuse the treated autologous cells. Each patient

TABLE XI
PATIENTS INCLUDED IN THE PHASE I I-RNA TRIAL

Patient	Diagnosis	Clinical course		Duration of response (months)	Present status
		Before I-RNA	After I-RNA		
1	Renal cell carcinoma	Lung mets ↑[a]	Lung mets gone	18	Alive, new lung mets[b]
2	Renal cell carcinoma	Lung mets ↑ Bone mets ↑ Scalene node ↑	Lung mets → Bone mets ↓ Scalene node ↓	10	Dead at 12 months
3	Renal cell carcinoma	Lung mets ↑ Liver mets ↑ Right atrium tumor thrombus	Lung mets → Liver mets ↓	8	Alive with disease
4	Renal cell carcinoma	Lung mets ↑	Lung mets →	4	Dead at 10 months
5	Renal cell carcinoma	Lung mets ↑	Lung mets →	3	Dead at 6 months
6	Renal cell carcinoma	Lung mets Brain mets ↑	I-RNA × 1 Brain mets ↓		Dead at 1 month
7	Recurrent melanoma	Inguinal-iliac-paraaortic nodes ↑	Nodal mets ↓		Dead at 8 months

[a] Mets, Metastases; ↑, progression; ↓, regression; →, stabilization.
[b] Patient will be retreated with I-RNA-exposed autologous lymphocytes.

underwent five treatments (every other day) and arteriovenous shunts were removed after the last autologous lymphocyte infusion.

Aliquots of the patient's peripheral blood lymphocytes (PBL) were frozen and stored at $-70°C$ in Weymouth's medium plus 10% dimethyl sulfoxide (DMSO) immediately before and after each *in vitro* immune RNA treatment. Serial peripheral blood lymphocyte specimens from each patient were simultaneously tested for evidence of change in their lymphocyte-mediated cytolytic effect at a later time. A scheme of the entire phase I treatment protocol is outlined in Fig. 11.

No toxicity was noted during or after the immune RNA treatments using RNA-sensitized autologous lymphocytes with every-other-day iv

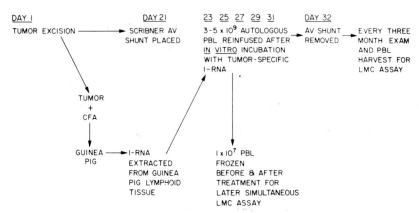

FIG. 11.   Protocol for phase I human I-RNA trial. CFA, Complete Freund's adjuvant; AV, arteriovenous.

injections consisting of $3-5 \times 10^9$ cells per injection. A single patient with renal cell carcinoma had complete resolution of multiple pulmonary metastases beginning 3 months after immune RNA treatment and is now in continued complete remission at 3 years. Two other patients with visceral metastases from renal cell carcinoma demonstrated a greater than 50% regression of measurable tumor, two patients showed stabilization of previously growing renal cell carcinoma pulmonary metastases, and one renal cell carcinoma patient and a single patient with widespread recurrent melanoma had no alteration in their rapidly progressive tumor courses.

All of the serial peripheral blood lymphocyte samples from individual patients were tested simultaneously for *in vitro* lymphocyte-mediated cytolysis against allogeneic renal cell carcinoma and melanoma targets. Lymphocyte-mediated cytolysis was boosted in peripheral blood lymphocyte samples after *in vitro* immune RNA treatment. A progressive increase in lymphocyte-mediated cytolysis was demonstrated in serial peripheral blood lymphocyte samples harvested from patients during immune RNA therapy (Table XII). As in earlier animal experiments, various assays for *in vitro* cytolytic effect were performed on the same samples, and the results were consistent (Table XIII). Increased lymphocyte-mediated cytolysis was found in peripheral blood lymphocyte samples harvested as long as 3–9 months after immune RNA therapy. Statistically significant boosts in the cytolytic effect of the lymphocyte samples harvested from treated renal cell carcinoma patients were restricted to renal cell carcinoma targets (Fig. 12). Similarly, only peripheral blood lymphocyte samples harvested during immune RNA treatment of the patient with

TABLE XII

SERIAL *in Vitro* LMC DURING I-RNA TREATMENT OF
PATIENT 2 (RENAL CELL CARCINOMA)

Time of PBL harvest	Effector: target ratio	Percentage of ^{51}Cr released on renal cancer targets (Pastor)	Cytotoxic effect[a]	Percentage of ^{51}Cr released on melanoma targets (S85A)	Cytotoxic effect[a]
Before first	100:1	37 ± 1[b]		50 ± 2	
I-RNA	30:1	39 ± 1		50 ± 3	
	10:1	47 ± 2		50 ± 2	
After first	100:1	53 ± 1	16[c]	47 ± 4	0
I-RNA	30:1	57 ± 3	17[d]	50 ± 2	0
	10:1	61 ± 1	14[c]	50 ± 1	0
Before second	100:1	54 ± 4	17[d]	49 ± 1	0
I-RNA	30:1	52 ± 2	13[c]	47 ± 3	0
	10:1	54 ± 1	7[d]	53 ± 8	3[e]
After second	100:1	52 ± 3	15[d]	43 ± 4	0
I-RNA	30:1	62 ± 5	23[f]	49 ± 1	0
	10:1	62 ± 6	15[f]	55 ± 4	5[e]

[a] Cytotoxic effect is calculated as the difference between mean percentage of ^{51}Cr released after exposure to I-RNA-treated PBL minus mean percentage of ^{51}Cr released after exposure to PBL harvested before the first I-RNA treatment.
[b] Mean ± SEM.
[c] Student's t test, $p < 0.001$.
[d] Student's t test, $p < 0.01$.
[e] Student's t test, not significant.
[f] Student's t test, $p < 0.05$.

melanoma showed increased lymphocyte-mediated cytolysis on the allogeneic melanoma targets (Table XIV). *In vitro* lymphocyte-mediated cytolytic activity was clearly boosted in all treated patients regardless of their clinical course after immune RNA therapy.

These results were felt to demonstrate that xenogeneic immune RNA therapy effective in an animal tumor model could be applied safely to humans. Despite the far-advanced tumors in the patients in this phase I trial, their clinical courses after immune RNA treatment were at least as promising as the results reported in earlier, nonrandomized human trials using xenogeneic immune RNA injected intravenously, despite probable deactivation by endogenous RNases. Previous B16 melanoma animal studies and the phase I human trial suggested that *in vitro* immune RNA exposure of autologous lymphocytes and reinfusion of treated lympho-

TABLE XIII

Cytotoxicity of Lymphocytes Harvested from Patient 5 (Renal
Cell Carcinoma) Before and After I-RNA[a]

PBL harvested	Effector: target ratio	Counts per minute on remaining renal cancer targets (A489)	Cytotoxicity index[b] (%)	Counts per minute on remaining melanoma targets (H130M)	Cytotoxicity index[b] (%)
Before fifth I-RNA	250:1	914.7 ± 93.9[c]		122 ± 14.2	
After fifth I-RNA	250:1	686.5 ± 288.7	25[d]	121 ± 9.7	0.8[e]
Before fifth I-RNA	125:1	1690.3 ± 119.9		136 ± 10.5	
After fifth I-RNA	125:1	993.3 ± 330.1	41[f]	132 ± 25.0	2.9[e]

[a] [125I]Iododeoxyuridine assay was performed using PBL obtained before and after the fifth I-RNA treatment.

[b] Cytotoxicity index = ([125I]iododeoxyuridine with PBL before fifth I-RNA − [125I]iododeoxyuridine with PBL after fifth I-RNA)/([125I]iododeoxyuridine with PBL before fifth I-RNA) × 100.

[c] Mean ± SEM.

[d] Student's *t* test, $p < 0.05$.

[e] Student's *t* test, not significant.

[f] Student's *t* test, $p < 0.001$.

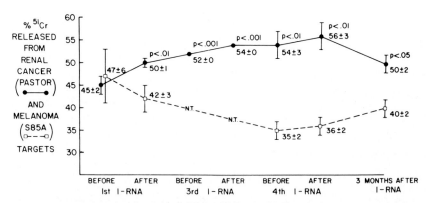

Fig. 12. Summary of serial *in vitro* LMC at effector:target ratio of 100:1 during I-RNA treatment of patient with renal cell cancer.

TABLE XIV

SERIAL *in Vitro* LMC AFTER I-RNA TREATMENT OF PATIENT 7 (MELANOMA)

Time of PBL harvest	Effector: target ratio	Percentage of ^{51}Cr released on renal cancer targets (Pastor)	Cytotoxic effect[a]	Percentage of ^{51}Cr released on melanoma targets (S85A)	Cytotoxic effect[a]
Before first	30:1	59 ± 2[b]	NT[c]	44 ± 3	NT
I-RNA	10:1	60 ± 2	—	40 ± 3	—
After first	30:1	66 ± 0	6[d]	NT	NT
I-RNA	10:1	59 ± 0	0	—	—
Before second	30:1	52 ± 5	0	49 ± 3	5[e]
I-RNA	10:1	55 ± 0	0	51 ± 4	11[f]
After second	30:1	56 ± 5	0	53 ± 2	9[f]
I-RNA	10:1	59 ± 2	0	43 ± 1	3[e]
Before third	30:1	63 ± 3	4[g]	46 ± 3	2[g]
I-RNA	10:1	55 ± 0	0	51 ± 2	11[f]
After third	30:1	63 ± 2	3[g]	51 ± 2	7[e]
I-RNA	10:1	57 ± 5	0	46 ± 4	6[e]

[a] Cytotoxic effect is calculated as the difference between mean percentage of ^{51}Cr released after exposure to I-RNA-treated PBL minus mean percentage of ^{51}Cr released after exposure to PBL harvested before the first I-RNA treatment.

[b] Mean ± SEM.

[c] NT, Not tested

[d] Student's t test, $p < 0.001$.

[e] Student's t test, $p < 0.05$.

[f] Student's t test, $p < 0.01$.

[g] Student's t test, not significant.

cytes might be a more effective method of influencing host antitumor immune response and achieving therapeutic benefit.

In contrast to the animal model data, no correlation was found between clinical course in the treated patients and serial *in vitro* lymphocyte-mediated cytolytic effect. However, the immune RNA treatment of C57BL/6J mice after B16 isograft excision was designed as an adjuvant immunotherapy model. In such a minimal residual disease setting, the effects of host lymphocyte-mediated cytolysis demonstrated by *in vitro* assay might have had a greater *in vivo* influence on tumor course. In contrast, all of the patients treated in the human phase I trial were chosen for their far-advanced disease state. Despite uniform success in manipulating a single immune parameter (*in vitro* lymphocyte-mediated cytolysis) in such patients with large tumor volumes, the likelihood of altering overall tumor course *in vivo* might be much less. This would be consistent with previous reports demonstrating the lack of clear-cut therapeutic benefit from immune RNA treatment of established tumor isografts despite evidence of increased *in vitro* lymphocyte-mediated cytolysis in treated animals.

Planned, prospective, randomized (phase III) studies should define rigorously any clinical immune RNA therapeutic efficacy. Ideally, the patients chosen for such a study should be treated when they have minimal tumor burden, a time of potential maximum correlation between *in vitro* and *in vivo* immune RNA effects, and in a setting with the best chance for obtaining long-lasting therapeutic benefits.

REFERENCES

Adler, F. L. (1976). *In* "Immune RNA and Neoplasia" (M. A. Fink, ed.), p. 9. Academic Press, New York.

Adler, F. L., and Fishman, M. (1975). *J. Immunol.* **115,** 129–134.

Aksenova, N. N., Bresler, V. M., Vorobyeu, V. I., and Olenov, J. M. (1962). *Nature (London)* **196,** 443–444.

Alexander, H. E., Koch, G., Mountain, I. M., and VanDamme, O. (1958). *J. Exp. Med.* **108,** 493–506.

Araujo, F. O., and Remington, J. S. (1974). *Immunology* **27,** 711–721.

Barr, M. L., Cabrera, E. J., Silverman , P. H., and Heidrich, J. E. (1977). *Cell. Immunol.* **33,** 447–451.

Bell, C., and Dray, S. (1970). *Science* **171,** 199–201.

Bell, C., and Dray, S. (1972). *Cell. Immunol.* **5,** 52–65.

Bell, C., and Dray, S. (1973). *Cell. Immunol.* **6,** 375–393.

Bernstein, I. D. (1977). *J. Immunol.* **118,** 1090–1128.

Bilello, P., Fishman, M., and Koch, G. (1976). *Cell. Immunol.* **23,** 309–319.

Bondevik, H., and Mannick, J. A. (1968). *Proc. Soc. Exp. Biol. Med.* **129,** 264–268.

Braun, D. P., and Dray, S. (1977). *Cancer Res.* **37,** 4138–4144.

Coates, M. R., and Pilch, Y. H. (1977). *Cancer Immunol. Immunother.* **3,** 145–152.

Cohen, A. M., Burdick, J. F., and Ketcham, A. S. (1971). *J. Immunol.* **107,** 895–898.

DeCarvalho, S. (1963). *Nature (London)* **197,** 1077–1080.

Deckers, P. J., and Pilch, Y. J. (1971). *Nature (London) New Biol.* **231,** 181–182.

Deckers, P. J., Wang, B. S., Stuart , P. A., and Mannick, J. A. (1975). *Transplant. Proc.* **7,** 259–263.

Deckers, P. J., Wang, B. S., and Mannick, J. A. (1976). *Ann. N. Y. Acad. Sci.* **277,** 575–591.

deKernion, J. B., Ramming, K. P., Brower, P., Skinner, D. G., and Pilch Y. H. (1975). *Am. J. Surg.* **130,** 575–578.

Ellem, K. A. O., and Colter, J. S. (1960). *Virology* **12,** 511–520.

Fishman, M. (1961). *J. Exp. Med.* **114,** 837.

Fishman, M., and Adler, F. L. (1964). *J. Exp. Med.* **17,** 595–602.

Fishman, M., and Adler, F. L. (1972). *Cell Immunol.* **8,** 221–234.

Fritze, D., Kern, D. H., Chow, N., and Pilch, Y. H. (1976). *Cancer Immunol. Immunother.* **1,** 245–250.

Garvey, J. S., Rinderknecht, H., Weliky, B. G., and Campbell, D. H. (1972). *Immunochemistry* **9**, 187–206.

Gierer, A., and Schramm, G. (1956). *Nature (London)* **177**, 702–703.

Gottlieb, A. A., Schwartz, R. H., and Waldman, S. R. (1972). *J. Immunol.* **108**, 719–725.

Greenup, C. J., Vallera, D. A., Pennline, K. J., Kolodziej, B. J., and Dogg, M. C. (1978). *Br. J. Cancer* **38**, 55–63.

Han, T., Pauly, J. L., and Mittelman, A. (1975). *Immunology* **28**, 127–132.

Herscowitz, H. B., and Stelos, P. (1970a). *J. Immunol.* **105**, 771–778.

Herscowitz, H. B., and Stelos, P. (1970b). *J. Immunol.* **105**, 779–782.

Honjo, T., Swan, D., Nau, M., Norman, B., Packman, S., Polsky, F., and Leder, P. (1976). *Biochemistry* **15**, 2775–2779.

Juras, D. S., and Abramoff, P. (1970). *J. Immunol.* **105**, 1244–1252.

Kern, D. H., and Pilch, Y. H. (1974). *Int. J. Cancer* **13**, 679–688.

Kern, D. H., and Pilch, Y. H. (1978). *J. Natl. Cancer Inst.* **60**, 599–603.

Kern, D. H., Drogemuller, C. R. and Pilch, Y. H. (1974). *J. Natl. Cancer Inst.* **52**, 299–302.

Kern, D. H., Fritze, D., Drogemuller, C., and Pilch, Y. H. (1976a). *J. Natl. Cancer Inst.* **57**, 97–103.

Kern, D. H., Fritze, D., Schick, P. M., Chow, N., and Pilch, Y. H. (1976b). *J. Natl. Cancer Inst.* **57**, 105–109.

Mannick, J. A. (1964). *Surgery* **56**, 249–255.

Mannick, J. A., and Egdahl, R. H. (1964). *J. Clin. Invest.* **43**, 2166–2177.

Meiss, H. K., and Fishman, M. (1972). *J. Immunol.* **108**, 1172–1178.

Mikami, H., Kawakami, M., and Mitsuhashi, S. (1971). *Jpn. J. Microbiol.* **15**, 169–174.

Mitsuhashi, S. (1967). *Subviral Carcinog. Int. Symp. Tumor Viruses* **1**, 265–272.

Mitsuhashi, S., Saito, K., Osawa, N., and Kurashige, S. (1967). *J. Bacteriol.* **94**, 907–913.

Nakamura, K. (1976). *Cell. Immunol.* **25**, 163–177.

Nedrud, J., Tauton, M., and Clark, W. R. (1975). *J. Exp. Med.* **142**, 960.

Niu, M. C., Cordova, C. C., and Niu, L. C. (1961). *Proc. Natl. Acad. Sci. U.S.A.* **47**, 1689–1700.

Paque, R. E. (1976). *Cancer Res.* **36**, 4530–4536.

Paque, R. E., and Dray, S. (1972). *Cell. Immunol.* **5**, 30–41.

Paque, R. E., and Dray, S. (1974). *Transplant Proc.* **6**, 203–207.

Paque, R. E., and Nealon, T. (1977). *Cell. Immunol.* **34**, 279–288.

Paque, R. E., and Nealon, T. (1979). *Cell. Immunol.* **43**, 48–61.

Paque, R. E., Meltzer, M. S., Zbar, B., Rapp, H. J., and Dray, S. (1973). *Cancer Res.* **33**, 3165–3171.

Paque, R. E., Ali, M., and Dray, S. (1975). *Cell. Immunol.* **16**, 261–268.

Pilch, Y. H., Veltman, L. L., and Kern, D. H. (1974). *Surgery* **76**, 23–34.

Pilch, Y. H., deKernion, J. B., Skinner, D. G., Ramming, K. P., Schick, P. M., Fritze, D., Brower, P., and Kern, D. H. (1976a). *Am. J. Surg.* **132**, 631–637.

Pilch, Y. H., Fritze, D., deKernion, J. B., Ramming, K. P., and Kern, D. H. (1976b). *Ann. N.Y. Acad. Sci.* **277**, 592–608.

Pilch, Y. H., Ramming, K. P., and deKernion, J. B. (1977). *Cancer* **40**, 2747–2757.

Ramming, K. P., and deKernion, J. B. (1977). *Ann. Surg.* **186**, 459–467.

Ramming, K. P., and Pilch, Y. H. (1968). *Transplantation* **7**, 296–299.

Reilly, E. B., and Garvey, J. S. (1978). *Cell Immunol.* **41**, 20–34.

Roelants, G. E., Goodman, J. W., and McDevitt, H. O. (1971). *J. Immunol.* **106**, 1222–1226.

Sabbadini, E., and Sehon, A. H. (1967). *Int. Arch. Allergy Appl. Immunol.* **32**, 55–63.

Saito, K., and Mitsuhashi, S. (1965). *J. Bacteriol.* **90**, 629–634.

Schaefer, A. E., Fishman, M., and Adler, F. O. (1974). *J. Immunol.* **112**, 1981–1986.

Schlager, S. I., and Dray, S. (1975). *Proc. Natl. Acad. Sci. U.S.A.* **72**, 3680–3682.
Schlager, S. I., Dray, S., and Paque, R. E. (1974). *Cell. Immunol.* **14**, 104–122.
Sell, S. (1976). *In* "Immune RNA and Neoplasia" (M. A. Fink, ed.), pp. 293–301. Academic Press, New York.
Singh, I., Tsang, K. Y., and Blakemore, W. S. (1977). *J. Natl. Cancer Inst.* **58**, 505–510.
Sondel, P. M., O'Brien, C., Porter, L., Schlossman, S. F., and Chess, L. (1976). *J. Immunol.* **117**, 2197–2203.
Steele, G., Jr., Wang, B. S., Richie, J., Wilson, R. E., Ervin, T., Yankee, R., Fallon, M., and Mannick, J. A. (1980). *Cancer Res.* **40**, 2377–2382.
Steele, G., Jr., Wang, B. S., Richie, J., Ervin, T., Yankee, R., and Mannick, J. A. (1981). *Cancer* **47**, 1286–1288.
Tohoku, J. (1966). *J. Exp. Med.* **89**, 307–314.
Veltman, L. L., Kern, D. H., and Pilch, Y. H. (1974). *Cell. Immunol.* **13**, 367–377.
Viza, D., Boucheix, C., Kern, D. H., and Pilch, Y. H. (1978). *Differentiation* **11**, 181–184.
Wang, B. S., and Deckers, P. J. (1976). *J. Surg. Res.* **20**, 183–194.
Wang, B. S., and Mannick, J. A. (1978). *Cell. Immunol.* **37**, 358–368.
Wang, B. S., and Mannick, J. A. (1979). *J. Immunol.* **123**, 1057–1061.
Wang, B. S., Stuart, P. A., and Mannick, J. A. (1974). *Cell. Immunol.* **12**, 114–118.
Wang, B. S., Deckers, P. J., and Mannick, J. A. (1978a). *Clin. Immunol. Immunopathol.* **9**, 218–228.
Wang, B. S., Onikul, S. R., and Mannick, J. A. (1978b). *Cell. Immunol.* **39**, 27–35.
Wang, B. S., Onikul, S. R., and Mannick, J. A. (1978c). *Science* **202**, 60–61.
Wang, B. S., Steele, G., Jr., Mannick, J. A., Fallon, M., and Onikul, S. R. (1979). *Cancer Res.* **39**, 1702–1707.
White, S. L., and Johnson, A. G. (1976). *Cell Immunol.* **21**, 56–69.
Williams, C. C., and Wu, W. G. (1971). *J. Immunol.* **107**, 163–171.
Yaun, L., and Campbell, D. H. (1972). *Immunochemistry* **9**, 1–8.

IMMUNOCHEMICAL LOCALIZATION AND
QUANTITATIVE ASSAYS

CHAPTER IV

FUNCTIONAL HISTOPATHOLOGY OF CANCER: A REVIEW OF IMMUNOENZYME HISTOCHEMISTRY*

F. JAMES PRIMUS AND DAVID M. GOLDENBERG

I. Introduction

For the majority of the past century, pathologists have utilized diverse methods of preparing and observing tissue sections to derive a precise tissue diagnosis based upon a static image at a point in time in what is otherwise a dynamic process. With the recent practical and conceptual advances in the biomedical sciences, other tools from the basic scientific disciplines of immunology, cell biology, and biochemistry are becoming increasingly available and of interest to the surgical pathologist. A case in point is the significant progress made in our understanding of non-Hodgkin's lymphomas, where views of this group of tumors from the histogenetic, functional, and clinical aspects have been dramatically altered by the addition of immunological methods to morphological studies (Lukes *et al.*, 1978).

* Some of our research reviewed in this chapter was supported by grants (CA-15799 and CA-24376) and a contract (CB-84257) from the National Cancer Institute, National Institutes of Health.

A major impetus for the use of antibodies to stain tissue components was the development of the fluorescent antibody method by Coons *et al.* (1941). Since then, immunoenzyme histochemical approaches have been developed and applied to problems of surgical pathology, and a number of excellent papers summarizing this progress have appeared in recent years (Taylor, 1978a; DeLellis *et al.*, 1979, 1981a; Heyderman, 1980; Mukai and Rosai, 1980). A diverse array of substances can be identified by these methods in routine and specially prepared tissue sections. Some of these substances, such as hormones, enzymes, blood group antigens, and immunoglobulins, are normally produced by adult cells and can be increased or decreased in the tissues or blood of patients with neoplasms derived from specific cells. Another group consists of substances which may serve as markers for particular cell types or tissues, such as particular hormones and filaments. A third category could include the so-called tumor-specific or tumor-associated antigens, depending upon the achievements of our tumor immunology efforts to identify the as yet elusive antigen distinct for cancer. Although not specific for cancer, α-fetoprotein (AFP) and carcinoembryonic antigen (CEA) have applications in the immunoenzyme histochemical analysis of tumors.

These immunohistochemical approaches have been recognized as potentially valuable adjuncts to the current techniques of diagnostic histopathology. However, there are other opportunities becoming evident, including the use of immunohistochemical and immunocytochemical techniques for studying the biochemical and morphological changes transpiring during the events preceding the development of neoplasia, the characterization of early and fully developed cancer, especially in the analysis of subpopulations expressing different marker substances. These applications have important clinical implications for aiding in early diagnosis, classification, prognostication, and prediction of response to therapy.

This chapter will not attempt to review all these aspects and applications, especially since a number of comprehensive papers (already cited) have appeared recently. Instead, we have chosen to consider a number of technical aspects of immunoenzyme histochemistry, and to provide a selected representation of the application of this methodology to problems of diagnostic pathology.

II. Immunoenzyme Methods

Immunohistological techniques using enzyme-labeled antibodies have rapidly grown in popularity and diversification since their introduction by

Nakane and co-workers (1966). Certain features of immunoenzyme techniques have made them as valuable as immunofluorescence, giving them desirable advantages over the latter in both investigative and diagnostic applications. Immunoenzyme methods are at least as sensitive as immunofluorescence (DeLellis *et al.*, 1979) and also provide stained specimens that are permanent and easily counterstained with routine histological stains, allowing direct morphological comparison with the immunological reaction. Furthermore, conventionally processed tissue specimens do not require special manipulation for immunoenzyme staining, and the same method is applicable at both the light and ultrastructural level. In this section, an overview of principles of immunoenzyme techniques, histochemical stains for peroxidase, specificity of staining reactions, tissue preparation and fixation, and dual staining procedures is presented, followed by two examples of staining protocols that we use. This overview will center on the use of immunohistochemistry at the light microscopic level. Earlier discussions of this topic can be found in Sternberger (1974), Mesa-Tejada (1977), Taylor (1978a,b), Bosman and Kruseman (1979), Heyderman (1979, 1980), Nadjii (1980), Pearse (1980), Petrusz *et al.* (1980), and DeLellis (1981b).

A. PRINCIPLES OF IMMUNOENZYME TECHNIQUES

Although *Escherichia coli* alkaline phosphatase (Avrameas, 1969; Mason and Sammons, 1978) and *Aspergillus niger* glucose oxidase (Kuhlmann and Avrameas, 1971; Suffin *et al.*, 1979) have been used as marker enzymes, horseradish peroxidase has received the most attention and is the basis for virtually all immunoenzyme staining procedures. Thus, most of the work cited will be based on the application of immunoperoxidase localization of tissue antigens. The choice of peroxidase as a marker enzyme is based on its having a lower molecular weight than the other enzymes. Its cytochemistry yields a relatively stable and nondiffusable reaction product, and its endogenous or pseudoactivity in mammalian tissues is restricted to macrophages, polymorphonuclear leukocytes, endothelial cells, and erythrocytes. The other enzymes may receive more use in future applications requiring simultaneous detection of two-antigen systems.

Two localization methods have been adopted for most immunoperoxidase studies. The simplest method is fashioned exactly after the indirect fluorescent antibody technique for tissue-antigen localization, whereby the site of the primary specific antibody reaction is demonstrated with an enzyme-labeled antiimmunoglobulin (anti-Ig) against the animal species providing the primary antibody (Fig. 1). The employment of an enzyme

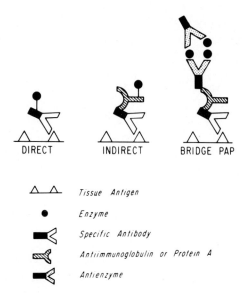

FIG. 1. Schematic representation of direct and indirect enzyme-labeled antibody techniques, and PAP bridge method.

histochemical reaction appropriate for the marker enzyme on the antibody discloses sites of antigen localization that are visualized by light microscopy. The indirect immunoenzyme technique is the method of choice over the direct procedure for two reasons. First, since the direct procedure requires coupling of the marker to the purified specific antibody, antibody purification may be difficult to achieve where the antiserum is limited in quantity or uneconomical in applications requiring several primary antisera. In the latter case, only a single preparation of labeled anti-Ig is needed for the indirect procedure as long as the primary antisera are from the same animal species. Second, the indirect method is more sensitive than the direct technique since the primary antibody serves as an intermediate antigen layer against which more than one labeled anti-Ig can react (Pearse, 1980).

Only a brief consideration of enzyme conjugation will be given since high-quality enzyme-labeled antibodies against IgG from most of the commonly used animal species are available commercially. Glutaraldehyde cross-linking or periodate oxidation are the two major contemporary methods of conjugating enzymes to antibodies, and the reader is referred to the following references concerning specific details: Avrameas and Ternynck (1971), Boorsma and Streefkerk (1979), and Nakane and Kawaoi (1974). Our preference is the low-pH periodate oxidation method

(Wilson and Nakane, 1978) for conjugating peroxidase or glucose oxidase to affinity-purified Ig (Hudson and Hay, 1980). The use of affinity-purified antibody reduces the amount of labeled irrelevant Ig in the preparation that can cause problems with background staining when labeled Ig is used at low dilution. The coupling efficiency for the periodate oxidation method is much higher than that of the glutaraldehyde procedure due to the small number of amino groups on the peroxidase molecule available for cross-linking (Sternberger, 1974). Use of the latter method necessitates more extensive purification of the conjugate to separate the large amount of unconjugated Ig which would compete with the labeled antibody for antigen binding sites, thereby reducing staining sensitivity. Enzyme–antibody conjugates prepared by periodate oxidation have predominantly a polymeric nature and, hence, decreased tissue penetration properties (Boorsma and Streefkerk, 1979). Optimal staining concentration of the labeled anti-Ig is determined by checkerboard titrations on tissue sections known to contain antigen and can vary between 30 and 500 μg of antibody protein/milliliter, depending upon the commercial source and method of conjugation.

The second immunoenzyme method is the unlabeled antibody or bridge technique introduced by Mason et al. (1969). This method is more complex than the labeled antibody procedure and places greater demands on one's knowledge of immunology. The original method involved the stepwise addition of primary specific antibody, anti-Ig antiserum, antienzyme antiserum raised in the same animal species as the primary antibody, and, finally, the free enzyme. The bridge method takes its name from the crosslinking of the primary specific and tertiary antienzyme antibodies, both raised in the same animal species, by the anti-Ig antibody. An important refinement in this method was the development of soluble immune complexes of enzyme and antienzyme by Sternberger et al. (1970) which are added to the tissue section after application of the primary and bridging antibodies (Fig. 1). The use of immune complexes not only reduces the time necessary to carry out the bridge method, but it also increases its sensitivity by eliminating Ig molecules from the antienzyme antisera that are irrelevant, denatured, or have low avidity, all of which would compete for the antigen binding sites of the bridging antibody (Sternberger, 1974). The peroxidase–antiperoxidase (PAP) bridge technique is rapidly replacing the labeled antibody method since it is generally accepted that it is more sensitive than both the labeled antibody and the immunofluorescence methods (Burns et al., 1974; Petrali et al., 1974; Sternberger, 1974; DeLellis et al., 1979). Electron microscopic studies have shown that the PAP complex typically consists of three molecules of enzyme and two of antibody, as depicted in Fig. 1 (Sternberger, 1974). Thus, for each primary antibody molecule bridged by a single anti-Ig molecule, three molecules of enzyme are deposited at the tissue-antigen site. Since most enzyme-labeled antibody preparations have a molar ratio of about 1, the PAP technique provides at least a threefold increase in potential sensitivity. The PAP procedure has gained wide acceptance since the complexes are stable and are now readily available commercially for several commonly used animal species.

The increased sensitivity of the PAP method allows the use of higher dilutions of primary antibody while retaining excellent localization, thus conserving specific antibody and minimizing background staining (Sternberger, 1979). When establishing a bridge procedure in the laboratory, it is important to carry out checkerboard titrations of both the primary and secondary antibodies on tissue sections containing antigen within the expected working range in order to determine their optimal dilutions. High concentrations of primary antibody can in fact inhibit staining as a consequence of antibody molecules reacting with tissue antigen in close proximity to one another (Bigbee et al., 1977). This increases the probability that both antigen-binding limbs of the bridging antibody are occupied by primary antibody and unavailable to react with the antienzyme antibody. On the other hand, some studies have suggested that increasing the primary antibody concentration can enhance staining of tissues having low antigen content (Heald et al., 1979; Limas and Lange, 1980).

Several variations of the bridge procedure have been described; among these, the labeled antigen (Sternberger and Petrali, 1977), self-sandwich (Hsu and Ree, 1980), and double immune complex (Vacca et al., 1980) techniques are depicted in Fig. 2. The latter two evolved with the intent to increase the sensitivity of the basic PAP method, but the general experience with them is too limited to ascertain whether the added sensitivity balances the extra time and tedium necessary to execute these procedures in routine practice. As expressed by the developers of these modifications, their value lies in the demonstration of small quantities of tissue antigen. This may have importance with antigens that are initially minute in concentration or are altered by tissue manipulation procedures. Immunohistochemical methods are basically semiquantitative at present and the primary motive behind the need to localize a particular tissue antigen is an important factor to weigh when addressing method sensitivity. In evaluating the diagnostic applications of certain tumor antigens, an increase in method sensitivity might be accompanied by a loss in specificity with substances that are produced in low amounts by normal tissues.

Other modifications of the standard PAP method can be developed in applications where the antienzyme antibody from the appropriate species is lacking or not readily available, as is the case with human or murine

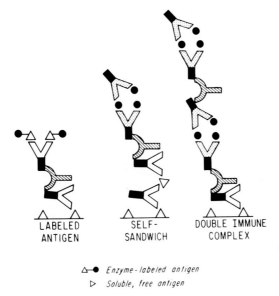

LABELED   SELF-   DOUBLE IMMUNE
ANTIGEN   SANDWICH   COMPLEX

△—● *Enzyme-labeled antigen*

▷ *Soluble, free antigen*

FIG. 2. Schematic representation of modified immunoenzyme bridge methods. Remainder of key the same as for Fig. 1.

primary antisera. Using murine monoclonal antibody as an example, the rabbit anti-mouse Ig can function as a second intermediate antigen layer after reacting with the murine antibody on the tissue section (Wahlström *et al.*, 1981). A swine anti-rabbit Ig can then serve as a bridging antibody linking the rabbit anti-mouse Ig with rabbit PAP.

B. VARIATIONS OF IMMUNOENZYME TECHNIQUES

1. *Staphylococcus aureus Protein A*

Protein A (PA) from *S. aureus* binds to the Fc portion of IgG molecules from a variety of animal species (Goding, 1978). Dubois-Dalcq *et al.* (1977) substituted peroxidase-labeled PA for enzyme-labeled anti-Ig and reported similar sensitivity but lower background staining with the PA reagent in demonstrating lymphocyte membrane markers or viral antigens on tissue-cultured cells. Human, goat, guinea pig, mouse, and rabbit primary antibodies could be used in conjunction with the labeled PA. Subsequent studies essentially confirmed these findings and, in addition, showed that PA could replace the bridging antibody in the standard PAP technique (Celio *et al.*, 1979; Trost *et al.*, 1980). However, the standard PAP procedure was more sensitive in detecting lower concentrations of primary antibodies (Celio *et al.*, 1979). The versatility and advantage of using PA as a second-step reagent have been summarized by Notani *et al.* (1979). Protein A is economical, can be used with primary antibodies from a variety of animal species, and can be used in combination with both fluorescent and enzyme-labeled reagents. Protein A does not react with Fc receptor-bearing cells, eliminating the need to use F(ab′)₂ fragments of anti-Ig antibodies, and peroxidase-labeled PA is comparable in molecular weight to that of enzyme-labeled Fab antibody fragments, indicating its potential usefulness for preembedding staining in ultrastructural immunohistochemical studies. These attributes of PA suggest that it will receive wider attention in the development of immunohistochemical techniques in the future.

2. Biotin–Avidin System

The high affinity of the egg white protein, avidin, for biotin, coupled with the ease by which these molecules can be introduced into functionally active substances and various markers, have made them ideally suited for localization techniques (Bayer and Wilchek, 1980). Guesdon *et al.* (1979) described two procedures based on the avidin–biotin system for the immunoenzyme localization of antigens (Fig. 3). The first, the bridged avidin–biotin technique (BRAB), involves the sequential addition of biotin-labeled antibody, free avidin, and biotin-labeled horseradish peroxidase. The quadrivalency of avidin and the high coupling efficiency with which antibodies and enzymes can be labeled with biotin without interfer-

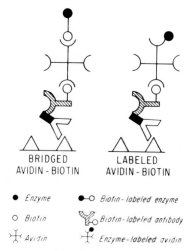

FIG. 3.   Schematic representation of bridged and labeled avidin–biotin systems.

ence with functional activity provide the basis for the technique. The BRAB technique gives slightly improved localization of lymphocyte cell-surface Ig than that obtained with peroxidase-labeled anti-Ig antibody. In the second procedure, termed the labeled avidin–biotin (LAB) technique, enzyme-labeled avidin is substituted for free avidin and biotin-labeled enzyme. Although the LAB procedure is simpler than the BRAB method, its sensitivity appears to be reduced. Both methods can be used with unlabeled primary antibodies in an indirect procedure, as depicted in Fig. 3. Warnke and Levy (1980) found that the detection of lymphocyte surface antigens with murine monoclonal antibodies was improved with an indirect LAB technique as compared to an indirect enzyme-labeled antibody method. Hsu *et al.* (1981) has compared the standard PAP method with the indirect BRAB and a procedure using preformed complexes of avidin and biotinylated peroxidase (ABC) analogous in principle to the preformed immune complexes used in the PAP technique. Immunostaining intensity and background staining were similar between the PAP and indirect BRAB methods, while the ABC technique yielded increased immunostaining intensity. Thus, these initial studies confirm the expectation that a bridged avidin–biotin system should equal or exceed the sensitivity of the standard PAP method based on the multivalency of avidin and the high biotin coupling efficiency. Since biotin-labeled anti-Ig antibodies and enzymes are now commercially available, these reagents should receive wider application in future immunohistochemical studies.

C. HISTOCHEMICAL STAINS FOR PEROXIDASE

The most widely used cytochemical reaction for peroxidase in immunoenzyme applications consists of diaminobenzidine (DAB) and H_2O_2, introduced by Graham and Karnovsky (1966). The brown reaction product is insoluble in organic solvents, allowing dehydration of stained preparations and the use of synthetic resin mountants. Mountants of this type have a better refractive index than that of aqueous mounting media, and stained preparations do not fade over a period of years (Taylor, 1978b). The $DAB-H_2O_2$ solution typically consists of freshly prepared 0.01–0.05% DAB tetrahydrochloride and 0.01–0.03% H_2O_2 in 0.05 M Tris buffer, pH 7.2–7.6. Although most immunostaining studies use Tris or phosphate buffer adjusted to the latter pH range, Weir *et al.* (1974a) found that a pH 5.0 citric-ammonium acetate buffer increased staining intensity, an observation confirmed and adapted by others (Straus, 1979; Vacca *et al.*, 1980). In addition to being closer to the pH optimum of horseradish peroxidase, the lower pH buffer may also enhance precipitation or stabilization of the oxidized reaction product. Incubations are carried out at room temperature for 10–30 minutes with the substrate solution protected from light to minimize light oxidation of the DAB. Since DAB is a potential carcinogen, care should be exercised in its use and disposal. The suspected carcinogenic properties of DAB have perhaps influenced the purity of commercially available DAB since we, as well as others (Pelliniemi *et al.*, 1980) have occasionally encountered inconsistent results when small amounts of DAB are weighed for individual experiments. Previous investigators circumvented this problem by storing frozen aliquots of DAB at 10 times the working concentration. Storage of the DAB in this manner for over 14 months did not alter its activity.

Other chromagens have been used for horseradish peroxidase histochemistry, some of which have received greater attention recently in search of suitable alternatives to DAB. Aminoethylcarbazole (Burstone, 1960) may be less hazardous than DAB, but its red reaction product is soluble in organic solvents, preventing dehydration of stained sections. Tubbs *et al.* (1979) reported comparable staining intensity and localization of human chorionic gonadotropin when the latter chromagen was substituted for DAB. The organic solvent-soluble chromagen, 4-chloro-1-napththol, is useful in combination with DAB for double staining techniques (Nakane, 1968; Sternberger and Joseph, 1979). Tetramethylbenzidine (Mesulam, 1978) and the Hanker–Yates reagent (Hanker *et al.*, 1977), consisting of phenylenediamine and pyrocatechol, are two other peroxidase chromagens that allow dehydration and mounting as permanent preparations. Mesulam and Rosene (1979) ranked tetramethylbenzidine as the most sensitive chromagen in a comparison of nine different methods for neurohistochemistry, where the Hanker–Yates reagent was the least sensitive in their hands. However, Reiner and Gamlin (1980) did not observe a comparable difference in sensitivity between the two techniques. They favor the Hanker–Yates reagent since its reaction product does not obscure cytologic detail and the method is not prone to the depositon of crystalline artifact characteristic of the tetramethylbenzidine procedure. Tubbs and Sheibani (1981) have modified the Hanker–Yates method for renal immunohistochemistry and found the results comparable to those obtained with DAB. While DAB still remains the most favored chromagen for immunoperoxidase studies, its potential hazard to laboratory personnel will require more investigators to focus their attention on the development of convenient, sensitive, and safer methods of peroxidase cytochemistry.

D. Specificity in Immunohistochemistry

The goal of immunohistochemical staining reactions is to achieve the greatest contrast between the specifically stained antigen under study and its surroundings. Background staining and authentic antigen localization are influenced by a variety of factors, some of which are inherent to the general immunological basis of the technique, whereas others are uniquely related to the principle of the method itself. As noted by Petrusz *et al.* (1980), a staining reaction should not occur in the absence of primary antibody (method specificity) or following absorption with antigen (antibody specificity) in order for it to be considered specific. Proof of method specificity is generally easier to attain than that of antibody specificity, and excellent discussions of these problem areas can be found in Sternberger (1974), Swaab *et al.* (1977), Heyderman (1979), Pearse (1980), and Petrusz *et al.* (1980).

1. Method Specificity

Method specificity is defined by the nonimmunological factors that can contribute to elevations in nonspecific background staining. This background staining in immunoperoxidase methods typically manifests itself as a diffuse stain of variable intensity of collagen and reticulum fibers, a cytoplasmic stain of epithelial cells, and the expression of endogenous or pseudoenzyme activity in the tissue section. Nonimmunological binding of immunoglobulin in the primary antiserum, secondary antiserum, and PAP immune complex to tissue sections will result in increased background staining. One factor perhaps not recognized by many workers that can cause nonspecific binding of immunoglobulins is incomplete removal of paraffin from tissue sections (DeLellis *et al.*, 1979). These investigators recommend that slides be heated to the melting point of the embedding medium before dewaxing in xylene to ensure efficient removal of paraffin. In other instances, certain proteins or substances in the tissue may interact with the immunoglobulin molecules (Pearse, 1980). One approach commonly used to minimize nonspecific immunoglobulin binding is preincubation of the tissue section with normal serum obtained from the animal species providing the bridging antibody or anti-Ig (Sternberger, 1974; Burns, 1975). Incorporation of normal serum in the various immunoreagents can further enhance blocking of immunoglobulin binding. The use of a blocking immunoglobulin is not always effective for a particular tissue type and may not be acceptable for different tissues. Reading (1977) could not reduce background connective tissue staining in the bronchus by using blocking immunoglobulin, whereas treatment of tissue sections with pepsin, but not collagenase, eliminated it. The method of tissue fixation is another factor needing consideration when one encounters background staining. Sim and French (1976) observed that liver Mallory bodies bound PAP by a protein-immunoglobulin binding mechanism in cryostat tissue sections that were unfixed or treated with chloroform–methanol or acetone. However, formaldehyde treatment of the tissue abolished PAP binding by the Mallory bodies.

In addition to nonspecific binding of immunoglobulin, free horseradish peroxidase and antibody-conjugated enzyme have been shown to bind to tissue-cultured glial cells (Palladini and Solheid, 1976), collagen fibers (Fan, 1980), and white blood cells (Sternberger, 1974). Preincubation with protein, extensive washing, or washing under slightly acidic conditions are steps that block or remove most of the tissue binding activity of the enzyme. Binding of PAP to white blood cells does not occur, apparently because binding sites on the enzyme are not exposed in the immune complex (Sternberger, 1974). Two other protein–protein interactions may occur in immunohistochemical reactions. First, staining of viable lymphoid or histiocytic cells in suspension may lead to nonspecific staining through interaction of Fc receptors on these cells with immunoglobulins in the antisera. The use of Fab or F(ab')$_2$ fragments of the various antibodies used in the immunological staining sequence is recommended to combat this problem. Slemmon et al. (1980) described a procedure for the preparation of PAP that uses the Fab portion of antiperoxidase antibody. Since this modified PAP complex retained its marker characteristics for localization, it may be adaptable to studies where Fc receptor-bearing cells are troublesome or where tissue penetration of the immune complex is a factor to consider in ultrastructural investigations. Second, the C1q component of complement may mediate nonspecific binding of immunoglobulins to certain cells, as reported by Buffa et al. (1979) in their studies of endocrine cells. Antisera deprived of complement by immunoprecipitation alleviated this problem, but the authors failed to determine whether simple heat treatment was equally effective.

One criterion that an enzyme marker must fulfill for staining purposes is that endogenous enzyme levels in tissues must be absent or low. Horseradish peroxidase is fairly ideal in this respect, since endogenous enzymes capable of showing cytochemical reaction with the disclosing reagents are restricted to myeloid leukocytes, macrophages, and central nervous system neurons (Pearse, 1980). Erythrocytes also show reactivity due to the peroxidase activity of hemoglobin. In many applications, the morphological recognition of endogenous enzyme activity is readily discriminated from specific immunological staining. However, in tissues containing large numbers of these cells or in preparations where a small number of isolated antigen-containing cells are being stained, endogenous enzyme staining may mask or interfere with the interpretation of specific localization. Streefkerk (1970) observed that fixation of tissues in methanol abolished endogenous peroxidase activity, whereas ethanol, formaldehyde, and glutaraldehyde were without effect. Straus (1971) subsequently reported that pretreatment of aldehyde-fixed tissue sections for 15 minutes at room temperature with methanol containing 0.074% HCl or methanol containing 1% sodium nitroferricyanide and 1% acetic acid abolished endogenous enzyme activity in leukocytes and erythrocytes. To avoid potential antigen denaturing problems caused by acid treatment, Streefkerk (1972) found that pretreatment with methanol, followed by dilute concentrations of H_2O_2, was also effective in inhibiting endogenous enzyme activity in leukocytes and erythrocytes. This latter method has been adapted to most staining protocols in which inhibition of endogenous activity is desirable (Taylor, 1978b; DeLellis, 1981b). However, for reasons unknown to us, this method is not uniformly efficient even on identical tissue specimens fixed in the same manner. Furthermore, these various pretreatment procedures can cause denaturation of antigens and antibodies (Fink *et al.*, 1979; Straus, 1979), and one needs to evaluate their effect on immunological activity when establishing the localization of a new antigen. Alternative procedures include postreatment with methanol–H_2O_2 after incubation with primary antibody (Fink *et al.*, 1979) or pretreatment with ethanol–HCl (Weir *et al.*, 1974b), phenylhydrazine (Straus, 1972, 1979), or periodic acid borohydride (Heyderman and Neville, 1977).

When establishing a staining procedure for the first time, one approach to evaluating method specificity is to substitute, in a comparable dilution range, normal or preimmune serum for the primary antiserum. This procedure will provide an overall analysis of nonspecific background staining. Omitting application of the antisera and enzyme marker to the tissue section will indicate the localization of endogenous enzyme activity and is a necessary control when the latter is not inhibited in staining protocols. Background staining due to immunoglobulin or enzyme marker binding is more difficult to discriminate since the immunoglobulin in antibody–enzyme conjugates or immune complexes may be mediating tissue binding rather than the enzyme. In actual practice, one is most concerned with delineating the efficacy of immunoglobulin-blocking steps in minimizing background staining that may arise from these sources. When using normal or preimmune serum to establish method specificity, it is important to realize that such sera may contain irrelevant natural antibodies against tissue antigens. Thus, some of the apparent background staining may not be nonspecific, but actually the result of a specific immunochemical reaction between antigen and antibody. Obviously, substitution of buffer for the primary antiserum does not resolve this question since it fails to control for nonspecific binding of immunoglobulin of the animal species providing the primary antiserum. Alternatively, Petrusz *et al.* (1980) recommend that tissue sections are stained with increasing dilutions of the primary antiserum until all staining disappears in order to establish method specificity. The reasoning behind this procedure is that nonspecific background staining is dilution independent, whereas specific staining is dilution dependent. Within certain limits this probably holds true. However, we and others (Swaab *et al.*, 1977) do not concur that this method provides an absolute estimate of background staining since some of the nonimmunologic factors (e.g., nonspecific immunoglobulin binding) contributing to background staining would also be dilution dependent. Nonetheless, either approach will give an investigator a reasonable evaluation of method specificity. Real problems in establishing method specificity are confronted when very low titer antisera are used, since it is then more difficult to block nonspecific binding of immunoglobulins and to differentiate staining due to irrelevant antibodies.

2. Antibody Specificity

Once the conditions of method specificity have been satisfied, one can focus attention on the most challenging question of immunohistochemistry, that of antibody specificity. All too often this question is given only token consideration, either because one places verification of antibody specificity in the hands of a commercial supplier of an antiserum or because verification is limited by the knowledge of the antigen under study, the resources of the investigator's laboratory, or the time and effort that one wishes to invest. Documentation of antibody specificity deals with two fundamental problems: (1) the presence of irrelevant antibodies in the antiserum that are not detectable by usual immunologic techniques but may reveal themselves immunohistochemically, and (2) the presence of cross-reactive antibodies that bind substances chemically unrelated or only partially related to the relevant antigen. The extent to which one can claim that an antiserum is free of irrelevant and cross-reactive antibodies in turn determines the extent of "monospecificity" of the antiserum. Since the various problems and approaches to verifying antibody specificity have been debated and reviewed by others (Petrusz *et al.*, 1976, 1977, 1980; Swaab *et al.*, 1977; Heyderman, 1979; Pearse, 1980), only a few points will be summarized here.

Conditions of antiserum absorption vary with the nature of the relevant and potential irrelevant antigens, in most cases requiring more than a superficial knowledge of immunology and protein chemistry. Procedures for antiserum absorption generally include immunoprecipitation, adsorption to cell-bound antigen or antigen insolubilized on a solid matrix, or competitive blocking prior to immunostaining. Removal of irrelevant antibodies is carried out by absorbing with preparations deficient in the relevant antigen and, in many instances, this is performed as a precautionary measure without evidence suggesting their presence. The antiserum is considered monospecific with respect to irrelevant antibodies and is operationally defined by the method of ancillary immunologic evaluation and/or the nature of the cross-absorbing antigen preparations. However, although the antiserum may be truly monospecific, the investigator has no guarantee that it is. The more exhaustive the investigator is in pursuing immunologic testing and absorption of the antiserum, the more definite one is of the certainty of antiserum monospecificity. Ideally, ultimate proof of antibody specificity can be gained by absorption of the antiserum with relevant antigen, which is then accompanied by a loss in staining reactivity. In our view, this procedure provides the only real proof for staining specificity. The major requirement here is the availability and purity of the antigen, since the emphasis placed on the absorption test as proof of specificity is only as solid as the quality of the antigen. Impurities in the immunogen that have elicited antibody would remove the latter if they were also present in the absorbing antigen. Consequently, the development of a monospecific antiserum may very rarely be realized, if at all, when one uses antisera prepared by conventional immunization. In this context, the application of hybridoma-derived monoclonal antibodies should eliminate problems associated with irrelevant antibodies, since they would be nonexistent in appropriately prepared monoclonal antibodies. However, monoclonal antibodies do not solve the second problem, that of defining antibody specificity, which concerns the presence of cross-reacting antibodies.

It is important to be reminded that antibodies recognize determinants, not antigens, and that these determinants can be expressed on unrelated substances that would also bind antibody. Since absorption with the immunogen would remove cross-reacting antibodies, abolition of staining following antiserum absorption with the immunogen does not necessarily mean that only the original antigen was recognized in immunohistochemistry. With a new antigen system, time and study will determine the uniqueness of a determinant(s) recognized by the primary antiserum. Different antibody populations in an antiserum may be realized due to differential staining of different tissues or cells (Petrusz et al., 1980), or by the separation of immunoreactive tissue components following protein separation techniques (Swaab et al., 1977). Once cross-reacting antibodies are identified, the ease with which they can be removed from the antiserum depends on the relative tissue distribution of the cross-reacting and relevant antigens, or how readily they can be separated from one another by fractionation techniques. Assuming that it is then possible to obtain the cross-reacting antigen free from the relevant antigen, the antiserum is first absorbed with the former, leaving behind those antibodies having a more restricted specificity for the relevant antigen.

The type of immunohistochemical techniques employed will have a bearing on antibody specificity (Sternberger, 1979). The greater sensitivity of the PAP and avidin–biotin methods allows the use of more dilute primary antisera. At higher dilutions, antibodies with higher affinities and, thus, specificities for the antigen would predominate in the staining reaction. Irrelevant and cross-reacting antibodies in low concentration would be undetected or only minimally active. Both the avidin–biotin system and the enzyme-conjugated, anti-Ig procedure also have an antibody specificity problem not inherent to the PAP method. If the anti-Ig antiserum contains tissue-reactive antibodies that are subsequently labeled with enzyme or biotin, background staining will be encountered due to an immunochemical reaction between the labeled antibody and tissue antigen. This is a method specificity problem unrelated to the primary antiserum and is not encountered in the PAP technique, since antitissue antibodies in the bridging antiserum would not react with the PAP complex, even though they may have reacted with tissue antigen. The use of affinity-purified anti-Ig antibody in the enzyme-labeled or biotin-labeled procedures would eliminate the specificity problem associated with these techniques.

E. Tissue Preparation and Fixation

The first question which arises when considering methods of tissue preparation is whether the tissue should be immediately fixed or frozen. According to Taylor (1978b), an ideal fixative for immunohistochemical studies should satisfy four criteria: (1) preservation of antigenic activity and prevention of diffusion or displacement of the antigen during subsequent manipulations, (2) maintenance of good morphology, (3) residual components of the fixative in the tissue should not interfere with the antigen–antibody reaction, and (4) the fixative should be readily available and, preferably, in common usage. It has been fortunate that many substances retain at least part of their antigenic activity after fixation in 4% formaldehyde, since this fixative is widely used in diagnostic histopathology. However, the best strategy to follow, particularly when establishing the detection of a new antigen–antibody system, is to test a variety of fixatives on cryostat sections of unfixed, frozen tissue in order to establish optimal fixation conditions (Feltkamp-Vroom, 1975; DeLellis, 1981b). To avoid ice crystal formation, which causes disruption of cell membranes and translocation of soluble materials, small pieces of tissue are rapidly frozen by quenching in liquid nitrogen or with a CO_2 expansion cooler (Pearse, 1980). Prior embedding of the tissue in 10–20% gelatin or other media (OCT Compound, Lab-Tek Products) facilitates handling of minute tissue samples and attachment of the block to holder while reducing tissue dehydration during storage (Miller and Hogg, 1980). Frozen tissue sections (4 μm) are then separately fixed at 4°C for 10 minutes with various fixatives: 85–100% ethanol, absolute acetone, absolute methanol, buffered 4% formaldehyde, buffered 1% paraformaldehyde, Bouin's fixative, and Zenker's fixative are examples of some of the more commonly used fixatives. Unfixed sections can be included for comparison but one must be cautious in interpreting staining reactions of unfixed sections due to diffusion or leaching of the antigen from the section. Once the optimal conditions for fixation are established, one can evaluate whether the antigen activity is retained following standard procedures for dehydration and embedding in paraffin or resin support media. If appreciable loss in immunologic activity is experienced after routine paraffin embedding, methods based on freeze-drying and freeze-substitution of tissue (Pearse, 1980), low-temperature dehydration and clearing (Saint-Marie, 1962), and frozen sectioning of fixed tissue blocks (Miller, 1972) can be explored. Immunohistochemistry is equally suitable for the study of surface and intracellular antigens of cells in suspension, cell smears, and monolayer tissue-cultured cells (Feltkamp-Vroom, 1975).

The availability of tissues fixed with 4% formaldehyde or Bouin's fixative facilitates the examination of antigens in retrospective immunohistochemical studies. However, if antigen activity is not adequately retained after treatment with cross-linking fixatives, it may be possible to enhance staining by enzyme digestion of the tissue sections. Trypsin (Huang et al., 1976; Curran and Gregory, 1978) and, to a lesser degree, Pronase (Denk et al., 1977) have been used for this purpose, mainly for the demonstration of immunoglobulins. The main problem that is encountered in the use of proteolytic enzymes is the difficulty in establishing optimal enzyme treatment conditions, since the ability to obtain consistent staining results is influenced by enzyme purity, type of tissue examined, method of tissue preparation, type of fixative, and duration of fixation (Curran and Gregory, 1978; Mepham et al., 1979). Another potential problem is that enzyme treatment may expose cross-reactive, cryptic determinants (Heyderman, 1979). An annoying problem that we have experienced using trypsin digestion according to the method of Huang et al. (1976) is the loss of sections from slides, necessitating the mounting of tissue sections on slides coated with a glue adhesive (Qualman and Keren, 1979).

F. SIMULTANEOUS ANTIGEN LOCALIZATION

In the area of cancer immunodiagnosis there is a growing interest in evaluating the diagnostic utility of measuring multiple antigenic or biochemical markers. Similarly, comparison of the presence and cytological distribution of multiple markers in tissue sections may provide an adjunctive tool for the functional classification of tumors by histopathologists. The staining of separate tissue sections for different markers is readily accomplished, but when the cellular proclivity of these markers in the same tissue is addressed, this approach would be laborious and, in many instances, difficult to determine without tedious comparison of serially sectioned specimens. Simple immunoenzyme procedures for the simultaneous detection of two or more antigens in the same tissue section would be a great asset in studies of this kind. Nakane (1968) first introduced simultaneous localization of three antigens in a single tissue section with peroxidase-labeled antibody techniques. His procedure involved the sequential application of three primary antisera raised in the same animal species, a common peroxidase-labeled anti-Ig against the latter animal species, and contrasting substrates for peroxidase. The tissue sections were first treated sequentially with one primary antiserum, enzyme-labeled anti-Ig, and DAB and H_2O_2, yielding a brown reaction product. Before proceeding to the second primary antiserum, it was necessary to remove the primary and secondary antibodies attached to the tissue section in the first-set reactions by acid elution, since they would supply antigenic sites and enzymatic activity, respectively, for the next staining reaction in the sequence. α-Naphthol–H_2O_2–pyronin was used as the chromagen for the second antigen system to yield a red reaction product. After acid elution to remove the immunoreagents from the second staining step, the third antigen was localized with 4-chloro-1-naphthol and H_2O_2 as the chromagen, providing a blue reaction product. Others then adapted this procedure for dual antigen staining with either the enzyme-labeled antibody method (Martin-Comin and Robyn, 1976) or the PAP technique (Erlandson et al., 1976; Vandesande and Dierickx, 1976), employing DAB and 4-chloro-1-naphthol as the contrasting chromagens. The DAB cytochemical reaction was performed first, since manipulations to remove the immunoreagents did not extract the DAB reaction product. These methods for dual staining have not received wide application, perhaps because of questions concerning incomplete removal of immunoreagents, which would then be a source of nonspecific color mixing, and the need to demonstrate that the antigens studied are resistant to the conditions of immunoreagent elution. Sternberger and Joseph (1979) made the fortuitous observation that immunoreagent removal is unnecessary when using the standard PAP method and a 0.025–0.05% DAB concentration. The interpretation of this finding is that excess bridging antibody completely saturates antigenic sites on the first primary antibody while excess PAP reagent, in turn, saturates all the free antigen-binding limbs of the bridging antibody. Furthermore, the presence of excess levels of the DAB substrate apparently ensures blockage of enzyme catalytic sites and immunoglobulin antigenic sites in the PAP complex by the polymerized DAB reaction product. This discovery by the previous investigators should generate more interest in simultaneous marker staining since elimination of the antibody removal step provides a more simplified approach for dual staining when both primary antisera are obtained from the same animal species.

Alternative methods exist for dual staining when the primary antisera are obtained from different animal species. Campbell and Bhatnagar (1976) studied the pituitary localization of luteinizing and growth hormone with rabbit and monkey primary antisera raised against the respective hormones. Peroxidase-labeled goat anti-rabbit immunoglobulin stained luteinizing hormone as a brown reaction product, while glucose oxidase-labeled goat anti-monkey immunoglobulin localized growth hormone as a blue reaction product, using glucose-Nitro Blue Tetrazolium (Nitro BT)-phenazine methosulfate as the disclosing reagent. This procedure uses primary antisera of different species origin with the appropriate antiimmunoglobulins against these species as well as different enzyme markers. Recently, we have obtained dual staining of two antigens with unlabeled antibody techniques consisting of PAP and immune complexes of glucose oxidase–antiglucose oxidase (Clark et al., 1982). The use of glucose oxidase as a second enzyme marker has two advantages: (1) its reaction product is stable to dehydration and mounting in synthetic resins, and (2) it is a microbial enzyme, thus eliminating problems associated with endogenous enzyme background staining. Unlabeled antibody techniques using peroxidase and alkaline phosphatase as the enzyme markers have also been applied to simultaneous antigen localization (Mason and Sammons, 1978). Dual staining procedures that use primary antisera from different animal species have one distinct advantage over the method introduced by Nakane (1968). The separate immunoreagents that are used in the different steps of the immunologic reaction sequence can be combined and incubated together. A requirement for these procedures, however, is that the anti-Ig antisera do not cross-react between the primary antibodies under staining conditions and cause nonspecific color mixing. Furthermore, the anti-Ig antisera must not cross-react with one another and, ideally, should be obtained from the same animal species. These requirements should not pose any serious problems due to the availability of a variety of anti-Igs raised in the same animal species. It is anticipated that more investigations will focus attention on dual labeling procedures based on the use of primary antisera from different animal species and, in particular, the application of biotinylated enzyme markers which already exist for peroxidase, glucose oxidase, and alkaline phosphatase.

G. Immunoperoxidase Staining Protocols

1. PAP Procedure

If paraffin-embedded tissues are used to establish staining conditions, tissue sections are deparaffinized and hydrated through xylene and a graded alcohol series. The slides are finally equilibrated against 0.05 M Tris buffer, pH 7.6, or 0.01 M phosphate-saline buffer (PBS), pH 7.2. Frozen sections are fixed with the appropriate fixative and washed with PBS. Our slides routinely have two sections per slide, one for the test antiserum, the other for the control serum.

1. Endogenous peroxidase activity is inhibited by incubating slides with 0.3% H_2O_2 in absolute methanol for 30 minutes at 22°C.

2. Wash slides two times with PBS, 5 minutes each wash.

3. Cover each section with 10% blocking normal serum (approximately 100 μl) and incubate in a moist chamber for 10 minutes at 37°C or 30 minutes at 22°C. The blocking normal serum is obtained from the same animal species supplying the anti-Ig used in step 7.

4. Blot excess blocking normal serum from slides.

5. Cover one section with diluted primary antiserum, the other section with antigen-neutralized primary antiserum or other appropriate control preparation and incubate in a moist chamber. With high titer antisera, we incubate for 20 minutes at 37°C using a 1:100–1:800 dilution. Prolonged incubations, 24–48 hours at 4°C, are recommended with highly diluted antisera. The primary antisera can be diluted in neat to 1% normal blocking serum to reduce background staining.

6. Wash slides two times with PBS, 5 minutes each wash. This represents a minimal washing cycle between all subsequent steps and should be extended in time and/or number of buffer changes depending upon nonspecific background staining levels. Agitation of the buffer by mixing or shaking also assists washing efficiency.

7. Incubate sections in a moist chamber for 20 minutes at 37°C or 30 minutes at 22°C with a 1:20–1:50 dilution of anti-Ig antiserum.

8. Wash slides as in step 6.

9. Incubate sections in a moist chamber for 20 minutes at 37°C or 30 minutes at 22°C with a 1:100–1:200 dilution of PAP (25–10 μg protein/ml), diluted in 1% blocking normal serum.

10. Wash slides as in step 6.

11. Incubate sections for 15 minutes at 22°C in the dark with 0.003% H_2O_2 and 0.01% DAB tetrahydrochloride in 0.05 M Tris buffer, pH 7.6.

12. Wash slides, counterstain lightly with hematoxylin, dehydrate, and mount.

The adjacent control section that received antigen-neutralized primary antiserum assesses nonspecific background staining resulting from endogenous enzyme activity and/or nonspecific binding of the immunoreagents. This technique is very reproducible and if the various reagents are made and applied correctly, the lack of positive staining usually indicating that the primary antiserum was of poor quality or that the antigen was not in the tissue specimen or was not adequately preserved. Once positive staining is obtained, a specimen known to be positive should be included as a control when testing unknown tissues. In the reading of slides, each investigator creates his/her own subjective intensity scale ranging from negative to a 4+ positivity.

2. Bridged Avidin–Biotin (BRAB) Procedure

The procedure outlined for the BRAB technique is based on the detection of a tissue antigen with murine monoclonal antibody that we have applied in the laboratory.

1–6. These steps are identical to those used for the PAP method. The appropriate dilution of the monoclonal antibody will depend upon its quality in terms of affinity and its concentration as dictated by method of production and purification. Negative controls can be irrelevant ascites fluid, purified myeloma or hybridoma protein of the same class or subclass specificity or, less desirably, normal mouse serum, unless the monoclonal antibody is diluted in the normal mouse serum.

7. Incubate sections in a moist chamber for 20 minutes at 37°C with 15–30 μg/ml of biotinylated goat anti-mouse IgG.

8. Wash slides two times with PBS, 5 minutes each wash.

9. Incubate sections in a moist chamber for 30 minutes at 22°C with 100 μg/ml of avidin, diluted in 0.05 M Tris, pH 8.6, + 0.15 M NaCl.

10. Wash slides as in step 8.

11. Incubate sections in a moist chamber for 30 minutes at 22°C with 25–50 μg/ml of biotinylated horseradish peroxidase.

12. Wash slides as in step 8.

13. Incubate sections for 15 minutes at 22°C in the dark with 0.003% H_2O_2 and 0.01% DAB tetrahydrochloride in 0.05 M Tris buffer, pH 7.6.

14. Wash slides, counterstain lightly with hematoxylin, dehydrate, and mount.

As an alternative enzyme marker, sections can be incubated with 25–50 μg/ml of biotinylated glucose oxidase. The disclosing reaction consists of 6.7 mg/ml β-glucose, 0.67 mg/ml Nitro BT, and 0.0167 mg/ml phenazine methosulfate, in 0.05 M Tris, pH 8.3. The glucose and Nitro BT are preheated to 37°C for 1 hour, at which point the phenazine methosulfate and the tissue sections are added. After further incubation for 1 hour at 37°C with light protection, the slides are washed, counterstained with nuclear fast red, dehydrated rapidly through alcohols and xylenes (no longer than 1 minute in each change), and mounted in Permount. In our experience, the color contrast between the blue reaction product of the glucose oxidase marker and red counterstain is superior to that obtained with horseradish peroxidase, providing an apparent increase in staining sensitivity (Clark *et al.*, 1982). Furthermore, the blocking-of-endogenous-enzyme step recommended for peroxidase procedures is not required with the glucose oxidase marker.

III. Selected Applications

A. Lymphoid Cell Markers

The use of immunological typing of B, T, and null lymphocytes has been of major importance for the classification of human lymphoid and myeloid malignancies, enabling a more precise classification of leukemia and lymphoma (Siegal and Good, 1977; Koziner *et al.*, 1978). The classification of the malignant cells as one of the lymphocyte types has been accomplished predominantly by certain functional tests on cell suspensions. For example, T lymphocytes rosette with sheep red blood cells and bind antisera specific for T cells. The availability of T-cell antibodies should permit the identification of T-cell malignancies by immunohistochemistry in addition to these other functional methods for typing lymphocytes. The latter approaches have identified such T-cell tumors as lymphoblastic lymphoma and acute lymphocytic leukemia, as well as the less common mycosis fungoids and its related Sézary syndrome. Null cells lack surface immunoglobulin (SIg) and T-cell markers, and are heterogeneous for Ia-like antigens and Fc and C3 receptors (Koziner *et al.*, 1978). This distinction is not always clear, and overlapping does occur. Thus, when cells lack the distinguishing markers for T and B lymphocytes, they are considered to be null-cell tumors.

The major applications of immunohistochemistry, however, have been in the identification of B lymphocyte-related neoplasms; the characterization of B cells has had a significant impact on the diagnosis and classification of lymphomas. The B lymphocytes express either cytoplasmic immunoglobulin (CIg) or SIg, as well as immunoglobulin Fc receptors, C3 receptors, and the HLA-D-related Ia-like antigens (see Taylor, 1980). The B-cell nature of lymphocytes is conveniently established by demonstrating the production of surface and/or cytoplasmic immunoglobulin by lymphoid cells. Taylor (1974, 1978c) described the use of the immunoperoxidase method to demonstrate the presence of CIg in fixed lymphoma tissue sections. Since then, most non-Hodgkin's lymphomas have been found to be of the B-lymphocytic type. Because individual differentiated lymphoid cells are believed to be restricted in their expression of immunoglobulin, their clonal derivatives are likewise considered to retain this restricted expression of a single variable segment of both heavy and light chains and a single light chain constant region of either the κ or λ type (see Warnke and Levy, 1981). The uniformity of the light chain in the specimen thus imparts a monoclonality, and this monoclonal pattern of Ig staining (i.e., only one light chain), as distinguished from a polyclonal staining in the cytoplasm, indicates both a lymphocytic origin and a neoplastic character. This property has been used to differentiate reactive and hyperplastic forms and plasmacytosis from true lymphoid malignancies, such as plasmacytoid lymphocytic lymphoma, plasmacytoma, immunoblastic sarcoma, and follicular cell lymphoma. Undifferentiated tumors showing a monoclonal Ig pattern can be classified as B-cell lymphoma, as opposed to undifferentiated or anaplastic carcinoma. Thus, B cells at a distinct stage of differentiation can be considered to be clonal progenitors of B-cell non-Hodgkin's lymphomas, expressing either a κ or λ light chain. As a result of combining such functional immunological studies and morphology, revised classifications of non-Hodgkin's lymphoma have evolved (Bennett et al., 1974; Dorfman, 1974; Gérard-Marchant et al., 1974; Lukes and Collins, 1974) and are expected to develop further as our repertoire of lymphoid markers and immunohistochemical capabilities expands. It has already been found that large-cell lymphomas are a very heterogeneous group of neoplasms, showing derivations from B cells, T cells, macrophages, or histiocytes, and sometimes even lacking the usual immunological markers (Warnke et al., 1980). The diffuse large-cell lymphomas are predominantly of B-cell nature, showing monoclonality, but various phenotypes can be observed on the basis of combinations of different immunological markers (Warnke et al., 1980).

The immunological phenotype not only contributes to lymphoid tumor classification and the interpretation of histogenesis, but it also may be related to prognosis. Bloomfield *et al.* (1976) examined the B-, T-, and null-cell surface marker characteristics of tumor-cell suspensions of non-Hodgkin's lymphoma and found that patients whose malignancies had B-cell markers survived much longer than those with null-cell characteristics. A better prognosis was recently claimed by Rudders *et al.* (1981) for patients with small cleaved follicle center cell lymphoma, whose tumor cells express C3 receptors and SIgD, than for patients with negatively reacting tumor cells. Yamanaka *et al.* (1981) reported that patients with T-cell-reactive non-Hodgkin's lymphoma had a shorter survival time than patients with B- or null-cell non-Hodgkin's lymphoma, thus supporting, in part, the view of Bloomfield and colleagues (1976). In a study of diffuse large-cell ("histiocytic") lymphomas, Warnke *et al.* (1980) found, in a retrospective analysis, that those who were Ig positive had more advanced disease and shorter survival periods. Presumably, the difference found between this finding and other studies cited is due to the different class of lymphoma studied. Additional studies, preferably of a prospective nature, are required before an understanding of the prognostic implications of immunological marker studies in diverse types of lymphoma is achieved.

In Hodgkin's disease, the presumed neoplastic cell is the Sternberg–Reed cell, the origin of which has been addressed in a number of studies utilizing immunohistochemical methods. By means of immunoperoxidase, IgG has been demonstrated in the cytoplasm of these cells (Garvin *et al.,* 1974; Taylor, 1974), suggesting that this cell is of B-lymphocyte origin. However, other reports have challenged this interpretation (Taylor, 1976; Papadimitriou *et al.,* 1978; Poppema *et al.,* 1978; Isaacson, 1979). Poppema (1980) has found that different types of Sternberg–Reed cells have different apparent origins. Sternberg–Reed cells (L and H types) of the nodular lymphocyte predominance type stained for IgG, J chain, and one type of light chain per cell, thus being interpreted as B immunoblasts. Typical- and lacunar-type Sternberg–Reed cells of mixed cellularity and nodular sclerosis subtypes, however, were found to contain IgG and both types of light chains per cell, with an α-1-antitrypsin reaction in some cells similar to that in histiocytes. The latter finding suggests that these Sternberg–Reed cells may be related to histiocytes. Thus, although much more work is needed to clarify this issue, the use of immunoperoxidase staining has suggested the presence of different types of Sternberg–Reed cells in different subtypes of Hodgkin's lymphoma.

Of particular importance has been the realization, by means of functional markers for lymphocytes, that tumors not previously believed to be derived or related to the lymphocyte do in fact have this association. Further, the various subtypes of non-Hodgkin's lymphoma are related to the variations of the B cell during transformation in lymph follicles and during differentiation to the plasma cell (i.e., small lymphocytic lymphoma, follicle center cell lymphoma, immunoblastic sarcoma, and plasmacytoma or myeloma). Thus, as more markers for different developmental stages of lymphoid cells become known and the corresponding antisera are generated, immunohistochemistry will provide further opportunities for classifying and understanding the geneology of lymphomas. However, as in the case of Ig staining, careful attention must be given to tissue fixation, which has been shown to affect adversely antigen detection (see Mason and Biberfeld, 1980), as well as other technical parameters discussed at the beginning of this chapter, with each new antigen–antibody system. An important consideration throughout the work related to Ig detection in lymphoid tumors has been whether the lymphoma cells accrete a component of interest instead of actually synthesizing it or having it as a cellular constituent. This has received considerable attention with regard to whether the Ig stained in lymphoma cells is taken up from the extracellular environment, and must be taken into consideration in the staining of lymphoid and other tumors (see Mason and Biberfeld, 1980).

B. Blood Group Antigens

The immunocytological localization of human ABH antigens in fetal, adult normal, and cancerous tissues has been a subject of investigation for over two decades (Glynn et al., 1957; Szulman, 1960, 1962, 1964, 1977; Davidsohn, 1979; Weinstein et al., 1981). Two forms of these antigens are present in tissues, one of which is probably a glycolipid, is alcohol soluble, and is a cell membrane component of vascular endothelium and a variety of epithelial cells. The other form of tissue blood group antigens exists as water-soluble glycoproteins of the mucous secretions. In the adult, the cell membrane antigens are found in endothelium as well as epithelium of the skin, upper gastrointestinal tract, ureters, bladder, uterine cervix, and vagina (Szulman, 1977). The ABH antigens of the gastrointestinal tract mucous secretions decrease in concentration caudally, such that the adult distal colon lacks ABH activity. The presence of blood group activity in secretions of the fetal distal colon, their absence in the adult, and their emergence in adenocarcinomas resemble developmental associations of other tumor antigens (Szulman, 1964; Cooper et al., 1980).

Examination of Table I reveals that loss of blood group antigens is a common finding in tumors derived from a variety of epithelial tissues, the loss being greater for tumors originating from non-mucus-secreting epithelium. Likewise, ABH antigens reemerge to a high incidence in adenocarcinomas of the distal colon. Despite this extensive knowledge of blood

TABLE I

DELETION OF BLOOD GROUP ANTIGEN EXPRESSION IN HUMAN TUMORS

Organ	Histopathology	Percentage of specimens antigen negative (%)	References
Oral mucosa	Squamous carcinoma	50–100	Prendergast et al. (1968); Liu et al. (1974)
Larynx	Squamous carcinoma	44–63	Dabelsteen et al. (1974); Lin et al. (1977)
Lung	Bronchogenic carcinoma	100	Davidsohn and Ni (1969)
	Squamous, oat, anaplastic adenocarcinoma	75	
Stomach	Adenocarcinoma	6–74 Mean, 52	Eklund et al. (1963); David-sohn et al. (1966, 1971a); Sheahan et al. (1971); Denk et al. (1974a); Slocombe et al, (1980); Kapadia et al. (1981)
Colon			
Proximal	Adenocarcinoma	55	Sheahan (1975)
Distal[a]	Adenocarcinoma	13–53 Mean, 46	Denk et al. (1974a,b); Cooper and Haesler (1978); Abdelfattah-Gad and Denk (1980)
Pancreas	Adenocarcinoma	83	Davidsohn et al. (1971b)
Breast	Intraductal carcinoma	100	Gupta and Schuster (1973); Strauchen et al. (1980)
Uterine cervix	Squamous carcinoma		
	In situ	69–86	Davidsohn et al. (1969, 1973); Bonfiglio and Feinberg (1976)
	Invasive	66–100	
Prostate	Adenocarcinoma	100	Gupta et al. (1973)
Bladder	Transitional cell carcinoma		
	In situ	88	Kay and Wallace (1961); Alroy et al. (1978); Em-mott et al. (1979, 1981); Weinstein et al. (1979); Limas and Lange (1980); Richie et al. (1980)
	Noninvasive	23–68 Mean, 52	
	Invasive	47–100 Mean, 85	

[a] Normal distal colon lacks blood group antigens. Therefore, about 54% of adeno-carcinomas of the distal colon reexpress these antigens.

group antigen alterations in human tumors, largely fostered by the pioneering studies of Davidsohn (1979) and co-workers, it has not proven to be a clinically useful tool, except perhaps in the urinary bladder. First, deletion or, as is the case in the distal colon, reexpression of ABH antigens in epithelial cells is not diagnostic of cancer, since similar perturbations in the expression of these antigens are observed in a variety of benign lesions (Table II). However, further careful study of this area is needed since histologically normal mucosa adjacent to invasive squamous cell carcinoma of the larnyx (Lin *et al.*, 1977), invasive adenocarcinomas of the proximal colon (Sheahan, 1975), and *in situ* bladder carcinoma (Weinstein *et al.*, 1979) lacked blood group antigens. Lin *et al.* (1977) also encountered four cases in which the initial biopsy specimens were histologically negative for carcinoma, negative for blood group antigen and, upon subsequent biopsy, positive for invasive squamous cell carcinomas of the larynx. Thus, can the loss of blood group antigens signify a potential for malignant transformation in otherwise morphologically normal cells, or identify subgroups of certain benign lesions that have a suspected proclivity for malignant conversion (Sheahan, 1979)? Second, blood group antigen expression does not correlate with histologic differentiation of tumors or clinical staging and, by itself, has not demonstrated any prognostic value in gastric, colon, or cervical cancer (Davidsohn *et al.*, 1969; Denk *et al.*, 1974a; Cooper and Haesler, 1978; Abdelfattah-Gad and Denk, 1980; Slocombe *et al.*, 1980).

   In contrast to other malignancies, several studies have suggested that loss of ABH antigens in low-stage transitional cell carcinomas of the bladder correlates quite well with subsequent invasive disease in these patients, whereas the persistence of antigen carries a more favorable prognosis (Decenzo *et al.*, 1975; Lange *et al.*, 1978; Emmott *et al.*, 1979; Limas *et al.*, 1979; Johnson and Lamm, 1980; Newman *et al.*, 1980; Richie *et al.*, 1980). This relationship between ABH expression and tendency for invasion appears to be independent of histologic grading, particularly for those tumors that are antigen positive (Davidsohn *et al.*, 1973; Alroy *et al.*, 1978; Lange *et al.*, 1978; Limas *et al.*, 1979; Emmott *et al.*, 1979; Newman *et al.*, 1980; Johnson and Lamm, 1980). It appears that certain morphological "look-alike" bladder tumors (Weinstein *et al.*, 1981) will manifest divergent biological behaviors that can be partially assessed at an early stage by their expression of ABH antigens. However, approximately 50% of patients with antigen-negative, lower grade tumors did not have invasive disease during the 5-year follow-up, demonstrating that on the basis of the data accumulated thus far, the absence of antigen does not warrant more aggressive therapy. Furthermore, Askari *et al.* (1981) could not demonstrate a difference between blood group antigen

TABLE II

BLOOD GROUP ANTIGENS IN BENIGN OR PREMALIGNANT HUMAN TISSUES

Organ	Histopathology	Blood group antigens	References
Oral mucosa	Leukoplakia with dysplasia	Diminished	
	Fibroepithelial polyps	Positive	Dabelsteen *et al.* (1975)
Lung	Chronic bronchitis	Positive	
	Squamous cell metaplasia	Positive	Davidsohn and Ni (1969)
Stomach	Intestinal metaplasia	Negative, diminished, or positive	Sheahan *et al.* (1971); Denk *et al.* (1974a); Slocombe *et al.* (1980); Kapadia *et al.* (1981)
Colon			
Proximal	Ulcerative colitis	67% positive	
	Crohn's disease	86% positive	
	Adenomas	21% positive	Sheahan (1975, 1979)
Distal[a]	Adenomas		
	Tubullo	39–44% positive	
	Villous	54–85% positive	Denk *et al.* (1975); Cooper
	Hyperplastic	Negative	*et al.* (1980)
Breast	Cystic disease	38–100% positive	
	Gynecomastia	Positive	
	Duct hyperplasia	Negative	
	Fibroadenomas	Positive	
	Sclerosing adenosis	Negative	Gupta and Schuster (1973);
	Duct papillamotosis	Negative	Strauchen *et al.* (1980)
Uterine	Squamous metaplasia	31% positive	
cervix	Dysplasia, slight to marked	Negative, diminished, or positive	Lill *et al.* (1976); Bonfiglio and Feinberg (1976)
Prostate	Hyperplasia	67% positive	Gupta *et al.* (1973)
Bladder	Cystitis cystica	Positive	
	Cystitis glandularis	Positive	
	Squamous metaplasia	Negative	Weinstein *et al.* (1979);
	Atypia	Negative	Emmott *et al.* (1981)

[a] Normal distal colon lacks blood group antigens. Therefore, 40–85% of adenomas of the distal colon regain blood group antigen expression.

expression and histologic grading in predicting eventual clinical outcome. Antigen positivity in stage O or A bladder cancer is not predictive of recurrence, since about an equal distribution of these patients have and do not have recurrences (Alroy *et al.*, 1978; Emmott *et al.*, 1979; Johnson and Lamm, 1980; Limas *et al.*, 1979; Newman *et al.*, 1980). Antigen negativity, however, is associated with a high recurrence frequency (average of 85%).

It is very likely that the method of antigen detection and evaluation accounts for a substantial portion of the difference and discrepancies noted in reported results for blood group antigen staining. Earlier studies used immunofluorescence techniques (Eklund *et al.*, 1963; Davidsohn *et al.*, 1966) that were quickly replaced by variations of the mixed-cell agglutination reaction (MCAR; also referred to as specific red cell adherence test, SRCA) adapted by Tönder *et al.* (1964) for the demonstration of antigens in tissue sections (Kovarik *et al.*, 1968; Alroy *et al.*, 1973; Davidsohn, 1979). The SRCA test is a simple procedure in which human anti-A or anti-B serum is first applied to tissue sections, followed by the addition of isologous indicator erythrocytes. Erythrocytes that do not specifically adhere to the tissue section via IgM anti-blood group antigen antibody linkage with the tissue antigen are removed by slide inversion. Although a few studies have used human natural anti-H antibody for the detection of H antigen in the SRCA test, most substitute *Ulex europeus* lectin for this purpose. For the detection of all three antigens, the SRCA test is simple yet very fragile, and one must exercise considerable care during manipulations to remove nonadherent indicator cells and during postfixation and counterstaining. Otherwise, specifically adhered cells can be removed and, in our experience, this occurs in a patchy fashion, giving the impression that the epithelial tissue stained contains antigen-positive and antigen-negative areas. This problem is more prevalent with tissues having a low-antigen content, such as the stratified epithelium of the cervix and bladder. The A and B detection system is fairly stable to artifactual removal of specifically adhered indicator cells, although we require that tests are performed in duplicate for confidence in staining interpretation. On the other hand, many investigators have encountered considerable difficulty in H detection using *Ulex* lectin (Davidsohn and Ni, 1969; Cooper and Haesler, 1978; Emmott *et al.*, 1979; Abdelfattah-Gad and Denk 1980; Johnson and Lamm, 1980; Strauchen *et al.*, 1980; Askari *et al.*, 1981) and we have abandoned the use of this procedure for demonstrating H antigen in tissue sections. Coon and Weinstein (1981) have concluded that the SRCA, as currently performed, is unsuitable for H detection in the bladder. Consequently, the validity of H antigen staining interpretations of previous studies is open to criticism, particularly since most of them did not provide an appraisal of staining performance.

Another problem that is not unique to the SRCA test is the criteria used to classify staining reactions in terms of positivity or negativity. For ABH detection with the SRCA test, negative specimens range from those that only have a few adherent cells (Weinstein et al., 1979) to those that have less than 30% of the expected reactive area covered with indicator cells (Lange et al., 1978; Newman et al., 1980). It is obvious that this represents a wide gap in the definition of staining negativity and should lead to differences in reported data by various investigators. Even a percentage cutoff is a very subjective assessment since it is based on a mental image formed by microscopic evaluation. This problem of classifying negative or positive reactions is also inherent to immunoenzyme techniques in which certain investigators have chosen to regulate staining intensity by low-power examination of stained specimens (Wiley et al., 1981). The correct interpretation and classification of specimens that show diminished or partial reactivity represent major problems in the standardization of immunocytological techniques applied to cancer biology and diagnosis investigations. As pointed out by Weinstein et al. (1981), blood group antigen expression in tumors is not an all-or-none phenomenon in that within many specimens, segregated areas of antigen positivity and negativity appear (Davidsohn et al., 1966, 1971a; Wiley et al., 1981). This property of blood group antigen expression is characteristic of other tumor antigens, such as CEA (Primus et al., 1981a), and in certain organ systems a similar mosaic in antigen expression of the corresponding normal tissues is reflected (Davidsohn et al., 1966; Sanders and Kent, 1970; Primus et al., 1981b). Gradation in antigen reactivity certainly provides a clue concerning the biology of a particular tumor, the ultimate significance of which could be lost if partially reactive tumors are arbitrarily grouped into antigen-negative or -positive categories.

The method of tissue preparation will also have some bearing on ABH detectibility. Early immunofluorescence studies by Glynn et al. (1957) demonstrated that ethanol treatment of frozen sections of gastric tumor specimens abolished staining reactivity. Thus it was thought that only ethanol-resistant, water-soluble ABH antigens would be preserved in formalin-fixed, paraffin-embedded tissues. Subsequent studies, however, have demonstrated that both alcohol-soluble and water-soluble ABH antigens are preserved in formalin–paraffin tissues and are detectable by immunofluorescence (Dabelsteen, 1972; Bonfiglio and Feinberg, 1976), immunoperoxidase (Dalelsteen, 1972; Bonfiglio and Feinberg, 1976; Berry and Amerigo, 1980), and SRCA (Kovarik et al., 1968; Davidsohn and Ni, 1969; Davidsohn et al., 1969; Lin et al., 1977). Although both types of ABH antigens are detectable in formalin–paraffin tissues, Limas and Lange (1980) have demonstrated improved antigen localization by the

SRCA test in frozen unfixed sections of bladder cancer compared to that of conventionally processed specimens. Six of 35 specimens previously negative in formalin–paraffin sections became positive in frozen tissue sections. These investigators also showed that positive staining of normal bladder mucosa could be achieved at a higher dilution of primary antiserum or *Ulex* lectin when compared to the dilution necessary to obtain comparable staining in tumors. The latter study further highlights how differences in immunocytological technique (reagent dilution) and tissue preparation have the potential to influence ABH detectibility in pathological specimens. A final potential problem is the influence of secretor status. Although nonsecretors synthesize reduced levels of immunocytologically demonstrable ABH antigens in normal tissues (Szulman, 1977), this question has been virtually ignored in studies of ABH detection in tumors. In retrospective studies where secretor status is not possible to assess, demonstration of blood group antigens in adjacent normal tissue would seem obligatory for correct interpretation of their absence in the tumor.

Immunoenzyme techniques have not been widely applied to ABH antigen detection although they offer several advantages: They provide enhanced morphological resolution of staining localization compared to the SRCA test, alternative approaches for reliable H antigen detection, and an indicator system that is adaptable for spectrophotometric quantitation of staining intensity. Dabelsteen (1972) and, later, Bonfiglio and Feinberg (1976) compared indirect immunofluorescence and immunoperoxidase procedures for the detection of A or AB antigens. They used human natural antibody, marker-labeled anti-human IgG, and formalin–paraffin sections of normal oral mucosa (Dabelsteen, 1972) or normal and dysplastic uterine cervix (Bonfiglio and Feinberg, 1976). Immunofluorescence was found more sensitive than immunoperoxidase in each study. Katoh *et al.* (1979) used similar procedures for AB antigen localization and enzyme-labeled *Ulex* lectin for H antigen detection in formalin–paraffin sections of normal bronchus. Appreciable staining positivity for all three antigens was observed only after trypsin treatment of the tissue sections. One interpretation of the low sensitivity of these immunoperoxidase procedures is that the enzyme-labeled anti-human IgG might have been of poor quality or had low potency toward IgM antibody. We have observed that certain anti-human IgG antibodies, containing both heavy and light chain specificities, do not work particularly well in the above systems in comparison to enzyme-labeled anti-human IgM antibodies (Clark and Primus, 1981). Recently, the standard PAP (Berry and Amerigo, 1980; Slocombe *et al.*, 1980; Weinstein *et al.*, 1981) and four-layer PAP variation (Wiley *et al.*, 1981) procedures were used to study ABH expression in formalin–

paraffin sections of vascular, gastric, colonic, and bladder tumors. Slocombe *et al.* (1980) used heterologous antisera against ABH antigens and found a lower percentage antigen deletion (18%) in gastric tumors than that typically reported with the SRCA test (50%, Table I), suggesting greater sensitivity of the PAP immunoperoxidase technique. In the study by Weinstein *et al.* (1981), human natural anti-A and anti-B antibodies were used in conjunction with chimpanzee PAP. Staining of bladder tumors revealed similar sensitivities for A detection by the SRCA test and the chimpanzee PAP technique. For H detection, Weinstein *et al.* (1981) used *Ulex* lectin followed by rabbit anti-*Ulex*, goat anti-rabbit Ig, and, finally, rabbit PAP. Detection of H in bladder tumors using this technique was more reliable and sensitive than the SRCA test. Thus, it appears that immunoenzyme procedures are suitable alternatives for the SRCA test and, as conveyed by Weinstein *et al.* (1981), discernment of positive staining reactions and cytological detail of reactive cells is easier with the former methods. It will be interesting to see if the correlation between blood group antigen expression and tumor behavior in bladder cancer is maintained or improved with immunoperoxidase detection methods.

C. CARCINOEMBRYONIC ANTIGEN

Carcinoembryonic antigen (CEA) can be localized by immunohistological procedures in a variety of gastrointestinal and extragastrointestinal epithelial malignancies (reviewed by Goldenberg *et al.*, 1976, 1978; Primus *et al.*, 1981a). Increasing CEA content tends to parallel cellular dedifferentiation in gastric, ovarian, cervical, and endometrial malignancies, while the inverse holds true for colonic and lung tumors. The presence of CEA in a tissue specimen does not indicate malignancy, especially in the large intestine where the antigen is synthesized by normal epithelium and benign tumors (Stenger *et al.*, 1979; Wagener *et al.*, 1978; Primus *et al.*, 1981b). Although the antigen is not present or is greatly diminished in normal tissues derived from the stomach, lung, ovary, uterine mucosa, uterine cervix, and breast, it is present to varying degrees in noncancerous diseased tissue, benign tumors, and atypical epithelium from these tissue sites. This may suggest that the appearance of CEA in these benign lesions signifies a premalignant change, but no evidence exists to support this supposition. Consequently, the immunohistological detection of CEA has virtually no value in differentiating benign and malignant lesions.

Carcinoembryonic antigen immunohistochemistry may have limited clinical utility in predicting cases that will have elevated blood levels of antigen and might benefit from regular monitoring of blood samples. Although several factors will influence blood levels of a tumor antigen other than its mere presence in the tumor (Goldenberg *et al.*, 1976), preliminary studies in colon (Pihl *et al.*, 1980; Goslin *et al.*, 1980), cervical (Rutanen *et al.*, 1978), and ovarian (van Nagell *et al.*, 1978) cancer patients suggest that CEA-positive primary tumors are frequently associated with antigen elevations in the blood. Carcinoembryonic antigen staining of regional lymph nodes (Fig. 4) may have some diagnostic value for detecting the presence and extent of micrometastases since metastatic tumor cells from antigen-positive primary tumors are almost always positive (Bordes *et al.*, 1973; van Nagell *et al.*, 1978, 1979; Shousha and Lyssiotis, 1978; O'Brien *et al.*, 1981). As yet, this application of immunohistochemistry has not detected involved lymph nodes that were unrecognized by conventional histologic stains (Sloane *et al.*, 1980; O'Brien *et al.*, 1981). It may be possible in questionable cases to discriminate between metastatic foci and histiocytosis by CEA staining of lymph nodes.

Most studies have not found a correlation between CEA staining of primary tumors and disease stage or prognosis, although measurement of blood antigen levels can aid in prognosis and monitoring of therapy. Preliminary reports in three different organ sites suggest that exceptions may exist. In medullary carcinoma of the thyroid, DeLellis *et al.* (1978) reported that CEA positivity was related to invasiveness. Shousha and Lyssiotis (1978) established a relationship between CEA staining of malignant breast tumors and their capacity to metastasize. Of the CEA-positive cases, 40% experienced nodal involvement compared with only 8% of the CEA-negative specimens. The absence of CEA staining in primary breast tumors appeared to correlate with a more favorable prognosis, and this correlation was independent of the presence or absence of metastasis, postoperative treatment, and histologic grade (Shousha *et al.*, 1979). Wiley *et al.* (1981) have compared the immunoperoxidase staining of CEA and AB blood

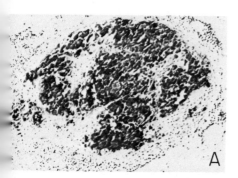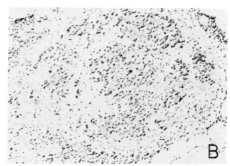

FIG. 4. Immunoglucose oxidase staining of CEA in lymph-node metastases of colonic adenocarcinoma. (A) Stained with anti-CEA antiserum; (B) stained with CEA-neutralized anti-CEA antiserum. Counterstained lightly with nuclear fast red. Magnification × 120.

group antigens in formalin–paraffin sections of Dukes' stage C or D colonic adenocarcinomas. Specimens were judged negative when less than 30% of the tumor area stained as visualized at 50× final magnification. Approximately 25% of the specimens were positive for both CEA and blood group antigens, positive for one antigen only, or negative for both irrespective of the site of the primary tumor and its histology. When both antigens were present, they rarely were found in the same tumor cell as previously observed by Denk *et al.* (1974a). A comparison of antigen staining with the development of metastatic recurrences revealed a significant increase in the incidence of metastases from tumors of the transverse and distal colon that were either blood group antigen negative or negative for both CEA and blood group antigens. A similar relationship was not found in adenocarcinomas arising in the proximal colon. These findings parallel similar observations of the relationship between blood group antigen negativity and invasion in transitional cell carcinomas of the bladder. Confirmation of these results is certainly warranted, as well as examination of lower stage tumors. However, the investigators did not correlate antigen staining and incidence of metastasis with histologic grade, nor did they specify the follow-up time for the patients studied, thus introducing a possible bias in their conclusions.

D. Human Chorionic Gonadotropin and α-Fetoprotein

The value of measuring blood levels of human chorionic gonadotropin (HCG) in gestational choriocarcinomas and α-fetoprotein (AFP) in hepatocellular carcinoma for monitoring therapy and prognosis is well recognized (Braunstein, 1979; Masseyeff, 1979; Waldmann and McIntire, 1979; Ruoslahti and Seppälä, 1979). Both of these markers are also associated with various forms of germinal tumors of the testis and ovary, providing valuable diagnostic tools for clinical staging and monitoring of therapy (Braunstein, 1979; Waldmann and McIntire, 1979). However, many patients with germ cell tumors and elevated blood levels of HCG and/or AFP will show a fall to normal levels of these markers following therapy, despite persistence of tumor, or will show discordance in their production following recurrence of tumor (Braunstein *et al.*, 1973; Sell *et al.*, 1976). The return of marker levels to normal in patients having persistent tumor reflects an interruption in marker production due to a block in synthesis or selective destruction of marker-producing cells, whereas discordance in AFP and HCG synthesis suggests that they are produced by different cells. Studies by Kurman and associates (reviewed in Kurman and Scardino, 1981) are an excellent example of how immunoperoxidase techniques have clarified our understanding of the appearance of blood AFP and HCG in the morphologically and histogenetically complex germ cell tumors. In the immunohistologic classification scheme proposed by these investigators, germinomas and primitive embryonal carcinomas, both lacking HCG and AFP, arise as two separate developmental pathways from a primordial germ cell. Embryonal carcinomas but not germinomas have the multipotential capacity to differentiate into endodermal sinus tumors, choriocarcinomas, or teratomas. Embryonal carcinoma cells, cytologically identical and AFP positive, are present in embryonal carcinomas and endodermal sinus tumors, but not in morphologically pure forms of the other germ cell tumors. The embryonal carcinoma cells, then, are the source of AFP and their presence in endodermal sinus tumors (yolk sac tumors) and embryonal carcinomas provides a biochemical and morphological developmental link between them and to the embryonic yolk sac that also produces AFP. Most endodermal sinus tumors and approximately 50% of pure embryonal carcinomas produce AFP. Focal positivity of cells and hyaline droplets are characteristic of both neoplasms. Human chorionic gonadotropin is found within syncytiotrophoblasts admixed with cytotrophoblast in nongestational choriocarcinoma or within isolated clusters of syncytiotrophoblastic giant cells, mainly found in embryonal carcinomas but also much less frequently in seminoma, endodermal sinus tumor, and teratoma. The preponderance of HCG-producing syncytiotrophoblasts within embryonal carcinomas supports a close developmental association between them and nongestational choriocarcinomas. Pure forms of teratomas are HCG and AFP negative, whereas marker production by mixed germ cell tumors will depend on their histologic composition. Thus, the immunohistologic classification of germ cell tumors should improve the histopathologic assignment of these tumors and correlation with marker blood levels. Greater precision in the pathologic classification of germ cell tumors is also required in the assessment of clinical prognosis and appropriate therapy (Beilly *et al.*, 1979). However, caution is needed in the interpretation of elevated blood markers, especially AFP, since AFP production can accompany hepatocyte proliferation (Ruoslahti and Seppälä, 1979). Javadpour (1980) has described a case of seminoma with moderately elevated serum AFP and HCG. Examination of retroperitoneal and liver masses did not reveal a nonseminomatous element, but did show histologic evidence of liver regeneration.

E. Prostatic Acid Phosphatase

Several studies have described the immunohistochemical localization of prostatic acid phosphatase in frozen, decalcified, or formalin–paraffin sections of human tissues (Jöbsis *et al.*, 1978; Stegehuis *et al.*, 1979;

Aumüller *et al.*, 1981; Manley *et al.*, 1981). Prostatic acid phosphatase is produced by the normal prostatic acinar or ductal columnar epithelial cells, whereas the basal cells are negative (Jöbsis *et al.*, 1978). All benign prostatic hyperplasia specimens, approximately 95% of primary prostatic adenocarcinomas, and 100% of their metastases are prostatic acid phosphatase positive. Nonprostatic normal tissues, carcinomas, and their metastases have been invariably prostatic acid phosphatase negative. Consequently, immunohistochemical staining for prostatic acid phosphatase should have diagnostic value in occult cases in discriminating between metastatic prostatic carcinoma and adenocarcinomas of different origin (Manley *et al.*, 1981). The latter has particular significance concerning the application of appropriate therapeutic modalities (Manley *et al.*, 1981). Prostatic acid phosphatase staining should also aid pathologists in distinguishing tumors within the prostate from prostatic or metastatic tumors from other tissue sites, particularly the bladder.

F. Intermediate Filaments

Intermediate filaments belong to a system of cytoplasmic filaments, intermediate in size between actin and myosin filaments, that can be biochemically and immunologically separated into five major classes (Lazarides, 1980): (1) keratin filaments in epithelial cells, (2) desmin filaments in muscle cells, (3) vimentin filaments in mesenchymal cells, (4) neurofilaments in neurons, and (5) glial filaments in glial cells. Schlegel *et al.* (1980a,b) have recently surveyed the immunoperoxidase localization of keratin in normal and neoplastic human tissues. In addition to the intracellular localization of keratin in epidermis, it was also demonstrated in normal epithelium of the bronchus, cervix, prostate, and bladder, as well as ductal epithelium of the salivary glands, breast, liver, and pancreas. Like actin (Bussolati *et al.*, 1980) and myosin (Sugano *et al.*, 1981), breast myoepithelial cells were keratin positive. Keratin was absent in glandular epithelium and in nerve, connective, and lymphoid tissues. Staining of various neoplasms generally followed that predicted by the staining pattern of the normal tissues (Schlegel *et al.*, 1980b). Thus, the detection of keratin proteins in metastatic tumors by immunoperoxidase techniques could contribute to the diagnosis of an occult epithelial tumor and in distinguishing poorly differentiated carcinomas from sarcomas and lymphomas. Strong reactivity would be suggestive of a squamous, urothelial, or mesothelial epithelium origin, whereas absence of reactivity would be much less specific, suggesting a brain, connective, lymphoid, or glandular epithelium tumor origin. Kapanci *et al.* (1981) have examined six cases of undifferentiated tumors in lymph node biopsies with antikeratin and anti-vimentin antibodies and accurately diagnosed their epithelial or mesenchymal origin. Furthermore, keratin staining may aid in the discrimination between thymoma and poorly differentiated or histiocytic lymphomas (Battifora *et al.*, 1980). It will be interesting to see if these preliminary studies are confirmed, since immunohistochemical detection of keratin, vimentin, and desmin filaments would certainly offer a less expensive and more rapid alternative to electron microscopy. Further work is also needed to determine if keratin staining correlates with differences in biological behavior of tumors (Schlegel *et al.*, 1980b). The cellular and tissue association of the various keratin polypeptides is another facet requiring further investigation (Löning *et al.*, 1980) which would be facilitated by the development of monoclonal antibodies (Gown *et al.*, 1981).

Glial fibrillary acidic (GFA) protein is produced by normal astrocytes, thus its presence does not indicate that a cell is neoplastic. However, immunohistochemical staining for GFA protein has been helpful in diagnosing glial components of mixed tumors, glioma metastasis in the leptomeninges, and reactive astrocytes secondary to inflammation or other brain tumors (reviewed by Bignami and Schoene, 1981). Astrocytomas, glioblastomas, ependymomas, and oligodendrogliomas are positive for GFA protein, whereas it is absent in Schwannomas, neurofibromas, and meningiomas.

IV. Conclusions

This article has attempted to address the current state of immunoenzyme methods and to provide a few examples of their applications in the diagnostic pathology of cancer. It is evident that this is a rapidly developing field which is experiencing methodological changes and increasing applications. The development of monoclonal antibodies by means of hybridization techniques has not only resulted in the availability of improved immunological reagents for immunoenzyme histochemistry, but the latter method is becoming a frequently used approach to assessing the tissue and cellular specificity of the monoclonal antibody reagents being developed. From the diagnostic and clinical viewpoints, we have discussed the use of immunoglobulin staining in providing a functional classification of certain lymphoreticular neoplasms, and for some degree of prognostication in certain non-Hodgkin's lymphomas. Immunoenzyme histochemistry can be applied to assessing the role of blood group antigen loss in reflecting the biological potentials of neoplasms, similar to what has been accomplished for urinary bladder cancer using other, more cumbersome approaches. Carcinoembryonic antigen and other tumor-associated markers demonstrated in tumor samples may serve to reflect or predict their use as blood markers to be followed as indicators of disease activity. Human chorionic gonadotropin and α-fetoprotein have together contributed to a reevaluation of the histogenetic relationships of germ cell neoplasms. Prostatic acid phosphatase and other tissue-specific markers can serve to differentiate certain tumors from morphologically similar lesions, and to identify the site of origin of isolated, morphologically obscure metastases. Finally, a variety of intermediate filaments can be used to identify the possible source and character of isolated metastases, to differentiate tumors of different histogenetic origins, and to aid in the classification of neoplasms derived from different cell types within the same organ.

It is thus apparent from these few examples that immunoenzyme histochemistry applied to the diagnostic pathology of cancer can offer the following advantages: (1) The cellular origin of a product can be identified; (2) the distribution of the product among certain or different cells within a heterogeneous population of tumor and normal cells can be demonstrated; (3) the presence of a new, modified, or ectopic product in a lesion can be documented; (4) the loss of a normal product or cellular constituent during or after the development of a neoplasm can be followed; and (5) the changes and interrelationships of multiple cellular products and substances can be assessed. These opportunities enable the pathologist to classify lesions according to functional cell types and to relate structure and function for an improved understanding of the histogenesis of cancer. Finally, as cell biological approaches begin to reveal etiological and pathogenetic aspects of neoplasia, the tools of immunohistochemistry will gain an even more significant role in the early diagnosis of cancer.

REFERENCES

Abdelfattah-Gad, M., and Denk, H. (1980). *J. Natl. Cancer Inst.* **64,** 1025–1028.
Alroy, J., Teramura, K., Davidsohn, I., and Weinstein, R. S. (1973). *Stain Technol.* **53,** 53–56.
Alroy, J. Teramura, K., Miller, A. W., Pauli, B. U., Gottesman, J. E., Flanagan, M., Davidsohn, I., and Weinstein, R. S. (1978). *Cancer* **41,** 1739–1745.
Askari, A., Colmenares, E., Saberi, A., and Jarman, W. D. (1981). *J. Urol.* **125,** 182–184.
Aumüller, G., Pohl, C., van Etten, R. L., and Seitz, J. (1981). *Virchows Arch. B* **35,** 249–262.
Avrameas, S. (1969). *Immunochemistry* **6,** 43–52.
Avrameas, S., Ternynck, T. (1971). *Immunochemistry* **8,** 1175–1179.
Battifora, H., Sun, T.-T., Bahw, R. M., and Rao, S. (1980). *Human Pathol.* **11,** 635–640.
Bayer, E. A., and Wilchek, M. (1980). *Methods Biochem. Anal.* **26,** 1–45.
Beilly, J. O. W., Horne, C. H. W., Milne, G. D., and Parkinson, C. (1979). *J. Clin. Pathol.* **32,** 455–461.

Bennett, M. H., Farrer-Brown, G., Henry, K., and Jelliffe, A. M. (1974). *Lancet* **2,** 405–406.

Berry, C. L., and Amerigo, J. (1980). *Virchows Arch. A: Pathol. Anat.* **388,** 167–174.

Bigbee, J. W., Kosek, J. C., and Eng, L. F. (1977). *J. Histochem. Cytochem.* **25,** 443–447.

Bignami, A., and Schoene, W. C. (1981). In "Diagnostic Immunohistochemistry" (R. A. DeLellis, ed.), pp. 213–226. Masson, Paris.

Bloomfield, C. D., Kensey, J. H., Brunning, R. D., Gajl-Peczalska, K. J. (1976). *Lancet* **2,** 1330–1333.

Bonfiglio, T. A., and Feinberg, M. R. (1976). *Arch. Pathol. Lab. Med.* **100,** 307–310.

Boorsma, D. M., and Streefkerk, J. G. (1979). *J. Immunol. Methods* **30,** 245–255.

Bordes, M., Michiels, R., and Martin, F. (1973). *Digestion* **9,** 106–115.

Bosman, F. T., and Nieuwenhuijzen Kruseman, A. C. (1979). *J. Histochem. Cytochem.* **27,** 1140–1147.

Braunstein, G. D. (1979). In "Immunodiagnosis of Cancer" (R. B. Herberman and K. R. McIntire, eds.), pp. 383–409. Dekker, New York.

Braunstein, G. D., McIntire, K. R., and Waldmann, T. A. (1973). *Cancer* **31,** 1065–1068.

Buffa, R., Solcia, E., Fiocca, R., Crivelli, O., and Pera A. (1979). *J. Histochem. Cytochem.* **27,** 1279–1280.

Burns, J. (1975). *Histochemistry* **43,** 291–294.

Burns, J., Hambridge, M., and Taylor, C. R. (1974). *J. Clin. Pathol.* **27,** 548–557.

Burnstone, M. S. (1960). *J. Histochem. Cytochem.* **8,** 63–70.

Bussolati, G., Botta, G., and Gugliotta, P. (1980). *Virchows Arch. B* **34,** 251–259.

Campbell, G. T., and Bhatnagar, A. S. (1976). *J. Histochem. Cytochem.* **24,** 448–452.

Celio, M. R., Letz, H., Binz, H., and Fey, H. (1979). *J. Histochem. Cytochem.* **27,** 691–698.

Clark, C. A., and Primus, F. J. (1981). *J. Histochem. Cytochem.* (submitted).

Clark, C. A., Downs, E. C., and Primus, F. J. (1982). *J. Histochem. Cytochem.* **30,** 27–34.

Coon, J. S., and Weinstein, R. S. (1981). *J. Urol.* **125,** 301–306.

Coons, A. H., Creech, H. J., and Jones, R. N. (1941). *Proc. Soc. Exp. Biol. Med.* **47,** 200–202.

Cooper, H. S., and Haesler, W. E., Jr. (1978). *Am. J. Clin. Pathol.* **69,** 594–598.

Cooper, H. S., Cox, J., and Patchefsky, A. S. (1980). *Am. J. Clin. Pathol.* **73,** 345–350.

Curran, R. C., and Gregory, J. (1978). *J. Clin. Pathol.* **31,** 974–983.

Dabelsteen, E. (1972). *Acta Pathol. Microbiol. Scand.* **80,** 847–853.

Dabelsteen, E., Mygind, N., and Henriksen, B. (1974). *Acta Oto-Laryngol.* **77,** 360–367.

Dabelsteen, E., Roed-Petersen, B., and Pindborg, J. J. (1975). *Acta Pathol. Microbiol. Scand. Sect. A* **83,** 292–300.

Davidsohn, I. (1979). In "Immunodiagnosis of Cancer" (R. B. Herberman and K. R. McIntire, eds.), pp. 644–669. Dekker, New York.

Davidsohn, I., and Ni, L. Y. (1969). *Am. J. Pathol.* **57,** 307–334.

Davidsohn, I., Kovarik, S., and Lee, C. L. (1966). *Arch. Pathol.* **81,** 381–390.

Davidsohn, I., Kovarik, S., and Ni, L. Y. (1969). *Arch. Pathol.* **87,** 306–314.

Davidsohn, I., Ni, L. Y., and Stejskal, R. (1971a). *Arch. Pathol.* **92,** 456–464.

Davidsohn, I., Ni, L. Y., and Stejskal, R. (1971b). *Cancer Res.* **31,** 1244–1250.

Davidsohn, I., Stejskal, R., and Lill, P. (1973). *Lab. Invest.* **28,** 382.

Decenzo, J. M., Howard, P., and Irish, C. E. (1975). *J. Urol.* **114,** 874–878.

DeLellis, R. A., ed. (1981a). "Diagnostic Immunohistochemistry." Masson, Paris.

DeLellis, R. A. (1981b). In "Diagnostic Immunohistochemistry" (R. A. DeLellis, ed.), pp. 7–16. Masson, Paris.

DeLellis, R. A., Wolfe, H. J., Rule, A. H., Reichlin, S., and Tashjian, A. H. (1978). *N. Engl. J. Med.* **299,** 1082.

DeLellis, R. A., Sternberger, L. A., Mann, R. B., Banks, P. M., and Nakane, P. K. (1979). *Am. J. Clin. Pathol.* **71**, 483–488.

Denk, H., Tappeiner, G., Davidovits, A., Eckerstorfer, R., and Holzner, J. H. (1974a). *J. Natl. Cancer Inst.* **53**, 933–938.

Denk, H., Tappeiner, G., and Holzner, J. H. (1974b). *Eur. J. Cancer* **10**, 487–490.

Denk, H., Holzner, J. H., and Obiditsch-Mayr, I. (1975). *J. Natl. Cancer Inst.* **54**, 1313–1317.

Denk, H., Radaszkiewicz, T., and Weirich, E. (1977). *J. Immunol. Methods* **15**, 163–167.

Dorfman, R. F. (1974). *Lancet* **1**, 1295–1296.

Dubois-Dalcq, M., McFarland, H., and McFarlin, D. (1977). *J. Histochem. Cytochem.* **25**, 1201–1206.

Eklund, A. E., Gullbring, B., and Lagerlöf, B. (1963). *Acta Pathol. Microbiol. Scand.* **59**, 447–455.

Emmott, R. C., Javadpour, N., Bergman, S. M., and Soares, T. (1979). *J. Urol.* **121**, 37–39.

Emmott, R. C., Droller, M. J., and Javadpour, N. (1981). *J. Urol.* **125**, 32–35.

Erlandsen, S. L., Hegre, O. D., Parsons, J. A., McEvoy, R. C., and Elde, R. P. (1976). *J. Histochem. Cytochem.* **24**, 883–897.

Fan, K. (1980). *Stain Technol.* **55**, 307–311.

Feltkamp-Vroom, T. M. (1975). *Ann. N.Y. Acad. Sci.* **254**, 21–26.

Fink, B., Loepfe, E., and Wyler, R. (1979). *J. Histochem. Cytochem.* **27**, 1299–1301.

Garvin, A. J., Spicer, S. S., Parmley, R. T., and Munster, A. M. (1974). *J. Exp. Med.* **139**, 1077–1083.

Gérard-Marchant, R., Hamlin, I., Lenvert, K., Rilke, F., Stansfeld, A. G., and van Unnik, A. M. (1974). *Lancet* **2**, 406–408.

Glynn, L. E., Holborow, E. J., and Johnson, G. D. (1957). *Lancet* **2**, 1083–1088.

Goding, J. W. (1978). *J. Immunol. Methods* **20**, 241–253.

Goldenberg, D. M., Sharkey, R. M., and Primus, F. J. (1976). *J. Natl. Cancer Inst.* **57**, 11–22.

Goldenberg, D. M., Sharkey, R. M., and Primus, F. J. (1978). *Cancer* **42**, 1546–1553.

Goslin, R. H., O'Brien, M. J., Steele, G. D., and Zamcheck, N. (1980). *Clin. Res.* **28**, 629a.

Gown, A. M., Vogel, A. M., and Benditt, E. P. (1981). *Fed. Proc. Fed. Am. Soc. Exp. Biol.* **40**, 832.

Graham, R. C., and Karnovsky, M. J. (1966). *J. Histochem. Cytochem.* **14**, 291–302.

Guesdon, J. C., Ternynck, T., and Avrameas, S. (1979). *J. Histochem. Cytochem.* **27**, 1131–1139.

Gupta, R. K., and Schuster, R. (1973). *Am. J. Pathol.* **72**, 253–260.

Gupta, R. K., Schuster, R., and Christian, W. D. (1973). *Am. J. Pathol.* **70**, 439–448.

Hanker, J. S., Yates, P. E., Metz, C. B., and Rustioni, A. (1977). *Histochem. J.* **9**, 789–792.

Heald, J., Buckley, C. H., and Fox, H. (1979). *J. Clin. Pathol.* **32**, 918–926.

Heyderman, E. (1979). *J. Clin. Pathol.* **32**, 971–978.

Heyderman, E. (1980). *J. R. Soc. Med.* **73**, 655–658.

Heyderman, E., and Neville, A. M. (1977). *J. Clin. Pathol.* **30**, 138–140.

Hsu, S-M., and Ree, H. J. (1980). *Am. J. Clin. Pathol.* **74**, 32–40.

Hsu, S-M., Raine, L., and Fanger, H. (1981). *J. Histochem. Cytochem.* **29**, 577–580.

Huang, S-N., Minassian, H., and More, J. D. (1976). *Lab. Invest.* **35**, 383–390.

Hudson, L., and Hay, F. C. (1980). "Practical Immunology," pp. 203–225. Blackwell, Oxford.

Isaacson, P. (1979). *J. Clin. Pathol.* **32**, 802–807.

Javadpour, N. (1980). *Cancer* **45**, 2166–2168.

Jöbsis, A. C., de Vries, G. P., Anholt, R. R. H., and Sanders, G. T. B. (1978). *Cancer* **41**, 1788–1793.

Johnson, J. D., and Lamm, D. L. (1980). *J. Urol.* **123,** 25–28.
Kapadia, A., Feizi, T., Jewell, D., Keeling, J., and Slavin, G. (1981). *J. Clin. Pathol.* **34,** 320–337.
Kapanci, Y., Barazzone, P., Franke, W., and Gabbiani, G. (1981). *Fed. Proc. Fed. Am. Soc. Exp. Biol.* **40,** 832.
Katoh, Y., Stoner, G. D., McIntire, K. R., Hill, T. A., Anthony, R., McDowell, E. M., Trump, B. F., and Harris, C. C. (1979). *J. Natl. Cancer Inst.* **62,** 1177–1185.
Kay, H. E. M., and Wallace, D. M. (1961). *J. Natl. Cancer Inst.* **26,** 1349–1365.
Kovarik, S., Davidsohn, I., and Stejskal, R. (1968). *Arch. Pathol.* **86,** 12–21.
Koziner, B., Mertelsmann, R., Siegal, F. P., and Filippa, D. A. (1978). *Clin. Bull.* **8,** 47–53.
Kuhlmann, W. D., and Avrameas, S. (1971). *J. Histochem. Cytochem.* **19,** 361–368.
Kurman, R. J., and Scardino, P. T. (1981). *In* "Diagnostic Immunohistochemistry" (R. A. DeLellis, ed.), pp. 277–298. Masson, Paris.
Lange, P. H., Limas, C., and Fraley, E. E. (1978). *J. Urol.* **119,** 52–55.
Lazarides, E. (1980). *Nature (London)* **283,** 249–256.
Lill, P. H., Norris, H. J., Rubenstone, A. I., Chang-To, M., and Davidsohn, I. (1976). *Am. J. Clin. Pathol.* **66,** 767–774.
Limas, C., and Lange, P. (1980). *Cancer* **46,** 1366–1373.
Limas, C., Lange, P., Fraley, E. E., and Vessella, R. L. (1979). *Cancer* **44,** 2099–2107.
Lin, F., Liu, P. I., and McGregor, D. H. (1977). *Am. J. Clin. Pathol.* **68,** 372–376.
Liu, P. I., McGregor, D. H., Liu, J. G., Dunlap, C. L., Jinks, W. L., Lin, F., Przybylski, C., and Miller, L. A. (1974). *Oral Surg. Oral Med. Oral Path.* **38,** 56–64.
Löning, T., Staquet, M. J., Thivolet, J., and Seifert, G. (1980). *Virchows Arch. A: Pathol. Anat.* **388,** 273–288.
Lukes, R., and Collins, R. (1974). *Cancer* **34,** 1488–1503.
Lukes, R. J., Parker, J. W., Taylor, C. R., Tindle, B. H., Cramer, A. D., and Lincoln, T. L. (1978). *Semin. Hematol.* **15,** 322–351.
Manley, P., Mahan, D. E., Bruce, A. W., and Franchi, L. (1981). *In* "Diagnostic Immunohistochemistry" (R. A. DeLellis, ed.), pp. 313–324. Masson, Paris.
Martin-Comin, J., and Robyn, C. (1976). *J. Histochem. Cytochem.* **24,** 1012–1016.
Masa-Tejada, R., Pascal, R. R., and Fenoglio, C. M. (1977). *Hum. Pathol.* **8,** 313–320.
Mason, D. Y., and Biberfeld, P. (1980). *J. Histochem. Cytochem.* **28,** 731–745.
Mason, D. Y., and Sammons, R. (1978). *J. Clin. Pathol.* **31,** 454–460.
Mason, T. E., Phifer, R. F., Spicer, S. S., Swallow, R. A., and Dreskin, R. B. (1969). *J. Histochem. Cytochem.* **17,** 563–569.
Masseyeff, R. F. (1979). *In* "Immunodiagnosis of Cancer" (R. B. Herberman and K. R. McIntire, eds.), pp. 117–130. Dekker, New York.
Mepham, B. L., Frater, W., and Mitchell, B. S. (1979). *Histochem. J.* **11,** 345–357.
Mesulam, M-M. (1978). *J. Histochem. Cytochem.* **26,** 106–117.
Mesulam, M-M., and Rosene, D. L. (1979). *J. Histochem. Cytochem.* **27,** 763–773.
Miller, E. P., and Hogg, R. M. (1980). *Med. Lab. Sci.* **37,** 93–94.
Miller, H. R. P. (1972). *Histochem. J.* **4,** 305–320.
Mukai, K., and Rosai, J. (1980). *Prog. Surg.* **1,** 15–49.
Nadji, M. (1980). *Acta Cytol.* **24,** 442–447.
Nakane, P. K. (1968). *J. Histochem. Cytochem.* **16,** 557–560.
Nakane, P. K., and Kawaoi, A. (1974). *J. Histochem. Cytochem.* **22,** 1084–1091.
Nakane, P. K., and Pierce, G. B. (1966). *J. Histochem. Cytochem.* **14,** 929–931.
Newman, A. J., Calton, C. E., and Johnson, S. (1980). *J. Urol.* **124,** 27–29.
Notani, G. W., Parsons, J. A., and Erlandsen, S. L. (1979). *J. Histochem. Cytochem.* **27,** 1438–1444.

O'Brien, M. J., Zamcheck, N., Burke, B., Kirkham, S., Saravis, C. A., and Gottlieb, L. S. (1981). *Am. J. Clin. Pathol.* **75**, 283–290.
Palladini, G., and Solheid, C. (1976). *Acta Histochem.* **57**, 87–92.
Papadimitrion, C. S., Stein, H., and Lenvert, K. (1978). *Int. J. Cancer,* **21**, 531–541.
Pearse, A. G. E. (1980). "Histochemistry: Theoretical and Applied." Churchill, London.
Pelliniemi, L. J., Dym, M., and Karnovsky, M. J. (1980). *J. Histochem. Cytochem.* **28**, 191–192.
Petrali, J. P., Hinton, D. M., Moriarity, G. C., and Sternberger, L. A. (1974). *J. Histochem. Cytochem.* **22**, 782–801.
Petrusz, P., Sar, M., Ordronneau, P., and DiMeo, P. (1976). *J. Histochem. Cytochem.* **24**, 1110–1112.
Petrusz, P., Sar, M., Ordionneau, P., and DiMeo, P. (1977). *J. Histochem. Cytochem.* **25**, 390–391.
Petrusz, P., Ordronneau, P., and Finley, J. C. W. (1980). *Histochem. J.* **12**, 333–348.
Pihl, E., McNaughtan, J., Ma, J., Ward, H. A., and Nairn, R. C. (1980). *Pathology* **12**, 7–13.
Poppema, S. (1980). *J. Histochem. Cytochem.* **28**, 788–791.
Poppema, S., Elema, J. D., and Halie, M. R. (1978). *Cancer* **42**, 1793–1803.
Prendergast, R. C., Toto, P. D., and Gargiulo, A. W. (1968). *J. Dent. Res.* **47**, 306–310.
Primus, F. H., Clark, C. A., and Goldenberg, D. M. (1981a). *In* "Diagnostic Immunohistochemistry" (R. A. DeLellis, ed.), pp. 263–276. Masson, Paris.
Primus, F. H., Clark, C. A., and Goldenberg, D. M. (1981b). *J. Natl. Cancer Inst.* **67**, 1031–1039.
Qualman, S. J., and Keren, D. F. (1979). *Lab. Invest.* **41**, 483–489.
Reading, M. (1977). *J. Clin. Pathol.* **30**, 88–90.
Reiner, A., and Gamlin, P. (1980). *J. Histochem. Cytochem.* **28**, 187–189.
Richie, J. P., Blute, R. D., and Waisman, J. (1980). *J. Urol.* **123**, 22–24.
Rudders, R. A., Ahl, T. A., DeLellis, R. A., and Begg, C. B. (1981). *Proc. Am. Assoc. Cancer Res. Am. Soc. Clin. Oncol.* **22**, 516.
Ruoslahti, E., and Seppälä, M. (1979). *Adv. Cancer Res.* **29**, 275–346.
Rutanen, E. M., Lindgren, J., Sipponen, P., Stenman, U. H., Saksela, E., and Seppälä, M. (1978). *Cancer* **42**, 581–590.
Sainte-Marie, G. (1962). *J. Histochem. Cytochem.* **10**, 250–256.
Sanders, E. M., and Kent, S. P. (1970). *Lab. Invest.* **23**, 74–78.
Schlegel, R., Banko-Schlegel, S., and Pinkus, G. S. (1980a). *Lab. Invest.* **42**, 91–96.
Schlegel, R., Banko-Schlegel, S., McLeod, J. A., and Pinkus, G. S. (1980b). *Am. J. Pathol.* **101**, 41–49.
Sell, S., Stillman, D., and Gochman, N. (1976). *Am. J. Clin. Pathol.* **66**, 847–853.
Sheahan, D. G. (1975). *Gastroenterology* **68**, A127,984.
Sheahan, D. G. (1979). *In* "Frontiers of Gastrointestinal Research" (L. vander Reis, ed.), pp. 51–64. Karger, Basel.
Sheahan, D. G., Horowitz, S. A., and Zamcheck, N. (1971). *Am. J. Dig. Dis.* **16**, 961–969.
Shousha, S., and Lyssiotis, T. (1978). *Histopathology* **2**, 433–447.
Shousha, S., Lyssiotis, T., Godfrey, V. M., and Scheuer, P. J. (1979). *Br. Med. J.* **1**, 777–779.
Siegal, F. P., and Good, R. A. (1977). *Clin. Haematol.* **6**, 355–422.
Sim, J. S., and French, S. W. (1976). *Arch. Pathol. Lab. Med.* **100**, 550–553.
Slemmon, J. R., Salvatura, P. M., and Saito, K. (1980). *J. Histochem. Cytochem.* **28**, 10–15.
Sloane, J. P., Ormerod, M. G., Imrie, S. F., and Coombes, R. C. (1980). *Br. J. Cancer* **42**, 392–398.

Slocombe, G. W., Berry, C. L., and Swettenham, K. V. (1980). *Virchows Arch. A: Pathol. Anat.* **387**, 289–300.

Stegehuis, F., de Vries, G. P., Jöbsis, A. C., and Meijer, A. E. F. H. (1979). *Histochemistry* **62**, 45–54.

Stenger, R. J., Chabon, A. B., Primus, F. J., and Wolff, W. I. (1979). *Mt. Sinai J. Med.* **46**, 185–189.

Sternberger, L. A. (1974). "Immunocytochemistry." Prentice-Hall, New York.

Sternberger, L. A. (1979). *J. Histochem. Cytochem.* **27**, 1657.

Sternberger, L. A., and Joseph, S. A. (1979). *J. Histochem. Cytochem.* **27**, 1424–1429.

Sternberger, L. A., and Petrali, J. P. (1977). *J. Histochem. Cytochem.* **25**, 1036–1042.

Sternberger, L. A., Hardy, P. H., Cuculis, J. J., and Meyer, H. G. (1970). *J. Histochem. Cytochem.* **18**, 315–333.

Strauchen, J. A., Bergman, S. M., and Hanson, T. A. S. (1980). *Cancer* **45**, 2149–2155.

Straus, W. (1971). *J. Histochem. Cytochem.* **19**, 682–688.

Straus, W. (1972). *J. Histochem. Cytochem.* **20**, 949–951.

Straus, W. (1979). *J. Histochem. Cytochem.* **27**, 1349–1351.

Streefkerk, J. G. (1970). *Neth. J. Zool.* **20**, 496–501.

Streefkerk, J. G. (1972). *J. Histochem. Cytochem.* **20**, 829–831.

Suffin, S. C., Muck, K. B., Young, J. C., Lewin, K., and Porter, D. D. (1979). *Am. J. Clin. Pathol.* **71**, 492–496.

Sugano, I., Nagao, K., Matsuzaki, O., Ide, G., and Toyota, N. (1981). *Acta Pathol. Jpn.* **31**, 35–44.

Swaab, D. F., Pool, C. W., and van Leeuwen, F. W. (1977). *J. Histochem. Cytochem.* **25**, 388–390.

Szulman, A. E. (1960). *J. Exp. Med.* **111**, 785–800.

Szulman, A. E. (1962). *J. Exp. Med.* **115**, 977–995.

Szulman, A. E. (1964). *J. Exp. Med.* **119**, 503–515.

Szulman, A. E. (1977). *In* "Human Blood Groups, 5th International Convocation for Immunology," pp. 426–436. Karger, Basel.

Taylor, C. R. (1974). *Lancet* **2**, 802–804.

Taylor, C. R. (1976). *Eur. J. Cancer,* **12**, 61–75.

Taylor, C. R. (1978a). *Oncology* **35**, 189–197.

Taylor, C. R. (1978b). *Arch. Pathol. Lab. Med.* **102**, 113–121.

Taylor, C. R. (1978c). *J. Histochem. Cytochem.* **26**, 496–512.

Taylor, C. R. (1980). *J. Histochem. Cytochem.* **28**, 777–787.

Tönder, O., Milgrom, F., and Witebsky, E. (1964). *J. Exp. Med.* **119**, 265–273.

Trost, T. H., Weil, H. P., Pullman, H., and Steigler, G. K. (1980). *Klin. Wochenschr.* **58**, 475–478.

Tubbs, R. R., and Sheibani, K. (1981). *J. Histochem. Cytochem.* **29**, 684.

Tubbs, R. R., Velasco, M. E., and Benjamin, S. P. (1979). *Arch. Pathol. Lab. Med.* **103**, 534–536.

Vacca, L. L., Abrahams, S. J., and Naftchi, N. E. (1980). *J. Histochem. Cytochem.* **28**, 297–307.

Vandesande, F., and Dierickx, K. (1976). *Cell Tissue Res.* **175**, 289–296.

van Nagell, J. R., Donaldson, E. S., Gay, E. C., Sharkey, R. M., Rayburn, P., and Goldenberg, D. M. (1978). *Cancer* **41**, 2335–2340.

van Nagell, J. R., Donaldson, E. S., Gay, E. S., Hudson, S., Sharkey, R. M., Primus, F. J., Powell, D. F., and Goldenberg, D. M. (1979). *Cancer* **44**, 944–948.

Wagener, C., Csaszar, H., Totovic, V., and Breur, H. (1978). *Histochemistry* **58**, 1–11.

Wahlström, T., Stenman, U-H., Lundquist, C., Tanner, P., Schröder, J., and Seppälä, M. (1981). *J. Histochem. Cytochem.* **29**, 864–865.

Waldmann, T. A., and McIntire, K. R. (1979). *In* "Immunodiagnosis of Cancer" (R. B. Herberman and K. R. McIntire, eds.), pp. 130–147. Dekker, New York.

Warnke, R., and Levy, R. (1980). *J. Histochem. Cytochem.* **28**, 771–776.

Warnke, R., and Levy, R. (1981). *In* "Diagnostic Immunohistochemistry" (R. A. DeLellis, ed.), pp. 203–211. Masson, Paris.

Warnke, R., Miller, R., Grogan, T., Pederson, M., Dilley, J., and Levy, R. (1980). *N. Engl. J. Med.* **303**, 293–300.

Weinstein, R. S., Alroy, J., Farrow, G. M., Miller, A. W., and Davidsohn, I. (1979). *Cancer* **43**, 661–668.

Weinstein, R. S., Coon, J., Alroy, J., and Davidsohn, I. (1981). *In* "Diagnostic Immunohistochemistry" (R. A. DeLellis, ed.), pp. 239–261. Masson, Paris.

Weir, E. E. Pretlow, T. G., II., Pitts, A., and Williams, E. E. (1974a). *J. Histochem. Cytochem.* **22**, 1135–1140.

Weir, E. E., and Pretlow, T. G., II, Pitts, A., and Williams, E. E. (1974b). *J. Histochem. Cytochem.* **22**, 51–54.

Wiley, E. L., Mendelsohn, G., and Eggleston, J. C. (1981). *Lab. Invest.* **44**, 507–513.

Wilson, M. G., and Kakane, P. K. (1978). *In* "Immunofluorescence and Related Staining Techniques" (W. Knapp, K. Holibar, and G. Wick, eds.), pp. 215–224. Elsevier, Amsterdam.

Yamanaka, N., Ishii, Y., Koshiba, H., Mikuni, C., Ogasawara, M., and Kikuchi, K. (1981). *Cancer* **47**, 311–318.

CHAPTER V

IMMUNOELECTRON MICROSCOPY

PAUL K. NAKANE

I. Introduction

Immunoelectron microscopy (IEM) is a technique designed to define sites of antigens and/or antibodies at the ultrastructural level. In this review, the scope will be limited to the localization of antigens within cells and tissues by transmission electron microscopy (TEM) and scanning electron microscopy (SEM).

The conditions required for a successful localization of antigens are many; some are general to immunohistochemistry, some are unique to transmission immunoelectron microscopy (TIEM) and scanning immunoelectron microscopy (SIEM). Those unique to IEM include the following: (1) The sites of antibody bound to intracellular antigens must be recognizable either by TEM or by SEM, (2) both the antigenicity and the ultrastructure must be preserved, (3) the antigen must remain fixed at its native habitat so that it can be accurately localized, and (4) the antigen(s) must be accessible to the antibody (which is true for any immunohistochemical procedure).

II. Antibody Markers

A. ELECTRON-DENSE MARKERS

For TIEM, the first requirement can be satisfied in either of two ways. First, the antibody can be labeled with an electron-dense material such as ferritin or colloidal gold. Ferritin is a molecule which has a diameter of 12 nm, a molecular weight of 650,000, and contains four micelles of iron at the center of the molecule which are responsible for its high electron density. Two methods for the conjugation of ferritin with antibodies are given in the Appendix, Section IX,A. Colloidal gold in complex with either immunoglobulin (Ig) or protein A from *Staphylococcus aureus* has been introduced more recently in immunoelectron microscopy (see review by Goodman *et al.,* 1980). They have high electron densities and their sizes may be manipulated during preparation (5–15 nm in diameter). Methods for the preparation of colloidal gold complexes are given in the Appendix, Section IX,B.

B. ENZYMATIC MARKERS

Second, the antibody can be labeled with an enzyme such as horseradish peroxidase (HRPO) (Nakane and Pierce, 1967). In this case, the enzyme sites are recognized histochemically by depositing reaction products which form an electron-dense material.

A variety of enzymes have been tried as markers. Our selection of an enzyme marker is based on the following conditions: (1) The enzyme must be available in relatively pure form from a commercial source; this condition avoids the often cumbersome procedures required for isolating a given enzyme in your own laboratory. (2) The enzyme can be localized by well-established histochemical means; again, this condition avoids the necessity of having to develop such methods. (3) The stability of the enzyme must be good; this allows one to use a single preparation of conjugated antibody over a period of years and avoids the problems encountered when one has an immunoglobulin labeled with inactive enzyme which will behave as an unlabeled antibody. (4) The enzyme should be as small as possible; this condition is necessary because often the enzyme-labeled antibody must be able to penetrate into tissue or tissue sections in order to localize an antigen deep within the cell or even within the nucleus of the cell. (5) The enzyme selected as a marker should have a relatively high turnover rate; this is important because one of the fundamental benefits of using the enzyme as a marker is the amplifying ability of the enzyme resulting in a more sensitive detection method. (6) The enzyme should be absent in generally used tissues such as mammalian tissues; this condition is desirable, although not mandatory, since endogenous enzyme activity can often be selectively abolished so that one will not confuse endogenous enzymatic activity with that of the enzyme which was used as a label.

Horseradish peroxidase meets all of these conditions, with the exception of the sixth. There is endogenous peroxidase activity in some tissues, particularly in leukocytes, erythrocytes, and the thyroid and mammary glands. However, several methods have been used to successfully abolish this endogenous activity (see Appendix, Section IX,K). Horseradish peroxidase is a heme-containing, glycoprotein enzyme which has a molecular weight of 40,000. The molecule consists of an outer shell of eight carbohydrate chains, which comprises 18% of the molecular weight of the molecule, and a heme–protein core consisting of approximately 300 amino acids. The carbohydrate shell is not essential for enzymatic activity. Horseradish peroxidase functions as a marker by catalyzing the oxidation of a hydrogen donor, usually 3,3'-diaminobenzidine (DAB), in the presence of hydrogen peroxide. This enzymatic reaction deposits polymers of diaminobenzidine at the site of the enzyme. Electron density is imparted by chelating the diaminobenzidine polymer with osmium tetroxide (Graham and Karnovsky, 1966). Three methods of labeling antibodies with peroxidase are given in the Appendix, Sections IX,C and D.

C. SCANNING ELECTRON MICROSCOPY MARKERS

Unlike TIEM, the most frequently employed markers for SIEM utilize the physical characteristics of size and shape rather than electron density for their localization. Examples of such markers are latex spheres, viruses, silicon particles, hemocyanin, etc. (Moldey *et al.*, 1975; DeHarven *et al.*, 1979; Peters *et al.*, 1976; Miller and Teplitz, 1978), which can be visualized using the secondary electron detection mode at the antigen sites. With improvements in the resolution capabilities of SEM, smaller markers such as ferritin, colloidal gold, and reaction products of enzymes are beginning to be utilized (Hattori *et al.*, 1976; Goodman *et al.*, 1979; Becker and DeBruyn, 1976; Carr and McGradey, 1974). The use of size- and shape-dependent markers is limited to localization of antigens on the surface. This limitation is imposed by either the inability of the marker-labeled antibody to penetrate into cells and tissues or the inability to detect these markers once below the surface. The ability to increase the secondary electron emission by the reaction product deposited at the antigen site by enzyme-labeled antibody has been described (Nakane and Hartman, 1980); however, this method suffers from a lack of sensitivity. More recently, other physical signals generated by the impact of the electron beam on the label have come into use. The detection of cathodoluminescence originating from fluorescein-labeled antibody has been reported; however, the instability of this marker under the electron beam limits its practicality (Springer *et al.*, 1974). The most widely used method for detection of intracellular enzymes or enzyme-labeled antibodies by SEM has been backscattered electron imaging (BSI) (Hartman and Nakane, 1981). Unlike secondary electrons which have a low energy level and are readily absorbed by surrounding tissue components such as the plasma membrane, backscattered electrons have a high energy level and can pass through these components and reach the detectors. Therefore, BSI can be used to detect substances beneath the surface of a specimen. With BSI, the signal intensity is proportional to the atomic number of the substance bombarded by the primary electron beam. Thus, one can use BSI to detect osmium tetroxide which is chelated to the diaminobenzidine polymers deposited at the site of the peroxidase-labeled antibodies.

III. Antibody Penetration

A. FACTORS AFFECTING PENETRATION

The choice of a marker for TIEM depends primarily upon the location of the sought antigen. Antigens can be localized within tissues or cells, upon cell surfaces, or upon the surfaces of ultrathin sections. If the antigen is to be localized within solid tissue or within cells, the antibody conjugate must be able to penetrate to the site of the antigen. The following factors affect the penetration of the conjugate:

1. The size of the conjugate, which is a function of both the size of the label and the size of the antibody. The smaller the conjugate, the more easily it can diffuse into cells, particularly through membranes. Thus, F(ab)' fragments (MW 46,000) of IgG diffuse more easily than whole IgG molecules (MW 156,000) (Nakane, 1975). The addition of the label to the antibody significantly retards its diffusibility. This effect is less with smaller labels. Antibodies labeled with peroxidase (MW 40,000) can penetrate tissue sections; in contrast, antibodies labeled with ferritin (MW 650,000) or peroxidase–antiperoxidase (PAP) complexes (MW 440,000) are useful only for surface staining due to their inability to penetrate well-fixed tissue. To minimize the size of the enzymatic marker, a heme octapeptide fragment of cytochrome c (MW 1500) with peroxidative activity has been used (Kraehenbuhl et al., 1974). However, this marker has not yet gained widespread usage.

2. The condition of the tissue, particularly the nature of the membranes. Since the plasma membranes of living cells are completely impermeable to immunoglobulins or their fragments, pores through the membranes must be created to allow antibody penetration into the cells. The simplest and most commonly used method of creating pores is by fixation. The size of the pore depends upon the type of fixative employed. It is generally agreed that the better the fixative is for ultrastructure, the smaller the pore it creates. In addition, a variety of other methods have been used to create pores, including the use of the following: detergents, such as Triton X-100 (Pickel et al., 1976), digitonin (Dales and Gomatos, 1965), and saponin (Graham et al., 1967; Seemen, 1967; Bohn, 1978); organic solvents, such as acetone, for lipid extraction; enzymes, such as trypsin, neuraminidase, hyaluronidase, and papain (Mazurkiewicz and Nakane, 1972; Kuhlmann et al., 1974); and means such as freeze-thawing, which causes mechanical damage to membranes (Morgan et al., 1961; Nakane, 1975). Although tissue penetrability by conjugates can be improved by the use of such physically or chemically induced membrane pores, there are disadvantages. Detergents and organic solvents often adversely affect the preservation of membrane morphology and extract some subcellular components. Enzymes have a variable effect on membranes, often producing patchy staining which may correlate poorly with antigen distribution (Kuhlmann et al., 1974), and freeze-thawing adversely affects the morphology of the entire tissue due to destruction caused by the formation of ice crystals (Nakane, 1975).

3. The physical environment of the antigen and antibody. This includes ambient temperature, duration of exposure to the antibody, and mechanical agitation of the sample during incubation with the antibody.

Because of a significant advantage in terms of minimum weight and size, peroxidase-labeled Fab or F(ab)' fragments are preferred for the localization of antigen in solid tissue or cells. An additional advantage of using Fab or F(ab)' fragments (which lack the Fc portion of the immunoglobulin molecule) is that these labeled antibodies will not bind to Fc receptors (Arali *et al.*, 1975; Itoh and Suzuki, 1977) or complement in tissues (Buffa *et al.*, 1979).

B. Surface Localization

There are two situations in which antigens are localized upon surfaces with TIEM. The first is the natural occurrence of antigens upon the surfaces of cells, such as immunoglobulins on the surfaces of lymphocytes (Hammond, 1970; Gonatas *et al.*, 1972). The only factors cited above which affect antigen accessibility in this instance are physical–environmental factors. The size of the conjugate and the nature of the membranes are not so important since antibodies need not penetrate the tissue or traverse membranes.

The second situation in which antigens are localized upon surfaces is the localization of antigens on ultrathin sections of either unembedded or embedded tissue. Although virtually no one at present localizes antigens on the surface of ultrathin sections of fresh tissues, antigens have been localized in ultrathin sections of fixed unembedded tissues (Leduc *et al.*, 1969). In handling ultrathin sections of embedded tissue, the antigens must first be made accessible on the surface of the sections by either "etching" or dissolving the embedding medium (Kawarai and Nakane, 1970). There are several factors which must be considered when localizing antigens on the surfaces of ultrathin sections of embedded tissues:

1. The effect of the embedding medium on antigenicity. In peptide hormone-producing cells, the hormones within secretion granules can be localized; however, antigens within the endoplasmic reticulum are not usually detectable. This is attributed to interference of the embedding media with antigens. There is evidence that the embedding medium can react with antigens and thereby decrease or abolish the antigenicity. For example, the antigenicity of immunoglobulin molecules embedded in styrene cannot be recovered by exposing the section to acetone, a solvent for

styrene. However, antigenicity can be recovered by exposing the section to protease, which enzymatically removes reacted styrene, thereby exposing antigenic sites (Vogt *et al.*, 1976). Another example is the different degree to which the antigenicity of different pituitary peptides is preserved in methacrylate or Epon (Nakane, 1971).

2. The effect of the embedding medium on the labeled antibody. For example, ferritin-labeled antibodies are not used to localize antigens on the surfaces of Epon-embedded tissues because of the high nonspecific affinity of ferritin for embedding media (Singer and McLean, 1963).

3. The type of embedding medium used. For example, embedding in methacrylate results in a greater loss of morphology, especially of membrane morphology, than does embedding in epoxy resins. However, antigenicity is often better preserved in methacrylate than in epoxy resin.

C. Methods of Choice

In summary, with TIEM, peroxidase-labeled antibodies or antibody fragments are best used for localizing antigens within tissues or within cells. In contrast, ferritin- or colloidal gold-labeled antibodies are best used for localizing antigens on cell surfaces or on ultrathin sections of unembedded tissues, and colloidal gold-labeled antibodies or PAP are best used for localizing antigens on ultrathin sections of embedded tissues. With SEM, the intracellular antigens are best localized with peroxidase-labeled antibodies when 3,3'-diaminobenzidine and H_2O_2 are used as substrate. On the surfaces of tissues and cells, antibodies which are labeled with morphologically recognizable particles, such as hemocyanin and virus particles, are recommended.

IV. Fixation

The first thing that one must consider before performing any type of immunohistochemistry is the preparation of tissues for immunocytochemistry. In this regard, there are several conditions which must be met. If an antigen is partially or completely soluble in aqueous media, one must be able to fix it as closely as possible to its native habitat. In accomplishing this we are faced with a paradox, since the majority of antigens we localize are proteins and the majority of fixatives involve the denaturation of proteins. Therefore, one is usually forced to select a midpoint where the proteins are fixed weakly enough to retain antigenicity, yet strongly enough to maintain cellular and tissue morphology and distribution.

Hence, the preservation of morphology in immunohistochemistry, in general, is somewhat mediocre when compared to routine electron microscopy.

A. HEAVY METAL FIXATIVES

There are two general categories of fixatives useful for IEM: heavy metal fixatives and cross-linking fixatives. Osmium is the only heavy metal fixative used for IEM. It fixes lipids and proteins by reacting at multiple sites. Advantages of using osmium as a fixative are that it is excellent at preserving morphology, it imparts electron density, and it can be removed from the tissue at a later time (Baskin *et al.*, 1979). Disadvantages are that the loss of antigenicity is often excessive and that it chelates free diaminobenzidine during the enzymatic reaction step when peroxidase is used as the tracer.

B. CROSS-LINKING FIXATIVES: THE ALDEHYDES

Among the cross-linking fixatives, the most commonly used group is the aldehydes, either alone or in combination with other reagents. Acrolein, a monoaldehyde, is the most reactive aldehyde; however, it is rarely used in IEM. Glutaraldehyde, a bifunctional dialdehyde, provides excellent preservation of morphology; however, it has the disadvantage of often decreasing or destroying antigenicity. This is especially true in the case of protein antigens because of the extensive cross-linking of amino groups. Formaldehyde, a monoaldehyde, cross-links proteins primarily between α and ϵ amino groups. Although antigenicity is not as severely affected as with glutaraldehyde, preservation of morphology is not as good as with glutaraldehyde. The combination of formaldehyde with other reagents has produced better fixatives. For example, formaldehyde, when combined with picric acid (Stefanini *et al.*, 1967), a protein precipitant, results in a fixative which retains the ultrastructural morphology and preserves adequate antigenicity for immunohistochemical localization for some antigens (Nakane, 1971). In addition, mixtures of formaldehyde and glutaraldehyde in low concentrations have also been successfully used for IEM (Pickel *et al.*, 1975).

Efforts in our laboratory directed at overcoming the problem of morphology versus antigenicity resulted in the development of the periodate–lysine–paraformaldehyde (PLP) fixative (McLean and Nakane, 1974). This fixative takes advantage of the fact that although most of the antibodies we use are directed against antigenic determinants which are protein in nature, many of these molecules are not pure proteins but are gly-coproteins. Because the carbohydrate portion of these molecules is not part of the antigenic site, one should be able to fix the antigen via the car-bohydrate portion of the molecule without loss of antigenicity. This can be done by oxidizing the carbohydrate moieties with sodium metaperio-date, which results in the formation of aldehyde groups. These newly formed aldehyde groups can then be cross-linked by a diamino compound such as lysine. While this type of fixation through carbohydrate moieties gives excellent retention of antigenicity, it by itself does not give adequate morphological preservation. However, by adding low concentrations of paraformaldehyde (1–2%) to the periodate–lysine solution, one can ob-tain good morphological preservation while retaining sufficient antigen-icity for immunohistochemical localization of most glycoprotein antigens. Other fixatives which fix by cross-linking but are not aldehydes include carbodiimide (Polak *et al.*, 1972) and diethyl malonimidate (McLean and Singer, 1970).

As should be clear by now, there is no single fixative of choice for IEM. The factor which most affects the choice of the fixative is the nature of the antigen. The degree of the loss of antigenicity with a given fixative varies considerably from one antigen to another. The antigenicity of peptide hor-mones appears to be one of the most resistant to destruction by fixatives and will frequently survive fixation in either osmium tetroxide (Kawarai and Nakane, 1970; Li *et al.*, 1977) or glutaraldehyde (Moriarty and Helmi, 1972). On the other hand, the antigenicity of immunoglobulins is easily lost and requires mild fixation by such compounds as PLP (McLean and Nakane, 1974; Brown *et al.*, 1976) or paraformaldehyde in low concentra-tions (Kraehenbuhl *et al.*, 1974).

C. SPECIAL FIXATIVES

Special fixatives must be used for lipids and steroids. Membrane lipids can be fixed either in OsO_4 in aqueous solution (Nielson and Griffith, 1979) or with a 0.2% solution of digitonin (digitonin stabilizes membranes by binding with cholesterol) in a 2.5% glutaraldehyde solution (Saland and Napolitano, 1977). Steroids have been localized for IEM with similar types of fixatives. For example, testosterone has been localized with 2% glutaraldehyde (Childs *et al.*, 1978), pregnenolone with a glutaraldehyde–digitonin mixture, and progesterone and corticosterone by a three-step process using glutaraldehyde, followed by sodium borohydride with digi-tonin, followed by PLP (Mukai and Nakane, 1976).

Additional factors which affect fixation and should also be considered are the manner in which the fixative is applied and the physical conditions of fixation. Although fixation by perfusion is theoretically ideal, fixation by immersion is usually adequate if the tissue is sufficiently small. The ambient temperature, pH, osmolarity of the fixative, and agitation of the specimen are important in determining the quality and rate of fixation.

V. Tissue Handling

A. Solid Pieces and Sections

The manner in which tissue is handled has a significant effect on the end result of IEM. Tissue can be handled as solid pieces, as sections mounted on slides, or as ultrathin sections. Pieces of solid tissue can be obtained in several different forms: (1) as small blocks hand-cut to minimum dimensions (Andres *et al.*, 1966); (2) as tissue sectioned to 35 to 150 μm in thickness by a tissue chopper (Smith and Farquhar, 1963); (3) as tissue sectioned to 10 to 100 μm by a Vibratome (Smith, 1970); and (4) as tissue sectioned to between 5 and 50 μm by a cryostat (Nakane and Pierce, 1966).

Tissue obtained by these means can be incubated in solutions of antibodies by immersion as free-floating blocks or sections. This approach avoids impairment of antigenicity by the embedding medium and allows access of the tissue to antibodies from all sides. However, there are several significant disadvantages. In practice, a significant amount of tissue is lost during the multiple steps involved in IEM. Also, it is difficult to orient the tissues, as well as to make an appropriate assessment of the specificity of the staining and of the penetration of the immunologic reagents into the tissues.

Alternatively, sections of fixed tissue from 5 to 30 μm in thickness obtained with either a Vibratome or a cryostat can be mounted on slides for immunostaining. If cryostat sections are used, the adverse effect on ultrastructural morphology resulting from freezing should be minimized by prior infiltration of the tissue with a cryoprotective agent such as 10% dimethyl sulfoxide, 10 to 80% sucrose, or 10 to 20% glycerol. In order to secure the sections to the glass slides, the slides must be coated with albumin or gelatin treated with glutaraldehyde (Mazurkiewicz and Nakane, 1972) or carbon (Hartman and Nakane, 1981) (see Appendix, Section IX,G).

The advantages of using sections mounted on slides are that the orientation of the tissue is maintained, the tissue can be sectioned sufficiently thin to ensure penetration of the immunologic reagents, the amount of reagents used is minimized, serial sections may be obtained and used for the variety of necessary controls for IEM, and the tissues may be examined conveniently with a light microscope during any step of processing for electron microscopy. The major disadvantage of this approach is that frequently the section shrinks or fragments during polymerization of the embedding medium due to adherence to the slide. This can be minimized by the use of smaller sections, by treating the sections with gelatin (Watanabe, personal communication), or by using an embedding medium such as Epon–Araldite instead of Epon alone.

B. ULTRATHIN SECTIONS

For the localization of antigens on ultrathin sections, two types are used: ultrathin sections of fixed, frozen tissue, or ultrathin sections of tissue embedded in a support medium, such as methacrylate or epoxy resin. When ultrathin sections of embedded tissue are used, the following characteristics of the embedding medium must be considered:

1. The effect of the medium on morphology (i.e., shrinkage of size or distortion of morphology)
2. The selective extraction of cellular constituents [i.e., secretory granules may dissolve and thereby be removed by infiltration with methacrylate (Kawarai and Nakane, 1970)]
3. Any impairment of antigenicity (the effect of embedding media on antigenicity has already been discussed)
4. The removability of the embedding medium to increase the accessibility of the antibodies to antigenic sites
5. Nonspecific absorption of labeled antibodies, such as ferritin-labeled antibodies which readily absorb nonspecifically to hydrophobic embedding media.

The following embedding media have been successfully used for immunohistochemical localization on ultrathin sections: glutaraldehyde-crosslinked albumin (McLean and Singer, 1970); a mixture of methyl and butyl methacrylate (Kawarai and Nakane, 1970); glycol methacrylate (Shahrabadi and Yamamoto, 1971); epoxy resins, including the Epon–Araldite mixture (Moriarty and Helmi, 1972; Nakane, 1971); and Spurr's medium (Moriarty, 1973). A disadvantage of all these media, except for crosslinked albumin, is that accessibility of antigenic sites to antibodies must be gained by "etching" the surface of the ultrathin sections of the embedded tissue. The following agents have been used for etching: a saturated aqueous solution of xylene or benzene for methacrylate (Kawarai and Nakane, 1970) and, for etching epoxy resins, a 0.1% solution of benzene in a 10% methanol or ethanol aqueous solution, a 10% hydrogen peroxide solution (Nakane, 1971), or a dilute solution of sodium ethoxide (Rodning *et al.*, 1978).

With ultrathin frozen sections, etching agents need not be used. These ultrathin sections are usually incubated in the antibody solutions using Marinozzi rings to support the tissue (Leduc *et al.*, 1969; Tokuyasu, 1973).

The first factor which affects the choice of a particular method for tissue handling is whether the orientation of the tissue is to be maintained. For example, a time sequence study of the movement of IgM and secretory components across gastrointestinal epithelium necessitates maintaining the orientation of the tissue (Brown *et al.*, 1976). In such a situation, large pieces of tissue must be used, for which the slide-mounted method is best.

If orientation need not be preserved, either ultrathin sections or solid tissue pieces can be used. The choice between these techniques depends upon the effect of the factors just identified. For example, if the embedding medium abolishes antigenicity, ultrathin sections of embedded tissue cannot be used.

C. Tissue for SEM

Methods of tissue preparation for SIEM are essentially identical to the slide-mounted method used for TIEM. The immunostained tissue sections may be embedded in Epon and sectioned at 1 to 2 μm in thickness and placed on a carbon- or indium-coated glass microscope slide and examined by a SEM (Hartman and Nakane, 1981). Since the reaction products of peroxidase can not be recognized readily with the secondary electron detection mode of SEM, it is essential that a backscattered electron mode of SEM be used (Becker and DeBruyn, 1976; Carr and McGradey, 1974). The intensity of detectable backscattered electrons is proportional to the atomic number and, as in TIEM, detection of the antigenic site is via detection of the osmium which has reacted with polymerized diaminobenzidine. In order to ground the surface of the glass slide, it is recommended that the surface be coated lightly with carbon by means of vacuum evaporation.

In addition to the use of immunostained tissue sections embedded in Epon, immunostained whole-cell or tissue sections may be examined by

SEM without the embedding steps. For this approach, the cells or tissue must be dehydrated either by the critical point drying method or by lyophilization. One major difference in tissue or cell preparation for this approach is the step of osmication. The concentration of osmium tetroxide should be reduced to 0.5–0.1% and the duration of osmication should be shortened to 2–10 minutes (Hartman and Nakane, 1981). The conditions of osmication used for TIEM will result in overosmication of general tissue and cell organelles, making it difficult to recognize osmicated DAB polymers from the other cellular structures.

The enzyme reaction product can be detected by SEM with the same degree of sensitivity as by light microscopy. When compared to TEM, the sensitivity again appears to be approximately equal, as judged by the ability of SEM to detect reaction product in ultrathin sections of Epon-embedded tissues. A major difference in comparison to TEM, however, is the lack of resolution. Under the conditions thus far employed, we are able to clearly resolve stained secretion granules of approximately 300 nm in diameter; however, the membrane surrounding the granules could not be resolved. Whether the backscatter mode will ever achieve the resolution obtainable with TEM is doubtful, though with improvements in instrumentation we may reach with backscatter imaging the resolution currently obtainable using the secondary electron mode. Observation by the secondary electron mode of the same area examined using the backscatter mode can be helpful in establishing the ultrastructural relationship between antigen location and surface topography.

VI. Nonspecific Staining

There are additional factors which must be considered in IEM. Nonspecific staining can result from two sources: endogenous peroxidase and nonspecific affinity of the antibodies for components in the tissue or embedding medium.

A. ENDOGENOUS PEROXIDASE ACTIVITY

Endogenous peroxidase-like compounds are normally present within red blood cells, neutrophils, eosinophils, monocytes, and histiocytes, including such tissue histiocytes as Kupffer cells. Unless the sought antigen occurs or is suspected to occur within one of these cell types, such endogenous peroxidase activity can usually be ignored since these cells can be readily identified. However, if the sought antigen occurs within one of these cell types, then the endogenous peroxidase activity must be removed prior to staining. There are a number of procedures which can be used to block the endogenous activity (see Appendix, Section IX,K).

B. NONSPECIFIC AFFINITY OF ANTIBODIES

Nonspecific affinity of antibodies can produce "false-positive" staining by several mechanisms:

1. Fc receptors and/or nonspecific Fc tissue interactions which are present in significant concentrations in the neuroglial tissue of the brain (Itoh and Suzuki, 1977) and on white blood cells (Buffa *et al.*, 1979) can bind whole immunoglobulin molecules. The use of Fab fragments obviates this problem.
2. Highly acidic tissues, such as placenta and necrotic tissue, can nonspecifically bind immunoglobulin.
3. Some embedding media, such as the methacrylates, have a stronger affinity for antibodies than such media as the epoxy resins. Most embedding media have a strong affinity for ferritin, which is a disadvantage of using ferritin-labeled antibodies on ultrathin sections of embedded tissue. Nonspecific binding of labeled antibodies to the embedding material can be significantly decreased by incubation of the sections with preimmune serum from the same animal species in which the labeled antibody was generated.
4. Antibodies can aggregate to form polymers, which have a greater nonspecific affinity for tissue. The use of immunoglobulin fragments and of all antibody solutions at the greatest possible dilutions which do not decrease staining intensity decreases the amount of antibody aggregation. Filtration of antibody solutions through Millipore filters before use can also remove large antibody aggregates.
5. Ferritin, regardless of whether it is conjugated to an antibody, has nonspecific affinity for intracellular components, particularly for membranes and for the endoplasmic reticulum (Parr, 1979). This can be a problem when using ferritin-labeled antibodies on ultrathin sections.

VII. False-Positive Reactions

There are several additional false-positive reactions which, since they cannot be practically or, perhaps, even theoretically circumvented limit the usefulness and applicability of IEM in certain situations.

A. Cross-Reactivity of Antibodies

The first type is a consequence of a similarity of antigenic determinants. Immunoelectron microscopy localizes antigenic determinants, not molecules. Hence, the smaller the antigenic determinants in the sought molecule, the greater the likelihood that there are different, perhaps functionally unrelated molecules which have identical antigenic determinants. These other molecules with common antigenic determinants will bind the antibody against the sought antigen and will thus result in false-positive localization of the sought antigen. Examples of molecules with common antigenic determinants are gastrin and cholecystokinin (Vaillant *et al.*, 1979) and vasoactive intestinal polypeptide (VIP) and VIP-like compounds in some colonic endocrine cells (Larson *et al.*, 1979).

B. Complex Binding to Antigen Receptors

The second type of false-positive reaction results from the binding of antigen–antibody complexes to antigen binding sites. Presumably, during immunization of an animal, antibodies are produced against the homologous antigen in the animal. If this antigen is a circulating substance, the serum of the immunized animal will contain antigen–antibody complexes. These antigen–antibody complexes cannot easily be detected and distinguished from free, noncomplexed antibodies by the usual methods of immunoglobulin isolation, especially if the antigen is small relative to the size of the antibody. The following are examples of binding sites which will localize the immune complex and thus produce false positivity: (1) enzymes for which the antigen is a substrate, (2) cell surface of cytoplasmic receptors, and (3) transport proteins specific to the antigen. In such cases, IEM will not have localized the antigen, but rather a binding site for the antigen. The presence in antisera of such immune complexes which may bind to antigen binding sites can be inferred if, upon addition of small aliquots of antigen, staining is not blocked but is increased. This technique has been used to identify luteinizing hormone-releasing hormone in the pituitary (Sternberger and Petrali, 1975; Sternberger *et al.*, 1978).

The existence of such sources of false positivity in IEM makes the performance of other confirmatory experiments to corroborate evidence obtained by IEM paramount.

VIII. Staining Methods

There are several sequences in the application of immunologic reagents for the localization of antigens. Examples are given using peroxidase as a

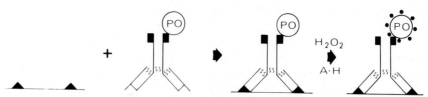

FIG. 1. The direct peroxidase-labeled antibody method.

marker. When other methods (i.e., ferritin or colloidal gold) are used, the histochemical steps are not necessary.

A. DIRECT ANTIBODY METHOD

One of the simplest methods used for immunohistochemical localization of antigens is the so-called "direct" method using whole immunoglobulins labeled with peroxidase (Fig. 1). An antibody labeled with peroxidase is reacted with tissue antigen, resulting in the formation of immune complexes with the antigen, and the sites of these immune complexes are then visualized histochemically through the deposition of reaction products at the enzyme sites (i.e., the antigen sites).

B. INDIRECT ANTIBODY METHOD

The indirect method involves one more step than the direct method (Fig. 2). An unlabeled antibody is allowed to form an immune complex with the tissue antigen. The antibody attached to the antigen is subse-

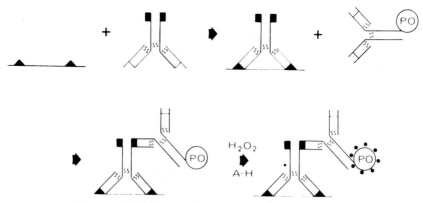

FIG. 2. The indirect peroxidase-labeled antibody method.

quently localized using a peroxidase-labeled antibody directed against the first antibody (antiantibody) or peroxidase-labeled protein A. Finally, the peroxidase is localized histochemically in the same manner as in the direct method.

C. BRIDGE METHOD

More recently, several steps of the procedure have been modified. The modification introduced by Spicer *et al.* (1976) is the so-called "bridge method" (Fig. 3). An unlabeled antibody is allowed to form an immune complex with tissue antigen as in the indirect method. Then antibody against the first antibody is reacted with the antibody. If an excess of antiantibody is used, one expects some antigen binding sites of the antiantibody to remain unoccupied. An antiperoxidase antibody which was produced in the same species as the first antibody is then reacted with the unoccupied antigen binding site of the antiantibody. Next the antibody against peroxidase is reacted with peroxidase and the peroxidase sites are finally visualized histochemically.

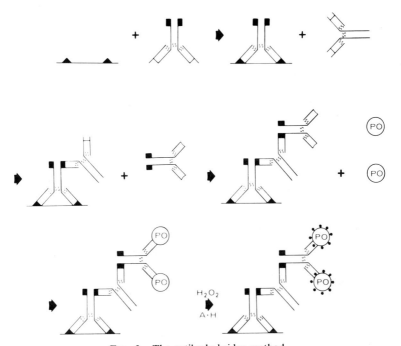

FIG. 3. The antibody bridge method.

200   PAUL K. NAKANE

The major advantage of this method is that it does not require a chemical conjugation of peroxidase to an immunoglobulin. However, when using this method, several aspects should be kept in mind. First, the antienzyme must be produced in the same species as the first antibody. Second, the antienzyme should not be admixed with other nonspecific antibodies. When there are other immunoglobulins admixed with the antienzyme, there is a dilution phenomenon since the other antibodies will bind equally well to the unoccupied antigen binding site of the antiantibody. Third, when the enzyme is coupled with an antienzyme, the activity of enzyme must be maintained. If this antibody inhibits the activity of the enzyme, the enzyme site (i.e., the antigen site) cannot be recognized.

D. PEROXIDASE–ANTIPEROXIDASE METHOD

To overcome this last problem, Sternberger *et al.* (1970) introduced another modification, the so-called peroxidase–antiperoxidase method (Fig. 4). Instead of sequentially applying antiperoxidase and peroxidase, they employed a soluble PAP immune complex. The use of isolated immune complexes avoids the problems arising in the bridge method from the admixing of nonspecific immunoglobulins. The deposition site of PAP is

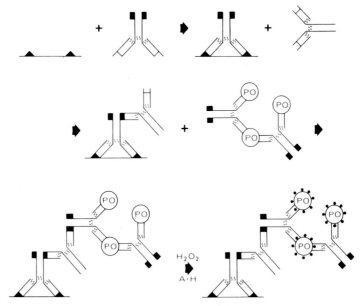

FIG. 4.   The peroxidase–antiperoxidase method.

then visualized histochemically as with the other methods. With this modification there is still the requirement that one antigen binding site of antiantibody must remain unoccupied prior to the application of the peroxidase–antiperoxidase complex.

In recent years, Fab or F(ab)' fragments of IgG have been utilized more frequently. The Fab or F(ab)' fragments of immunoglobulin can be labeled directly with peroxidase. In this way, the monovalent antibody will bind to the antigen and the enzyme on the Fab is subsequently localized histochemically. A similar method can be used in an indirect manner. In this case, Fab of the first antibody is used and then followed with peroxidase-labeled Fab of antiantibody. Finally, the peroxidase is localized histochemically. There are two reasons for the use of Fab or F(ab)' fragments (Nakane, 1975). First, the use of Fab or F(ab)' results in a drastic reduction in the nonspecific binding of immunoglobulin to tissues. Second, the reduction in the size of immunoglobulin and its conjugates results in an increased tissue penetrability.

IX. Appendix

A. PREPARATION OF FERRITIN-LABELED ANTIBODIES

1. Two-Step Toluene 2,4-Diisocyanate Coupling Procedure (Singer and Schick, 1961)

1. To 5.0 ml of a 1.5% horse spleen ferritin solution in 0.1 M phosphate buffer, pH 7.5, at 0°C, add 0.1 ml of toluene 2,4-diisocyanate and vigorously stir in an ice bath at 0°C for 25 minutes.

2. Centrifuge for about 0.5 hour at a speed sufficient to pellet the unreacted diisocyanate without sedimenting any appreciable amount of ferritin, approximately 1000 g, and carefully remove the supernatant and allow it to stand for 1 hour at 0°C.

3. Add 5.0 ml of a 1.5% solution of γ-globulin in 0.1 M borate buffer, pH 9.5, at 37°C, and maintain at 37°C for 1 hour.

4. Dialyze against 0.1 M $(NH_4)_2CO_3$.

2. Two-Step Glutaraldehyde Coupling Procedure (Otto et al., 1973)

1. Dissolve 50 to 80 mg of horse spleen ferritin in 1.0 ml of a 0.02–0.2% glutaraldehyde solution (obtained as a 25% solution, freshly diluted before use in 0.1 M phosphate buffer, pH 7.0).

2. React the ferritin and glutaraldehyde for 2 hours at 37°C under gentle agitation.

3. Separate the unreacted glutaraldehyde from glutaraldehyde-bound ferritin by fractionating the solution through a Sephadex G-25 fine column (25 × 1.6 cm) with the 0.1 M phosphate buffer and collect only the middle section of the ferritin peak (can be seen as brown).

4. To the ferritin solution add 10 to 16 mg of γ-globulin dissolved in approximately 1 ml of 0.1 M phosphate buffer.

5. Let the reaction mixture stand 12 to 24 hours at 37°C without stirring.

6. Add 1 ml of 0.01 M lysine to stop further cross-linkage between ferritin and γ-globulin and to block the remaining aldehydes. The final approximate concentration of ferritin should be 15 mg/ml, and of γ-globulin, 3 mg/ml.

7. Unreacted ferritin and free globulin are separated from the ferritin-labeled antibodies by preparative electrophoresis in the Geon block with barbital buffer, pH 8.6, and ionic strength 0.05.

With the above method, approximately 50 and 70% of the ferritin conjugated with γ-globulin when 0.1 and 0.125% glutaraldehyde was used, respectively (Otto et al., 1973).

B. PREPARATION OF COLLOIDAL GOLD

Colloidal gold can be prepared either as a sol of particles of similar diameter (monodisperse) or as particles with a heterogeneous diameter (polydisperse).

1. Monodisperse Suspension of Colloidal Gold (Diameter About 150 Å) (Frens, 1973)

One hundred milliliters of a $10^{-2}\%$ aqueous solution of $HAuCl_4$ (from Merck, Darmstadt, Federal Republic of Germany) is heated in a siliconized Erlenmeyer flask, and when the solution begins to boil, 4 ml of a 1% aqueous solution of Na_3-citrate is rapidly added. The reduction of gold chloride is complete after 5 minutes of boiling, as indicated by a color change to brilliant red. The pH is adjusted to 6.9 by addition of 0.2 N K_2CO_3. For pH measurement, an aliquot of the colloid (about 5 ml) is mixed with 10 drops of a 1% aqueous solution of polyethylene glycol (MW 20,000; from Merck, Darmstadt, Federal Republic of Germany) and the pH is controlled with a pH electrode. The 5-ml aliquot is discarded after each pH measurement.

2. Polydisperse Suspension of Colloidal Gold (Diameter between About 30 Å and 120 Å) (Zsigmondy and Thiessen, 1925)

Of a 0.6% aqueous solution of $HAuCl_4$ 2.5 ml is added to 60 ml of distilled water in a siliconized Erlenmeyer flask. An ether solution of white phosphorus (0.5 ml) is added to this stirred solution. The mixture is shaken for 15 minutes at room temperature and then heated over an open flame until a wine-red color appears. The pH of the colloid is adjusted to 6.9 by addition of 0.2 N K_2CO_3, as above. The ether solution consists of four parts of diethyl ether and one part of ether-saturated phosphorus. All glassware used for preparation of the colloidal suspensions has to be siliconized and must be carefully cleaned. The distilled water should be doubly distilled and the different solutions should be filtered with Millipore filter systems (0.45 μm pore size). The aqueous solution of $HAuCl_4$ is stable at 4°C.

C. PREPARATION OF THE pAG COMPLEX*

Protein A (0.5 ml) (from Pharmacia Fine Chemicals, Uppsala, Sweden) dissolved in 0.1–0.2 ml of distilled water is placed in a plastic centrifuge tube and 10 ml of the colloidal gold is added with shaking. After 2–3 minutes, 1 ml of a 1% aqueous solution of polyethylene glycol (MW 20,000) is added. After about 15 minutes, the mixture is centrifuged at 60,000 g (150 Å gold particles, according to Frens) or at 105,000 g (gold particles, according to Zsigmondy and Thiessen) for 1 hour at 4°C. The colorless supernatant is discarded and the dark-red sediment is resuspended to 1.5 ml with phosphate-buffered isotonic saline (PBS), pH 7.2, containing 0.2 mg of polyethylene glycol (MW 20,000) per ml. This stock solution can be stored for several months at 4°C. The working solution in the pAG technique is usually a 10- to 20-fold dilution of the pAG stock solution.

D. PREPARATION OF PEROXIDASE-LABELED ANTIBODIES

1. Periodate Oxidation Method (Recent Modification by Fogleman and Nakane, 1981, and Wilson and Nakane, 1978)

1. Dissolve 4 mg HRPO [RZ† > 3, commercially available peroxidase may require further purification (i.e., chromatographic separation by a

---

* Roth et al. (1978, 1980).
† RZ: $OD_{403\ nm}/OD_{280\ nm}$. This value reflects the ratio of hemin to protein in the sample. Peroxidase samples having an RZ < 3 are usually not usable.

Sephacryl 5-200 column)] in 1 ml distilled water and, while stirring, add 0.05 ml of freshly prepared $NaIO_4$ (38.5 mg/ml) and continue stirring for 20 minutes at room temperature.

2. Chromatograph on a Pharmacia PD-10 column which has been previously equilibrated with 0.001 M acetate buffer, pH 4. Collect the colored peroxidase eluate.

3. Immediately titrate the peroxidase to pH 9.5 with 0.2 M NaOH, then add 10 mg IgG or 5 mg F(ab)' in 1 ml 0.01 M sodium carbonate buffer, pH 9.5. Stir 2 hours at room temperature.

4. Add 100 μl of 4 mg/ml $NaBH_4$ in distilled water. Leave at 4°C for 2 hours.

5. (Optional) Dialyze overnight versus PBS.

6. Chromatograph on Sephacryl S-200 (2.5 × 30-cm column or equivalent) 40 ml/hour. Collect 2-ml fractions with PBS.

7. Read OD_{280} and OD_{403} and select the 90,000-MW peak for F(ab)' or the 200,000-MW peak for IgG.

8. The fractions comprising the desired conjugate peak are pooled, bovine serum albumin is added to a final concentration of 10 mg/ml, and aliquots are quick-frozen and stored at −20°C or −80°C.

2. Two-Step Glutaraldehyde Coupling Procedure (Avrameas and Ternynck, 1971)

1. Dissolve 15 mg of peroxidase in 0.2 ml of a 1% glutaraldehyde solution in 0.1 M phosphate buffer, pH 6.8.

2. Leave the preparation for 18 hours at room temperature.

3. Fractionate through a Sephadex G-25 fine column (0.9 × 60 cm) equilibrated with 0.15 M NaCl in order to remove the free glutaraldehyde. The brown-colored fractions containing the peroxidase are pooled and, if required, concentrated to 1 ml with a Diaflo using a PM10 membrane.

4. To the peroxidase solution add 1 ml of a 0.15 M NaCl solution containing either 5 mg of γ-globulin or 2.5 mg of Fab previously dialyzed against 0.15 M NaCl.

5. Add 0.2 ml of 1 M carbonate–bicarbonate buffer, pH 9.5.

6. Maintain at 4°C for 24 hours.

7. Add 0.2 ml of 1 M lysine solution, pH 7.

8. After 2 hours, dialyze the mixture overnight against PBS at 4°C.

9. Filter through a sterile Millipore membrane (0.11 μl) and add an equal volume of glycerol.

10. Conserve the conjugate at 4°C.

This method does not remove the unreacted peroxidase. If removal of the peroxidase is required, following step 8 the conjugate may be fractionated through a Sephadex G-100 or G-200 column.

E. Preparation of PAP Complexes*

1. To 6.0 ml of a 0.4% solution of peroxidase (freshly prepared by dissolving 128 mg of lyophilized peroxidase in 32 ml of saline) add an amount of antiperoxidase serum needed to precipitate 16 mg of peroxidase.

2. Mix and allow to stand at room temperature for 1 hour.

3. Centrifuge at 1,000 g for 20 minutes at 4°C and discard the supernatant.

4. Resuspend the pellet in a small volume of cold saline and wash by adding 200 ml of saline. Centrifuge and discard the supernatant. Repeat this step three times.

5. Resuspend the precipitate in 24 ml of the 0.4% solution of peroxidase (left over from step 1) and, with mild continuous stirring, lower to pH 2.3 at room temperature with HCl (0.01 to 1.0 N).

6. Neutralize to pH 7.4 at room temperature with NaOH (1.0 to 0.01 N).

7. Add 2.4 ml of an aqueous solution containing 0.08 N sodium acetate and 0.14 N ammonium acetate, chill in an ice bath, and centrifuge at 37,000 g for 10 minutes at 4°C.

8. While stirring at 4°C add to the supernatant an equal volume of NH_4SO_4 saturated at 4°C, stir for 25 minutes, and centrifuge at 37,000 g for 15 minutes at 4°C.

9. Dialyze the pellet in the dark against three changes of sodium ammonium acetate saline (13.5 liters saline, 1.5 liters water, 75 ml 1.5 N sodium acetate, and 75 ml of 3 N ammonium acetate solution).

10. Centrifuge at 37,000 g for 15 minutes and discard the supernatant.

F. Preparation of Special Fixatives

1. Preparation of Paraformaldehyde–Picric Acid (Stefanini et al., 1967)

1. Add 20 gm of paraformaldehyde to 150 ml of a doubly filtered saturated aqueous solution of picric acid.

2. Heat to 60°C and alkalinize with drops of 2.52% NaOH in water to dissociate the paraformaldehyde into formaldehyde.

3. Cool, filter, and make the volume up to 1 liter with phosphate buffer (3.31 gm $NaH_2PO_4 \cdot H_2O$) and 33.7 gm $Na_2HPO_4 \cdot 7 H_2O$ in 1 liter of water). The final osmolarity is 900 mOsm, pH 7.3. The fixative is very stable and can be stored at room temperature for 12 months.

---

* Sternberger *et al.* (1970).

2. Preparation of Periodate–Lysine–Paraformaldehyde (PLP) (McLean and Nakane, 1974)

Stock A = 0.1 M lysine–0.05 M sodium phosphate, pH 7.4

1. Dissolve 1.827 gm L-lysine–HCl in 50 ml H_2O (0.2 M lysine–HCl).
2. Adjust pH to 7.4 with 0.1 M Na_2HPO_4.
3. Make up to 100 ml with 0.1 M sodium phosphate buffer, pH 7.4. Osmolality should be approximately 300 mOsm.
4. Store at 4°C for a maximum of 10 days.

Stock B = 8% paraformaldehyde

1. Mix 8 gm of paraformaldehyde in 100 ml H_2O.
2. Heat to 60°C with stirring.
3. Slowly add 1–3 drops of 1 N NaOH until clear.
4. Filter.
5. Store at 4°C.

Just before use, combine three parts (A) with one part (B) and add sodium metaperiodate to 0.01 M (i.e., 21.4 mg $NaIO_4$/10 ml). The final composition is, therefore, 0.01 M $NaIO_4$, 0.075 M lysine, 0.0375 M sodium phosphate buffer, and 2% paraformaldehyde. The final pH will be approximately 6.2 and osmolality around 700 mOsm.

G. PREPARATION OF COATED SLIDES

1. Albumin-Coated Slides

1. Clean glass microscope slides in 1% HCl–70% EtOH by immersion and agitation for several minutes.
2. Dip slides in 100% acetone and allow them to air dry.
3. Combine one egg white and 1 ml concentrated NH_4OH with 500 ml distilled water. Stir 10 minutes. Filter through a paper towel or six layers of gauze.
4. Place cleaned slides into freshly made egg albumin solution for 1 minute. Drain off excess solution on a paper towel and place slides in racks to dry.
5. Dry at 60°C for 2 hours to overnight.
6. Up to 500 slides can be coated from the above egg mixture and they can be kept indefinitely.

*7. Slides are immersed in 2% glutaraldehyde overnight at 4°C.

*8. They are then washed from 30 to 60 minutes in multiple changes of distilled water, allowed to air dry, and used within 12 hours.

2. Glutaraldehyde-Gelatin-Coated Slides (For Tissue Sections to Be Studied by EM)

1. Make a 6% solution of gelatin in distilled water. Boil with gentle stirring in an Erlenmeyer flask until dissolved. Set in 60°C water bath.

2. Dip acid-cleaned microscope slides into the warm gelatin for about 5 minutes. Drain on a paper towel and place in wooden boxes.

3. Dry in 60°C oven overnight. Dried slides may be stored indefinitely.

4. Glutaraldehyde coating should be done the night before the slides will be used. Set slides in 25% glutaraldehyde (practical grade) at 4°C overnight.

5. Wash in several changes of distilled water over approximately 30 minutes. Air dry.

6. Pick up frozen tissue section onto a dry glutaraldehyde-gelatin-coated slide and immediately place in PBS–10% sucrose.

H. Immunoelectron Microscopy of Sections Mounted on Slides Using the Peroxidase-Labeled Antibody Method

1. Six- to 12-μm-thick frozen or 10- to 50-μm-thick Vibratome sections of fixed tissue well washed in PBS containing 10% sucrose (PBS-S) are cut, placed on albumin-coated slides, and allowed to dry.

2. Wash in PBS-S 3 × 10 minutes.

3. Make a moist chamber. (We use baking dishes lined with moist paper towels secured by tape inverted on a moist paper surface).

4. Wipe excess PBS-S from around the section with gauze. With a capillary pipet apply about 20 μl of antibody solution (this technique is a direct technique using peroxidase-labeled immunoglobulin fragments; if an indirect technique is used, repeat steps 4 through 6 for the second antibody) to the section.

5. Mix the antibody solution thoroughly with residual PBS-S, which is still over the tissue, being careful not to scratch the section. Place in the moist chamber for 3 to 24 hours. Keep the chamber moist and do not let the section dry until embedding.

---

* Steps 7 and 8 are optional. These steps are especially useful in improving the adherence of Vibratome sections to slides.

6. Rinse conjugate off the slides with PBS-S. Wash in PBS-S 3 × 10 minutes.

7. Incubate in a solution of 2% glutaraldehyde in PBS-S for 30 minutes.

8. Wash in PBS-S 3 × 10 minutes.

*9. Immerse slides in 1% gelatin in 0.1 M phosphate buffer, pH 7.4, for 5 to 10 minutes.

*10. Dry rapidly with compressed air.

*11. Immerse slides again in 2% glutaraldehyde in PBS-S for 15 minutes.

*12. Wash in PBS-S 3 × 10 minutes.

13. Incubate in DAB solution containing 10% sucrose for 30 minutes.

14. Incubate in DAB–H_2O_2 solution containing 10% sucrose for 2 to 8 minutes.

15. Wash in PBS-S 3 × 10 minutes. At this point the slides may be briefly examined for staining under a light microscope, taking care not to let the tissue dry out.

16. Incubate in 2% OsO_4–0.1 M sodium phosphate buffer, pH 7.2, for 1 to 2 hours.

17. Wash in PBS-S 3 × 10 minutes.

18. Dehydrate in graded ethanols (10 minutes each) to 100%.

19. Embed by inverting a gelatin capsule of fresh Epon–Araldite over each section.

20. Polymerize the Epon by incubating at 37°C overnight and at 60°C for 24–48 hours. The block and its tissue section can then be removed from the slide by briefly heating the slide over a Bunsen burner flame.

I. IMMUNOELECTRON MICROSCOPY OF ULTRATHIN SECTIONS OF EMBEDDED TISSUES USING THE PEROXIDASE–ANTIPEROXIDASE METHOD†

1. Place ultrathin Araldite- or Epon-embedded sections on nickel or gold grids.

2. Etch the sections by flotation for 3 minutes at room temperature on drops of 5% aqueous solution of hydrogen peroxide. Wash with a "spray" of saline from a spray bottle and blot by holding edgewise on filter paper. In steps 3 through 8, the grids are floated on single drops of the respective solutions.

3. Float the grid on normal serum diluted 1:30 in 0.05 M Tris saline, pH 7.6, for 5 minutes at room temperature. Blot, but do not wash.

---

* Steps 9 through 12 are optional. They may improve morphology.

† From Sternberger (1979).

4. Float the grid on the primary antiserum, diluted in 0.05 M Tris saline, pH 7.6, containing 1% normal serum (preimmune serum of the animal in which the "link" antiserum was generated) for 48 hours at 2–5°C, permitting the dishes to reequilibrate to room temperature for the last 1–2 hours. Wash with Tris saline, pH 7.6, and blot.

5. Float the grid on normal serum, diluted 1 : 30 in Tris saline, for 5 minutes at room temperature. Blot, but do not wash.

6. Float the grid on the link antiserum, diluted 1 : 10 in 0.05 M Tris saline, pH 7.6, for 5 minutes at room temperature. Wash with Tris saline, pH 7.6, and blot.

7. Float the grid on normal serum, diluted 1 : 30 in Tris saline, for 5 minutes at room temperature. Blot, but do not wash.

8. Float the grid on PAP diluted to 0.066 mg antiperoxidase per ml in 0.05 M Tris buffer, pH 7.6, containing 1% normal serum, for 5 minutes at room temperature (this concentration of antiperoxidase is usually attained by a 1 : 40 to 1 : 50 dilution of PAP). Wash with 0.05 M Tris buffer, pH 7.6, but do not blot.

9. The grids are held in forceps and immersed for 3 minutes at room temperature into a beaker containing a freshly prepared solution of 0.0125% diaminobenzidine tetrahydrochloride and 0.0025% hydrogen peroxide in 0.05 M Tris buffer, pH 7.6. This solution is kept under agitation over a magnetic stirrer at 50 to 80 rpm.

10. Suspend the grids in water for 30 minutes under agitation. Wash each grid with a spray of water.

11. Incubate a 4% solution of aqueous osmium tetroxide in porcelain depression dishes for 10–25 minutes. Wash again in water.

J. THE PROTEIN A–COLLOIDAL GOLD METHOD*

This staining procedure is performed on thin sections of aldehyde-fixed and Epon-embedded material placed on Parlodion and carbon-coated nickel or gold grids (150 mesh). The fixation protocol with glutaraldehyde or formaldehyde, mixtures of both aldehydes, or other fixatives depends on the antigen studied.

1. Nonetched thin sections are floated for 5 minutes at room temperature on drops of a 1% ovalbumin–PBS solution, pH 7.4, and then transferred to the antiserum.

2. The sections are floated on drops of the specific antiserum (whole antiserum or affinity-purified antibodies can be used) in a moist chamber

* From Roth *et al.* (1978, 1980).

for 2 hours at room temperature or for 12–18 hours at 4°C. In each case, the antibody dilution which gives intense specific and low background staining has to be determined empirically. The antiserum is diluted in 1% ovalbumin–PBS, pH 7.4, or in 1% ovalbumin–0.05 *M* Tris saline, pH 7.4. The sections are then "jet-washed" by a spray of PBS from a plastic spray bottle, placed in PBS for about 2 minutes, jet-washed a second time with PBS and, finally, blotted by holding them edgewise on filter paper.

3. The sections are floated on drops of the diluted pAG solution for 1 hour at room temperature in a moist chamber. They are then jet-washed with PBS for about 1 minute, immersed for 5 minutes with PBS in porcelain depression dishes, jet-washed a second time and immersed in PBS, and, finally, jet-washed with distilled water. Finally, the sections are stained with 5% aqueous uranyl acetate for 10–20 minutes and Reynold's lead citrate for 2–5 minutes. During the staining procedure the grids are never allowed to dry completely.

K. Technique to Decrease Staining Due to Endogenous Peroxidase Activity*

1. Before exposing the sections on glass slides to antisera, incubate them in a 0.005 *M* solution of periodic acid in distilled water, pH 2.5 (adjusted with citric acid phosphate), for at least 5 minutes to oxidize the pseudoperoxidase compounds.

2. Incubate the sections in a 0.003 *M* solution of sodium borohydride in distilled water for 30 minutes to reduce the aldehyde groups formed in the preceding step.

ACKNOWLEDGMENTS

This work was supported in part by grants AI-09109, CA-09157, and CA-15823 from the National Institutes of Health and by a gift from R. J. Reynolds Industries, Inc.

REFERENCES

Aarli, J. A., Aparicio, S. S., Lumsden, C. E., and Tönder, O. (1975). *Immunology* **28,** 171.
Andres, G. A., Accinni, L., Hsu, K. C., Zabriskie, J. B., and Seegal, B. C. (1966). *J. Exp. Med.* **123,** 399.
Avrameas, S., and Ternynck, T. (1971). *Immunochemistry* **8,** 1175.
Baskin, D. G., Erlandsen, S. L., and Parsons, J. A. (1979). *J. Histochem. Cytochem.* **27,** 867.
Becker, R. P., and DeBruyn, P. P. H. (1976). *Scanning Electron Microsc.* **II,** 172–178.
Bohn, W. (1978). *J. Histochem. Cytochem.* **26,** 293.
Brown, W. R., Isobe, Y., and Nakane, P. K. (1976). *Gastroenterology* **71,** 985.

* From Isobe *et al.* (1977).

Buffa, R., Crivelli, O., Fiocca, R., Fontana, P., and Solcia, E. (1979). *Histochemistry* **63**, 15.
Carr, K. E., and McGradey, J. (1974). *J. Microsc.* (*Oxford*) **100**, 323–330.
Childs, G. V., Hon, C., Russell, L. R., Gardner, P. J. (1978). *J. Histochem. Cytochem.* **26**, 545.
Dales, S., and Gomatos, P. J. (1965). *Virology* **25**, 193.
DeHarven, E., Pla, D., and Lampen, N. (1979). *Scanning Electron Microsc.* **III**, 611–618.
Fogleman, D., and Nakane, P. K. (1981). In preparation.
Frens, G. (1973). *Nature* (*London*) *Phys. Sci.* **241**, 20.
Gonatas, N. K., Antome, J. C., Stieber, A., and Avrameas, S. (1972). *Lab. Invest.* **26**, 253.
Goodman, S. L., Hodges, G. M., Trejdosiewicz, L. K., and Livingston, D. C. (1979). *Scanning Electron Microsc.* **III**, 619–628.
Goodman, S. L., Hodges, G. M., and Livingston, D. C. (1980). *Scanning Electron Microsc.* **II**, 133.
Graham, R. C., and Karnovsky, M. J. (1966). *J. Histochem. Cytochem.* **14**, 291.
Graham, R. C., Karnovsky, M. J., Schafer, A. W., Glass, E. A., and Karnovsky, M. L. (1967). *J. Cell Biol.* **32**, 629.
Hammond, E. (1970). *Exp. Cell Res.* **59**, 359.
Hartman, A. L., and Nakane, P. K. (1981). *Scanning Electron Microsc.* **II**, 32–44.
Hattori, A., Matsukura, Y., Ito, S., Fugita, T., and Tokunaga, J. (1976). *Arch. Histol. Jpn.* **39**, 105–115.
Isobe, S. T. C., Nakane, P. K., and Brown, W. R. (1977). *Acta Histochem. Cytochem.* **10**, 161.
Itoh, G., and Suzuki, I. (1977). *J. Histochem. Cytochem.* **25**, 259.
Kawarai, Y., and Nakane, P. K. (1970). *J. Histochem. Cytochem.* **18**, 161.
Kraehenbuhl, J. P., Galardy, R. E., and Jamieson, J. D. (1974). *J. Exp. Med.* **139**, 208.
Kuhlmann, W. D., Avrameas, S., and Ternynck, T. (1974). *J. Immunol. Methods,* **5**, 33.
Larsson, L. I., Polak, J. M., Buffa, R., Sundler, F., and Solcia, E. (1979). *J. Histochem. Cytochem.* **27**, 936.
Leduc, E. H., Scott, G. B., and Avrameas, S. (1969). *J. Histochem. Cytochem.* **17**, 211.
Li, J. Y., Dubois, M. P., and Dubois, P. M. (1977). *Cell Tissue. Res.* **181**, 545.
McLean, I. W., and Nakane, P. K. (1974). *J. Histochem. Cytochem.* **22**, 1077.
McLean, J. D., and Singer, S. J. (1970). *Proc. Natl. Acad. Sci. U.S.A.* **65**, 122.
Mazurkiewicz, J. E., and Nakane, P. K. (1972). *J. Histochem. Cytochem.* **20**, 969.
Miller, M. M., and Teplitz, R. L. (1978). *Scanning Electron Microsc.* **II**, 893–898.
Molday, R. S., Dreyer, W. J., Rembaum, A., and Yen, S. P. S. (1975). *J. Cell Biol.* **64**, 75–88.
Morgan, C., Hsu, K. C., Rifkind, R. A., Knox, A. W., and Rose, H. M., (1961). *J. Exp. Med.* **114**, 833.
Moriarty, G. C. (1973). *J. Histochem. Cytochem.* **21**, 855.
Moriarty, G. C., and Helmi, N. S. (1972). *J. Histochem. Cytochem.* **20**, 590.
Mukai, K., and Nakane, P. K. (1976). *J. Cell Biol.* **70**, 176a.
Nakane, P. K. (1971). *In* "*In Vitro* Methods in Reproductive Cell Biology" (E. Diczfalusy, ed.), pp. 190–204. Bogtrykkeriet Forum, Copenhagen.
Nakane, P. K. (1975). *Ann. N.Y. Acad. Sci.* **254**, 203.
Nakane, P. K., and Hartman, A. L. (1980). *Histochem. J.* **12**, 435–447.
Nakane, P. K., and Pierce, G. B. (1966). *Int. Congr. Electron Microsc. 6th* **II**, 51.
Nakane, P. K., and Pierce, G. B. (1967). *J. Cell Biol.* **33**, 307.
Nielson, A. J., and Griffith, W. P. (1979). *J. Histochem. Cytochem.* **27**, 997.
Otto, H., Takamiya, H., and Vogt, A. (1973). *J. Immunol. Methods.* **3**, 137.
Parr, E. L. (1979). *J. Histochem. Cytochem.* **27**, 1095.

Peters, K. R., Gschwender, H. H., Holler, W., and Rutter, G. (1976). *Scanning Electron Microsc.* **II**, 75–83.
Pickel, V. M., Joh, T. H., and Reis, D. J. (1975). *Proc. Natl. Acad. Sci. U.S.A.* **72**, 659.
Pickel, V. M., Joh, T. H., and Reis, D. J. (1976). *J. Histochem. Cytochem.* **24**, 792.
Polak, J. M., Kendall, P. A., Heath, C. M., and Pearse, A. G. E. (1972). *Experientia* **28**, 368.
Rodning, C. B., Erlandsen, S. L., Coulter, H. D., and Wilson, I. D. (1978). *J. Histochem. Cytochem.* **26**, 223.
Roth, J., Bendayan, M., and Orci, L. (1978). *J. Histochem. Cytochem.* **26**, 1074.
Roth, J., Bendayan, M., and Orci, L. (1980). *J. Histochem. Cytochem.* **28**, 55.
Saland, L. C., and Napolitano, L. M. (1977). *J. Histochem. Cytochem.* **25**, 280.
Seeman, P. (1967). *J. Cell Biol.* **32**, 55.
Shahrabadi, M. S., and Yamamoto, T. (1971). *J. Cell Biol.* **50**, 246.
Singer, S. J., and McLean, J. D. (1963). *Lab. Invest.* **12**, 1002.
Singer, S. J., and Schick, A. F. (1961). *J. Biophys. Biochem. Cytol.* **9**, 519.
Smith, R. E. (1970). *J. Histochem. Cytochem.* **18**, 590.
Smith, R. E., and Farquhar, M. G. (1963). *Nature (London)* **200**, 691.
Spicer, S. S., Phifer, R. F., Garvin, A. J., and Zehr, D. (1976). *In* "First International Symposium on Immunoenzymatic Techniques INSERM Symposium" (G. Feldman, P. Druet, J. Bignon, and S. Avrameas, eds.), No. 2, pp. 59. North-Holland Publ., Amsterdam.
Springer, E. L., Riggs, J. L., and Hackett, A. J. (1974). *J. Virol.* **14**, 1623–1626.
Stefanini, M., de Martino, C., and Zamboni, L. (1967). *Nature (London)* **216**, 173.
Sternberger, L. A. (1979). *In* "Immunocytochemistry" (L. A. Sternberger, ed.), Chap. 5. Wiley, New York.
Sternberger, L. A., and Petrali, J. P. (1975). *Cell Tissue Res.* **162**, 141.
Sternberger, L. A., Hardy P. H., Jr., Cuculis, J. J., and Meyer, H. G., (1970). *J. Histochem. Cytochem.* **18**, 315.
Sternberger, L. A., Petrali, J. P., Joseph, S. A., Meyer, H. G., and Mills, K. R. (1978). *Endocrinology* **102**, 63.
Tokuyasa, K. T. (1973). *J. Cell Biol.* **57**, 551.
Vaillant, C., Dockray, G., and Hopkins, C. R. (1979). *J. Histochem. Cytochem.* **27**, 932.
Vogt, A., Takamiya, H., and Kim, W. A. (1976). *In* "First International Symposium on Immunoenzymatic Techniques INSERM Symposium" (G. Feldman, P. Druet, J. Bignon, and S. Avrameas, eds.), No. 2, p. 109. North-Holland Publ., Amsterdam.
Wilson, M. B., and Nakane, P. K. (1978). *In* "Immunofluorescence and Related Staining Techniques" (W. Knapp, K. Holubar, and G. Wick, eds.), pp. 215–224. Elsevier, Amsterdam.
Zsigmondy, R., and Thiessen, P. A. (1925). "Das Kolloidale Gold." Akademische Verlagsgesellschaft, Leipzig.

CHAPTER VI

ENZYME IMMUNOASSAYS: APPLICATIONS IN CANCER RESEARCH

CURTIS C. HARRIS, ROBERT H. YOLKEN, AND IH-CHANG HSU

I. Introduction

The specificity that antibodies exhibit against antigens is one of the most remarkable achievements of biological evolution. Minor modifications of complex macromolecules can be recognized by the humoral immunological system. In addition, immunoglobulins can be used to measure small molecules. Cancer researchers have utilized this remarkable property of antibodies to measure a variety of antigens, including tumor-specific antigens, ectopic hormones, viruses, chemical carcinogens, and, more recently, carcinogen–DNA adducts.

Enzyme immunoassay (EIA) is a relatively new immunological approach in which the antibody–antigen reaction is amplified by measuring the activity of an enzyme linked to the antibody–antigen complex through conjugation either with antibody or with antigen. The rapid rate of enzymatic

ISBN 0-12-147680-4

conversion of substrate to product, usually thousands of molecules per minute, serves as the basis of this amplification. Rapid and sensitive EIAs have been developed to measure either antigen or antibody. These immunoassays have substantial potential as methods for cancer research.

II. Principles of EIAs

Enzyme immunoassays are based on the labeling of an immunoreactant with an enzyme. Following a series of antigen–antibody reactions, the quantity of labeled reactant involved in the reaction is quantitated by the addition of enzyme substrate. The amount of substrate conversion is measured either by determining the accumulation of product or by kinetic measurements (Voller *et al.*, 1980; Engvall and Perlmann, 1972; Wisdom, 1976; Avrameas and Ternynck, 1971; Pesce *et al.*, 1976). The inherent magnification of the enzyme–substrate reaction allows for the measurement of small quantities of immunoreactants. The sensitivity of an EIA is determined by the kinetics of the enzyme–substrate reaction and by the physical–chemical properties of the product [i.e., the quantity of product which can be detected by the use of the appropriate instrumentation (Bullock and Walls, 1977)]. The specificity of EIA reactions is determined largely by the specificity of the antigen–antibody reaction and by the efficiency of the technique used to separate reacted from unreacted label (Yolken, 1980; Pesce *et al.*, 1978).

In general, EIA systems require the separation of enzyme-labeled immunoreactant which has participated in the antigen–antibody reaction from that which has not. This separation can be accomplished by a number of techniques, including centrifugation, immunoprecipitation, and gel diffusion (Yolken, 1980). However, for the performance of a large number of assays, it is convenient to bind one of the immunoreactants to a solid phase. The reactant which participates in the antigen–antibody interaction can be separated from that which does not by means of washing the solid phase with an excess of buffer solution. This technique allows for the accurate performance of a large number of determinations without the need for expensive equipment. A number of solid phases have been used for this purpose. These include polyacrylamide beads, filter papers, controlled-pore glass, nylon beads or powders, and a number of plastic materials. One particularly convenient plastic material is a microtitration plate containing 96 wells (Pesce *et al.*, 1977; Lehtonen and Viljanen, 1980). The use of such a receptacle allows for the performance of a large number of reactions under controlled conditions with a minimum of manipulation. The availability of equipment capable of performing the necessary washing steps and measurement of the enzyme–substrate reactions in microtiter plates allows for extensive automation of reactions performed in this manner.

In addition, there have been EIAs designed which do not require the use of a solid phase. Such assays, which are known as homogeneous assays, are based on the exclusion of substrate by steric hindrance (Rubenstein, 1978; Ngo and Lenhoff, 1980). In such assays labeled antigen will not react with substrate if it is a part of an antigen–antibody complex, whereas it will react with the substrate if it is uncomplexed (Fig. 1). Homogeneous assays have the advantage of not requiring any separation step, thus avoiding the time delay required for the performance of this washing as well as the problems of variable interaction of reagents with the solid phase. However, current homogeneous assays are limited as to the size of the antigen which can be measured, with most assays involving aggregates with molecular weights of less than 1000 (Rubenstein, 1978).

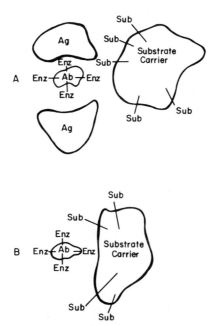

FIG. 1. Homogeneous EIA for viral and bacterial antigens. (A) If antigen (Ag) is present in a specimen, it will react with the antibody (Ab)–enzyme conjugate. When the macromolecular substrate is added, it will be prevented from reacting with the antigen–antibody enzyme complex by steric hindrance. (B) Uncomplexed antibody will react with available substrate to produce a measurable product. The amount of product is inversely proportional to the amount of antigen in a specimen.

Such assays are thus not applicable for larger molecular weight antigens such as protein hormones, viruses, bacteria, or toxins.

Solid-phase immunoassays for the measurement of these larger molecules can be formulated in either a competitive or a noncompetitive manner (Yolken, 1980). Competitive assays make use of the blocking of labeled antigen or antibody from the solid phase by means of antigen in the test specimen. Competitive assays can be established utilizing either labeled antigen (Fig. 2) or labeled antibody (Fig. 3). Competitive assays have the advantage of involving few incubation steps and, if nonequilibrium conditions are used, the assays can be performed in a short period of time. However, the labeled antigen competitive assay has the disadvantage of requiring purified antigen in sufficient quantity so that it can be labeled with the enzyme. While this is not a problem if the antigen is a synthetic substance such as a drug, it is often difficult to obtain a sufficient quantity of other antigens, such as infectious agents and hormones,

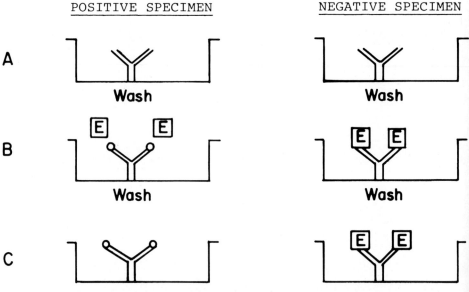

Fig. 2. Competitive EIA for antigen measurement—labeled antigen method. (A) Antibody (Y) is bound to the solid phase. Unbound antibody is removed in the washing step. (B) The specimen is added. If it contains antigen (○), it will bind to the solid-phase antibody. Enzyme-labeled antigen (E) is then added. This will react with antibody sites not occupied by antigen from the specimen. (C) Unbound enzyme-labeled antigen is removed by washing and the amount of bound enzyme-labeled antigen is quantitated by the addition of the appropriate substrate. The amount of substrate product is inversely proportional to the amount of antigen in the test specimen.

POSITIVE SPECIMEN   NEGATIVE SPECIMEN

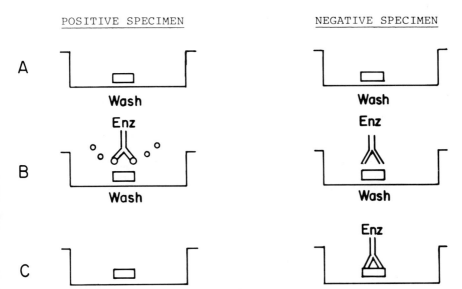

FIG. 3. Competitive EIA for antigen measurement—labeled antibody method. (A) Antigen (▭) is bound to the solid phase. Unbound antigen is removed in a washing step. (B) The specimen is reacted with enzyme-labeled antibody (Å) and the mixture is added to the solid phase. If the specimen contains antigen (○) it will react with the enzyme-labeled antibody, thus preventing the enzyme-labeled antibody from reacting with the solid phase. (C) Unbound enzyme-labeled antibody is removed in a washing step and the bound enzyme is quantitated by the addition of substrate. The amount of substrate product is inversely proportional to the amount of antigen in the specimen. Unlabeled antibody can also be used in place of the enzyme-labeled antibody. In this case, enzyme-labeled antiglobulin or staphylococcal Protein A is used to quantitate the antibody bound to the solid phase.

to provide for an efficient label for these assays (Fisher, 1980; Hunter, 1973). The labeled antibody method depicted in Fig. 3 is thus more practical for these antigens since it is usually more feasible to obtain sufficient quantities of an antibody to an antigen than it is to obtain such quantities of the antigen itself. This is due to the fact that a small quantity of antigen can be utilized to produce a large quantity of antibody, either by the immunization of a laboratory animal or by the production of monoclonal antibodies by means of a hybridoma system (Davies, 1973; Kohler and Milstein, 1975). However, competitive-labeled antibody systems have an inherent disadvantage: namely, endogenous antibody will compete with the labeled antibody, thus yielding a false-positive reaction. This is especially a problem with the measurement of infectious antigens in serum and other body fluids since these fluids may often contain antibodies to the antigen measured (Yolken, 1980; Berg et al., 1980; Yolken and Stopa, 1980). It is thus necessary to denature the antigen or to remove it from the reaction milieu prior to the performance of the antigen–antibody reactions.

Because of these difficulties, noncompetitive methods are often used for the measurement of large protein antigens in body fluids (Yolken *et al.*, 1980). The simplest noncompetitive method involves the use of enzyme-labeled antibody directed against the antigen to be measured. In this type of assay, usually called a direct noncompetitive EIA (Fig. 4), unlabeled antibody is first bound to the solid phase. Then, the specimen is added. Antigen present in the specimen will bind to the antibody while unreacted material will be removed by means of a washing step. Enzyme-labeled antibody is then added. This antibody will bind to antigen bound in the previous steps, while unreacted antibody will be removed. The amount of bound antibody is measured by adding a substrate solution and measuring the formation of substrate products by kinetic or accumulation methods. One disadvantage of this direct noncompetitive system is that it requires a separate enzyme-labeled antibody for each antigen to be measured. It is thus more convenient to perform an indirect assay as depicted in Fig. 5. In this form of assay system, unlabeled antibody (Ab$_2$) is added

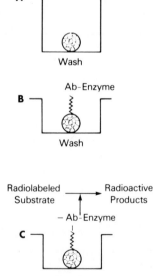

Fig. 4. Noncompetitive direct USERIA for antigen measurement. (A) Antigen is adhered to the well of a microtiter plate. Wash. (B) Enzyme-labeled antibody directed against the antigen adhered to the solid phase. Wash. (C) A radiolabeled substrate is added. The enzyme adhered to the well will convert the substrate to radioactive products which are separated from the substrate by chromatography. The amount of radioactive products is proportional to the amount of antigen in the test material.

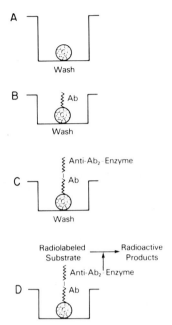

Fig. 5. Noncompetitive indirect USERIA for antigen measurement. (A) Antigen is adhered to the well of a microtiter plate. Wash. (B) Unconjugated antigen-reactive antibody (Ab) is added. This will react with antigen that is adhered to the solid phase. Wash. (C) Enzyme-labeled antibody directed against the IgG globulin subclass of the animal source of Ab₂ is added. Wash. (D) A radiolabeled substrate is added. The enzyme adhered to the well will convert the substrate to radioactive products which are separated from the substrate by chromatography. The amount of radioactive products is proportional to the amount of antigen in the test material.

in place of the enzyme-labeled antibody. Following a reaction of this antibody with the antigen bound to the solid phase, unreacted Ab₂ is removed by washing and enzyme-labeled antiglobulin directed at the animal species of Ab₂ is added. This will bind to the solid phase and convert substrate as described above. In this system the only labeled reactant required is a labeled antiglobulin, and the same labeled antiglobulin can be used for the measurement of any antigen provided that Ab₂ is in the appropriate animal species (Yolken et al., 1980). Alternatively, enzyme-labeled staphylococcal Protein A can be utilized as long as the antibody used to coat the solid phase is of an immunoglobulin subclass which will not react extensively with it. (Engvall, 1978).

One inherent problem in the noncompetitive assays involves the nonspecific binding of materials in the specimen with the immunoreactants. One major nonspecific reactant is an antiglobulin or rheumatoid-like factor. Such antiglobulins will bind with the antibody used to coat the solid phase and the labeled immunoreactants, leading to a false-positive determination in the absence of the specific antigen (Yolken *et al.*, 1979a). Such immunoglobulins are common during the course of acute infections and also may be present in body fluids such as stool or joint fluids (Salonen *et al.*, 1980). The effect of these antiglobulins can be minimized by the dilution of reactants with an excess of antibody without specific activity for the antigen to be measured. This will allow for the absorption of the nonspecific antiglobulins without interference with the specific antigen–antibody reaction. Since most of the antiglobulin activity is directed at the Fc portion of the antibody molecule, Fc fragments can also be utilized (Yolken, 1980; Winchester, 1980; Kato *et al.*, 1979). However, antiglobulins can be present in such high concentrations that they cannot be totally absorbed by such techniques. It is thus advisable to perform a control reaction consisting of the testing of the specimen in a solid phase coated with nonimmune serum of the same species and at the same concentration as the immune serum. A specific activity is then calculated for each specimen by subtracting the activity of the specimen reacted with nonimmune solid phase from that of the solid phase coated with specific antibody. Since an antiglobulin will result in equal binding to both the immune and nonimmune solid phases, a specimen containing nonspecific immunoglobulins will not yield a net positive specific activity. Using this system a number of specimens known not to contain this specific antigen are assayed in each test run. A specific activity is calculated for each and an unknown specimen is considered to be positive for the antigen if it yields a specific activity which is two standard deviations greater than the mean of the known negative controls (Yolken, 1980).

LIMITS OF ANTIGEN DETECTION

The sensitivity of EIAs is determined both by the kinetics of the enzyme–substrate reaction and the interactions of the antigen and the antibody. The detection limit of the enzyme–substrate reaction is determined both by the specific activity of the enzyme bound to the immunoreactant as well as by the detectability of the substrate products (Bullock and Walls, 1977; Yolken, 1980; Pesce *et al.*, 1978). Properties of enzymes commonly used in EIAs are depicted in Table I. Alkaline phosphatase and peroxidase are two enzymes which have attained widespread usage in EIA systems since they both offer high turnover rates and a variety of suitable substrates. Glucose oxidase and β-galactosidase have also been utilized although they offer turnover rates somewhat slower than that of

TABLE I
COMPARISON OF ENZYMES AVAILABLE FOR EIA[a]

Enzyme	Source	Uses	pH optimum	Specific activity (units/mg)	Molecular weight	Practical methods of conjugation	Practical substrates available		
							Visual	Fluorescent	Radioactive
Alkaline phosphatase	Calf intestine	EIA	8–10	400	100,000	Glutaraldehyde 1 step	NP-PO$_4$	MU-PO$_4$	[³H]AMP
Peroxidase	Horseradish	EIA	5–7	900	40,000	Glutaraldehyde 1 step; Glutaraldehyde 2 step; Sodium m-periodate	H$_2$O$_2$ + 5AS; H$_2$O$_2$ + OPD; H$_2$O$_2$ + ABTS	NADH; HPA	NA
β-Galactosidase	Escherichia coli	EIA	6–8	400	540,000	Glutaraldehyde 1 step; p-Benzoquinone NN'-OPLD	NP-Gal	MU-Gal	[³H]GalP
Glucose oxidase	A. niger	EIA; HIST	4–7	200	160,000	Glutaraldehyde 1 step	Glu + 5AS; Glu + NBT; Glu + MTT	NADH; HPA	[³H]Glu
Catalase	Calf liver	EIA	6–8	40,000	250,000	Glutaraldehyde 1 step (SPA)	H$_2$O$_2$[b]	NA	NA

[a] NP-PO$_4$, nitrophenyl phosphate; MU-PO$_4$, methylumbelliferyl phosphate; FM-PO$_4$, fluorescein methyl phosphate; H$_2$O$_2$, hydrogen peroxide; 5AS, 4,5-aminosalicylic acid; OPD, o-phenylenediamine; HPA, α-hydroxyphenylacetic acid; NA, none available; ABTS, 2,2-azino-di-(3-ethylbenzothiazolin sulfone-6) diammonium salt; NP-Gal, nitrophenylgalactose; MU-Gal, methylumbelliferylgalactose; [³H]GalP, tritium-labeled β-galactose phosphate; N,N'-OPLD, N,N'-o-phenylenedimaleimide; HIST, enzyme-mediated histochemical procedure; [³H]Glu, tritium-labeled glucose; NBT, nitro blue tetrazolium chloride; MTT, thiazolyl blue; SPA, enzyme-labeled staphylococcal Protein A.

[b] Measured spectrophotometrically at $A_{240\ nm}$.

the other two enzymes (Pesce *et al.*, 1976; Zidoni and Kramer, 1974; Haining and Legan, 1972). Catalase has the theoretical advantage of having a greater specific activity than the other enzymes. However, the use of catalase has been limited since it is difficult to maintain activity following conjugation with immunoreactants and also because it is difficult to measure the enzyme–substrate reaction utilizing reactions which can be monitored in the visible range (Haining and Legan, 1972).

Most EIA systems utilize substrates which produce visibly colored products (Table I). Such substrates are convenient in that they can be monitored with the naked eye or measured by simple instrumentation. In the case of microtiter plates, the availability of instrumentation capable of reading 96 reactions in a short period of time has increased the scope of large-scale EIA testing. However, colorimetric substrates have the disadvantage that relatively large amounts of substrate are required for the measurement of the products by standard spectrophotometric instrumentation. For example, the minimum amount of nitrophenyl phosphate, the commonly used substrate for alkaline phosphatase, which can be detected is 10^{-8} mole. Assuming a turnover rate of 10^5 molecules per minute of the enzyme, the minimum amount of enzyme which can be detected in a 10-minute period is 10^{-14} mole. However, smaller quantities of alkaline phosphatase can be detected by the use of either fluorescent or radioactive substrates. For example, the fluorescent molecule, 4-methylumbelliferon, can be detected at a level of 10^{-11} mole, thus allowing for the measurement of 10^{-17} mole of alkaline phosphatase in a 10-minute period (Yolken *et al.*, 1979b; Shalev *et al.*, 1980). An even more sensitive system is provided by the use of [^{3}H]adenosine 5'-monophosphate (AMP) as a substrate for alkaline phosphatase (Harris *et al.*, 1979). The substrate product, [^{3}H]adenosine, can be separated from the parent compound by means of ion-exchange chromatography (Fig. 6) and detected at levels of 10^{-13} mole by standard liquid scintillation-counting instrumentation. The use of this substrate allows for the detection of 10^{-19} mole of enzyme in a 10-minute period. Phenyl phosphate (^{3}H labeled) has recently proven to be an even better substrate for alkaline phosphatase (Harris *et al.*, unpublished results). It should be noted that the theoretical detection limit of EIA systems can be improved by the use of longer substrate times. It is thus theoretically possible to detect even smaller amounts of enzyme provided that sufficiently long substrate incubation times are used and provided that the conditions can be adequately controlled.

However, the sensitivity of EIA systems is based not only on the kinetics of the enzyme–substrate reactions but also on the interactions of the antigen and antibody. In the noncompetitive assay system the interactions can be expressed by the law of mass action, as shown in Table II

TABLE II
INTERACTIONS IN NONCOMPETITIVE EIA

Law of mass action[a]

$$\frac{[AgAb]}{[Ag][Ab]} = K_a$$

Theoretical equilibrium values

K_a	$[Ab]^b$	Fraction of antigen bound
10^{-8} (High-affinity Ab)	10^{-7}	0.90
	10^{-8}	0.50
	10^{-9}	0.09
	10^{-10}	0.01
10^{-6} (Low-affinity Ab)	10^{-7}	0.09
	10^{-8}	0.01
	10^{-9}	0.001
	10^{-10}	0.0001

Attainable solid-phase antibody concentrations[b]

	% Ab	[Ab]
Monoclonal	100	10^{-7}
Affinity purified	30	3×10^{-8}
Hyperimmune	10	10^{-8}
Postinfection	1	10^{-9}

[a] [AgAb], Concentration of antigen–antibody complex (mole/liter); [Ag], concentration of unbound antigen; [Ab], concentration of unbound antibody; K_a, affinity constant of antigen–antibody reaction.

[b] Assuming a maximum binding capacity of 10 μg/ml and a molecular weight of 100,000.

(Ekins, 1980). The binding of enzyme-labeled antibody is thus determined by the concentration of antibody used and the affinity constant of the antibody. Commonly achievable concentrations of antibody result in the binding of a significant fraction of antigen in a specimen. However, in practice the sensitivity is also affected by the nonspecific interactions of the enzyme-labeled antibody with the solid phase. These interactions are shown in Table II. The limiting amount of antigen which can be detected is thus proportional both to the affinity constant of the antibody and to the affinity constants of the nonspecific interactions. To achieve the extreme degree of sensitivity promised by the use of highly sensitive substrates, it

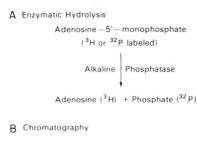

A Enzymatic Hydrolysis

Adenosine – 5' – monophosphate
(^{3}H or ^{32}P labeled)

Alkaline | Phosphatase

Adenosine (^{3}H) + Phosphate (^{32}P)

B Chromatography

Reaction Mixture

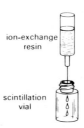

ion-exchange resin

scintillation vial

FIG. 6. Chromatographic separation of radioactive products. The reaction mixture from the enzymatic hydrolysis is added to the column containing positively charged ion-exchange resin. While AMP and phosphate, which have negative charges, are retained, adenosine flows freely through the resin into the scintillation vial. By altering the ionic strength of the eluate, phosphate can be eluted. After adding scintillator, the radioactivity is measured in the eluted material.

is thus necessary that the nonspecific interactions be minimized and that the antibodies of high affinity be utilized.

III. Practical Aspects of EIA for Measurement of Carcinogen–DNA Adducts

A. REAGENTS AND MATERIALS

Benzo[*a*]pyrene (B[*a*]P) (Baum, 1978) and (7β,8α)-dihydroxy-(9α,10α)-epoxy-7,8,9,10-tetrahydrobenzo[*a*]pyrene [(±)-BPDE I] (Sims *et al.*, 1974) used for preparation of both B[*a*]P–DNA and (7*R*)-BPDE I-deoxyguanosine (dG) (Poirier *et al.*, 1980) were supplied by the Standard Chemical Carcinogen Reference Repository, DCCP, National Cancer Institute, Bethesda, MD. Goat anti-rabbit IgG alkaline phosphatase conjugate, methylated bovine serum albumin (BSA), and Freund's adjuvants were purchased from Miles, Elkhart, IN; calf thymus DNA and p-nitrophenyl phosphate from Sigma Chemical Co., St. Louis, MO; polyvinyl microtiter plates from Dynatech Lab., Inc., Alexandria, VA; horse serum and fetal calf serum from Grand Island Biological Co., Grand Island, NY; and diethylaminoethyl (DEAE)-Sephadex A-25 from Pharmacia Fine Chemical, Piscataway, NJ. Calf thymus DNA was modified *in vitro* with (±)-BPDE I to a level of 1.4% (1.4 adducts per 100 nucleotides) for immunization and 0.2% for ultrasensitive enzymatic radioimmunoassay (USERIA), as previously described (Jeffrey *et al.*, 1977). Denatured B[*a*]P–DNA was prepared by heating the (±)-BPDE I-modified calf thymus DNA at 100°C for 5 minutes and then cooling quickly at 4°C. For immunization, either native or denatured BPDE I–DNAs were complexed electrostatically to equal amounts (w/w) of methylated BSA in a 0.9% NaCl solution (Plescia *et al.*, 1964). The BPDE I–DNA-methylated BSA was emulsified with an equal volume of complete Freund's adjuvant, and an amount equivalent to 1 mg of BP-modified DNA was injected intramuscularly (im) into the hindquarters of New Zealand white rabbits. Four initial injections, 1 week apart, were followed by five booster injections at monthly intervals. Each rabbit received a total of 75 μg of (7*R*)-BPDE I-dG. Rabbits were bled from the ear veins at regular intervals beginning 8 weeks after the first injection.

For preparation of antiserum against 2-acetylaminofluorene (AAF)–DNA adducts (Poirier *et al.*, 1977), guanosine and *N*-acetoxy-AAF (*N*-Ac-AAF) (Midwest Research Institute), each at 4.6 m*M* in 30% ethanol, were incubated for 24 hours at 37°C. The resultant *N*-(guanosine-8-yl)acetyl-aminofluorene (G-8-AAF) (Miller *et al.*, 1966; Kriek, 1972) was separated from the reaction mixture using a 20–100% methanol gradient on Sephadex LH-20 (Pharmacia) and rechromatographed until it gave a characteristic absorption spectrum (Kriek *et al.*, 1967). The purified product (9 mg) was coupled to BSA (35 mg; Sigma) by $NaIO_4$ oxidation followed by $NaBH_4$ reduction (Erlanger and Beiser, 1964), yielding 3.5 mg of covalently bound G-8-AAF (A_{305} 1.5 × 10⁴). Three rabbits were immunized with G-8-AAF–BSA, initially in complete and then in incomplete Freund's adjuvant at weeks 0, 1, 3, 12, 15, 17, and 23. Injections of 0.3 mg hapten were given im in the hind legs. Blood was taken from the ear veins before immunization, at 1 and 2 months, and weekly between 2 and 5 months. All three rabbits produced high levels of antibody by 4 months when assayed by radioimmunoassay (RIA) (Poirier, 1980).

[³H]AMP (generally ³H-labeled, 15 Ci/mmole, New England Nuclear; 1 Ci = 3.7 × 10¹⁰ becquerels) was purified by column chromatography with DEAE-Sephadex (A-25, Pharmacia; Fig. 6) in a stepwise manner as follows: (1) 2 mCi of [³H]AMP in 0.2 ml of distilled water was applied to a disposable column (Isolab, Akron, OH) containing 2 ml of DEAE-Sephadex; (2) the contaminating [³H]adenosine was eluted with distilled water and discarded; (3) [³H]AMP was eluted with 0.1 M ammonium carbonate; and (4) after lyophilization to remove the ammonium carbonate, the [³H]AMP was dissolved in 50% (v/v) ethanol. The column-purified [³H]AMP contained less than 0.2% [³H]adenosine and was stable at $-20°C$ for at least 3 months (Harris *et al.*, 1979). Dulbecco's phosphate-buffered saline (PBS), Dulbecco's PBS–Tween (10 mM phosphate buffer, pH 7.4, with 0.05% Tween 20), and 1 M diethanolamine buffer, pH 9.6, were supplied by the National Institutes of Health media unit.

Bronchial specimens obtained from immediate autopsy samples were cut into approximately 1 × 1-cm squares and cultured for 1 week before use (Harris *et al.*, 1976). The bronchial explants were then exposed to a culture medium containing 1 μg/ml of [³H]B[a]P (3.4 Ci/mmole) for 2 days with medium changes every 12–14 hours, and the DNA was isolated from the bronchial mucosa as previously described (Hsu *et al.*, 1978). Two-day-old primary cultures of BALB/c mouse epidermal cells were grown in 150-mm dishes (Yuspa and Harris, 1974) and exposed to BPDE I at concentrations of 10^{-5}, 10^{-6}, and 10^{-7} M for 1 hour. DNAs were prepared on CsCl gradients as previously described (Hsu *et al.*, 1978) and heat denatured after dialysis and before assay by USERIA or RIA. [9-¹⁴C]N-Ac-AAF (40.6 mCi/mmole) and nonradioactive N-Ac-AAF were supplied by the National Cancer Institute Chemical Carcinogen Repository.

B. SELECTION AND PRETREATMENT OF MICROTITER PLATES

The quality of microtiter plates affects both the accuracy and the sensitivity of the assays. We have tested 96-well plates from several manufacturing companies. Differences in plates are found among the various companies as well as among different lot numbers of plates from a single company. Polyvinyl microtiter plates bind most macromolecules to the solid phase better than polystyrene plates. For measurements of carcinogen–DNA adducts, the background values in the assays are generally lower in polyvinyl U-bottom plates than in V-bottom plates. Since the outer rows of wells tend to give inconsistent results, perhaps due to the casting temperature, the peripheral wells of microtiter plates are not generally used. In addition, variation in the activity can be minimized by pretreating the plates with DEAE-dextran. The optimal amount of DEAE-dextran varies with the type of macromolecule to be bound to the solid phase and has to be determined experimentally. To coat B[a]P–DNA, we pretreated the microtiter plates with 6 ng/well of DEAE-dextran in 0.2 ml carbonate buffer, pH 9.6, for 16–24 hours; the variation in the quadruplicate wells is usually less than 10%.

C. Coating of the Microtiter Plates with either Antigen or Antibody

When nanogram to microgram per milliliter amounts of protein in 0.1 M carbonate buffer, pH 9.6, are incubated in the microtiter wells, a large portion of the protein will be adsorbed by the wells. The adhered molecules generally retain their immunological properties and can be detected by the subsequent antigen–antibody reactions. The mechanisms of the attachment are unexplainable by simple charge differences (Cantarero *et al.*, 1980). When methylated [*methyl*-^{14}C]globulin (0.1–1 µg/ml) was dissolved either in PBS, pH 7.4, or carbonate buffer, pH 9.6, and incubated at 37°C in polyvinyl U plates, greater than 80% of the radioactivity remained adsorbed to the plates even after five washes with PBS–Tween. Neither PBS, pH 7.4, nor carbonate buffer, pH 9.6, caused any further release of radioactivity from the solid phase.

To measure carcinogen–DNA adducts by solid-phase EIA (Hsu *et al.*, 1981), the DEAE-dextran-pretreated polyvinyl U microtiter wells are first coated with DNA, either with or without carcinogen modification. Nanogram amounts of DNA dissolved in 60 µl of Dulbecco's PBS buffer are added to microtiter wells and allowed to dry overnight in a 37°C incubator. B[*a*]P metabolite bound to calf thymus DNA is stable at 37°C for several days without change of antigenicity. DNA can also be adhered to the plates by dissolving it in 0.1 M carbonate buffer, pH 9.6, and incubating at 37°C. However, we find that Dulbecco's PBS gives more reproducible results.

D. Antigen–Antibody Reaction in Microtiter Plates

The adhered carcinogen–DNA adducts will specifically absorb only their own antibodies, which will then react with alkaline phosphatase conjugated to IgG of a second antibody against the first antibodies. These reactions are carried out in PBS–Tween with 1% fetal calf serum at 37°C. Binding of the specific antibodies and alkaline phosphatase-conjugated IgG to the adhered carcinogen–DNA on the solid phase reaches maximum after 1 to 2-hour incubation at 37°C (Fig. 7). The amount of either the primary antiserum or the alkaline phosphatase-conjugated IgG is adjusted (1) to achieve a high signal-to-noise ratio, and (2) to obtain enzyme activities in the wells that will release enough product to be detected in a rea-

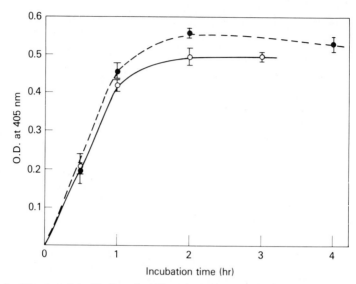

F<small>IG</small>. 7.   Kinetics of the binding of rabbit antiserum (●) or alkaline phosphate IgG conjugate (○) that was specifically bound to the solid phase during the assay procedure. B[*a*]P–
DNA for coating was 5 ng/well, the concentration of rabbit antiserum was 1:5 × 10⁴ dilution, and alkaline phosphatase IgG conjugate 1:500 dilution.

sonable time period. More dilute antisera are required for USERIA as
compared to enzyme-linked immunosorbent assay (ELISA) (Engvall and
Perlmann, 1972).

E. E<small>NDPOINT</small> M<small>EASUREMENT OF</small> A<small>NTIGEN</small>–A<small>NTIBODY</small> R<small>EACTIONS</small>

The specific antigen–antibody reactions are quantitated by measuring
the alkaline phosphatase activities on the solid phase. We use [³H]AMP as
the substrate in USERIA (Harris *et al.*, 1979) and *p*-nitrophenyl phosphate as substrate for EIA (Engvall and Perlmann, 1972). Alkaline phosphatase in 1 *M* diethanolamine buffer, pH 9.8, will hydrolyze *p*-nitro-
phenyl phosphate to *p*-nitrophenol, which can be detected in the microtiter plates by a spectrophotometer, such as a Multiscan (Flow Labs), at
405 nm. In addition, the enzyme will release [³H]adenosine from
[³H]AMP in a 0.1 *M* diethanolamine buffer, pH 9. The hydrolyzed
[³H]adenosine, after separation from [³H]AMP by a DEAE-Sephadex A-
25 column 1-ml bed volume, is measured in a liquid scintillation counter
and is linear for enzyme concentrations of 10^{-17}–10^{-21} mole (Fig. 8). As
low as 10^{-21} mole of alkaline phosphatase in 0.1 ml of pH 9 buffer can be
measured in 90 minutes with [³H]AMP as substrate, whereas 10^{-17} mole of

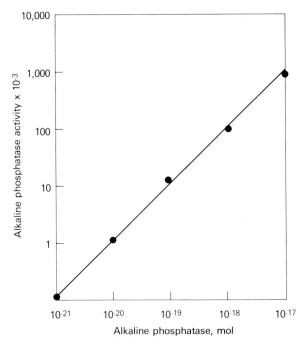

FIG. 8. Determination of the sensitivity of the assay. Various dilutions of alkaline phosphate (10^{-17}–10^{-21} mole) were included in 0.1-ml reaction volumes of 10 mM diethanolamine buffer, pH 9, containing 100 pmole of [^{3}H]AMP as substrate. The products were isolated by DEAE-Sephadex column chromatography. The activity is expressed as adenosine (dpm) released in 90 minutes.

the same enzyme is required under the conditions necessary to generate enough p-nitrophenol from p-nitrophenyl phosphate for detection.

IV. Measurements of Carcinogen–DNA Adducts

In recent years, considerable progress has been made in the use of immunological approaches to measure carcinogen binding to DNA (Poirier et al., 1980; Muller and Rajewski, 1980; Haugen et al., 1981). Procedures to measure DNA adducts of B[a]P and AAF by RIA, ELISA, and USERIA will be discussed.

A. DETERMINATION OF B[a]P BINDING TO DNA

Native and denatured calf thymus DNA were modified in vitro with (±)-BPDE I (Sims et al., 1974; Poirier et al., 1980). This modified DNA was then allowed to complex to equal amounts (w/w) of methylated BSA, emulsified with complete Freund's adjuvant, and injected im into New Zealand white rabbits (Poirier *et al.*, 1980). To determine the titer, sensitivity, and specificity of the rabbit serum, RIA was performed by competing BPDE I-[³H]dG against BPDE I–DNA nucleotides or B[*a*]P derivatives for antiserum. In an RIA with BPDE I-[³H]dG, the greatest sensitivity (50% inhibition at 5 pmole) was obtained when BPDE I-modified DNA was used as an unlabeled competitor (Poirier *et al.*, 1980). After denaturation and hydrolysis with S_1 nuclease, the BPDE I–DNA was a less efficient competitor (50% inhibition at 15 pmole) when assayed by RIA. The authentic deoxyguanosine adducts (7*R*)-BDPE I-dG or BPDE II-dG were both recognized equally, giving 50% inhibition at about 40 pmole. The following compounds showed no competition with BPDE I-[³H]dG in the RIA: 5–22 μg native or denatured unmodified DNA; 17–35 μg denatured and S_1-hydrolyzed unmodified DNA; 300–3000 pmole of tetrol derived from BPDE I–tetrol; and 100–1000 pmole dG-8-AAF. Also, when 10 μg DNA and 5.5 μg BP were added simultaneously to the assay tubes, no competition was observed.

To compare the sensitivity and specificity of RIA and solid-phase EIAs, the same serum was used in the following noncompetitive and competitive EIAs and USERIAs (Hsu *et al.*, 1981). For noncompetitive USERIA or EIA, microtiter plates were coated with either control DNA or (±)-BPDE I-modified DNA (0.2% modification) by drying 60 μl per well of the DNA solution in Dulbecco's PBS, pH 7.4, for 16–24 hours at 37°C. The plates were washed five times with PBS–Tween. To prevent nonspecific binding of antibody to the wells, each well was exposed to 0.2 ml of 1% goat serum in PBS–Tween for 1 hour at 37°C and then washed five times with PBS–Tween. Diluted rabbit antiserum to B[*a*]P–DNA (0.1 ml/well) dissolved in PBS containing 1% fetal calf serum was added and the plates were incubated at 37°C for 1.5 hours. The plates were then washed five times with PBS–Tween and incubated with 0.1 ml per well of goat anti-rabbit IgG alkaline phosphatase conjugate (1:400 dilution for ELISA, 1:2000 for USERIA) dissolved in PBS containing 1% fetal calf serum. The plates were washed five more times with PBS–Tween and then twice with 0.1 *M* diethanolamine buffer, pH 9.6, before adding the enzyme–substrate in diethanolamine buffer. The activity of alkaline phosphatase bound to the solid phase by the above reactions was determined either by radiometric measurement of [³H]adenosine (USERIA) (Harris *et al.*, 1979) or by spectrophotometric assay of *p*-nitrophenol at 405 nm (EIA) (Engvall and Perlmann, 1972). Only B[*a*]P–DNA-coated wells reacted specifically with rabbit antiserum to B[*a*]P–DNA, as determined by the activities of alkaline phosphatase conjugated to goat anti-rabbit IgG bound to the solid phase. Normal rabbit serum did not specifically react with either calf thymus DNA or B[*a*]P–DNA.

The enzyme activity of alkaline phosphatase goat anti-rabbit IgG conjugate that bound to the plates increased proportionally with increasing amounts of B[*a*]P–DNA coated on the plates (Fig. 9A). However, the enzyme activity reached maximum at approximately 100 ng per well of B[*a*]P–DNA adducts that can be measured in 10 ng DNA by a noncom-

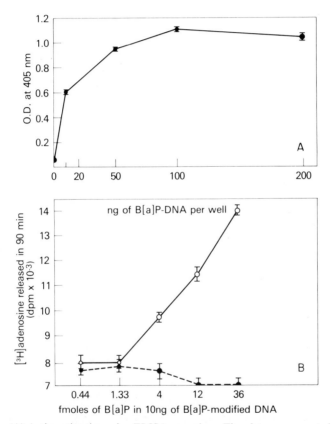

FIG. 9. (A) Antigen titration using ELISA procedure. The plates were coated with various amounts of B[*a*]P–DNA and the subsequent antigen–antibody reactions were determined by spectrophotometric measurement of the enzymatic product, *p*-nitrophenol. (B) Dose–response curve of noncompetitive USERIA. The plates were coated with 10 ng calf thymus DNA per well containing 0, 0.44, 1.33, 4, 12, and 36 fmole of B[*a*]P–DNA adducts. The methodology for USERIA is described in the text; assays were incubated with [³H]AMP for 90 minutes. Experimental values (○) were determined from wells coated with various amounts of B[*a*]P–DNA; control values (●) were determined from wells coated with 10 ng calf thymus DNA only.

petitive USERIA procedure. Various amounts of BPDE I-modified DNA were mixed with calf thymus DNA. When a total of 10 ng of the mixture was added to each well and the antigen–antibody reaction was measured by noncompetitive USERIA, as few as 3 fmole of B[a]P–DNA adducts in 10 ng DNA could be determined (Fig. 9B). This is equivalent to one molecule of the B[a]P–DNA adduct per 30,000 nucleotides.

Competitive USERIA was performed by antibody competition of B[a]P–DNA attached to the solid phase and free B[a]P–DNA in the reaction mixture. The plates were coated with either B[a]P–DNA or DNA (control) (6 ng/well for EIA and 1 ng/well for USERIA) and incubated with 0.2 ml of 1% horse serum in PBS–Tween for 1 hour at 37°C to block the nonspecific binding of antibody, as described above. Standard curves for the competition assays were determined by mixing serial dilutions of B[a]P–DNA with diluted rabbit antiserum (5×10^4-fold dilution for EIA and 2.5×10^5-fold dilution for USERIA) and adding 0.1 ml of the mixtures to each well containing a standard amount of B[a]P–DNA bound to the solid phase. After a 1.5-hour incubation at 37°C, the plates were treated with goat anti-rabbit IgG alkaline phosphatase conjugate. The enzymatic substrates were finally added to determine the alkaline phosphatase activity bound to the wells, as described in noncompetitive assays. As shown in Fig. 10, the amounts of B[a]P–DNA adducts in 1 μg of DNA that showed a 50% inhibition were 5300 fmole for RIA, 55 fmole for EIA, and 1 fmole for USERIA. In addition to a 500-fold increase in sensitivity for USERIA as compared to RIA, the optimal amount of rabbit antiserum used in the assay was also 500-fold less than that used in RIA. (7R)-BPDE I-dG, as competitor, did not compete as efficiently as B[a]P–DNA against the coated B[a]P–DNA. Unmodified single-stranded DNA had very little effect on the results of the competitive assay (Table III).

To determine the efficiency of USERIA for measuring carcinogen–DNA binding in biological samples, DNA was extracted from (1) cultured human bronchial explants exposed to 4×10^{-6} M B[a]P (Harris *et al.*, 1976), and (2) mouse epidermal cells exposed to ($\pm$)-BPDE I (10^{-5}, 10^{-6}, or 10^{-7} M) (Yuspa and Harris, 1974). As shown in Fig. 10 (—○—), B[a]P-modified cellular DNA from human bronchus (20 fmole B[a]P/μg DNA, or 1 molecule of adduct in 2×10^5 nucleotides, as determined by radiochemical methods) competed against B[a]P–DNA absorbed to the wells. At a DNA concentration of 4 μg/0.1 ml reaction mixture, a competition curve with B[a]P metabolite-modified human cellular DNA as the competitor was established; 1 μg of the DNA per 0.1 ml reaction mixture caused 52% inhibition, corresponding to 13 fmole/μg DNA. The three immunoassays were also applied to measure B[a]P–DNA adducts in mouse epidermal cells exposed to increasing concentrations of ($\pm$)-BPDE I in the

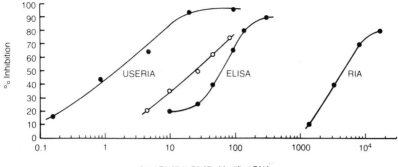

fmol B[a]P in B[a]P - Modified DNA

FIG. 10. Percentage inhibition curves from competitive assays for detection of B[a]P metabolite bound to DNA. For USERIA, the microtiter plates were coated with 1 ng of B[a]P–DNA per well. The 0.1 ml competition mixture containing rabbit antiserum (2.5 × 10⁵-fold dilution) was mixed with serial dilutions of 0.2% (±)-BPDE I-modified DNA (●, standard curves), or DNA isolated from [³H]B[a]P-treated bronchial mucosa in culture (○). The final concentration of DNA in this solution was adjusted with calf thymus DNA to 1 μg/0.1 ml. [³H]AMP was added for 90 minutes. For ELISA (○, human bronchial DNA: 1 adduct per 2 × 10⁵ bases) the plates were coated with 6 ng of B[a]P–DNA per well. The reaction mixture contained rabbit antiserum (5 × 10⁴-fold dilution) with serial dilution of B[a]P–DNA. The detailed methodologies of RIA, USERIA, and ELISA are described in the text. For RIA (●), 1.4% (±)-BPDE I-modified DNA competed with [³H](7R)-BPDE I-dG for antibody in 0.4 ml of reaction solution, as described previously (Poirier et al., 1980).

TABLE III

IMPROVEMENT OF USERIA SENSITIVITY BY INCREASING THE AMOUNT OF FREE DNA IN THE COMPETITIVE REACTION SOLUTION

μg DNA (fmole nucleotides) in 0.1 ml competitive solution	Femtomole B[a]P–DNA adducts mixed in the calf thymus DNA	[³H]adenosine released (dpm × 10⁻³)	Percentage inhibition
1 (2.9 × 10⁶)	34	17.3	71.1
	0	59.8	
5 (14.5 × 10⁶)	34	17.6	71.5
	0	61.75	
25 (7.5 × 10⁷)	34	17.2	74.6
	0	67.7	
10 (2.9 × 10⁷)[a]	34	15.5	75.5
	0	63.4	

[a] Double-stranded DNA.

TABLE IV

COMPARISON OF RIA, ELISA, AND USERIA FOR DETECTION OF BPDE I-dG IN DNA
FROM CULTURED MOUSE EPIDERMAL CELLS EXPOSED TO BPDE I

	Concentration of BPDE I in the medium of epidermal cell cultures (M)	Content of BPDE I-dG (fmole per μg DNA)		
		RIA	ELISA	USERIA
Expt. 1	10^{-5}	558 ± 36^a	442 ± 8	479 ± 57
Expt. 1	10^{-6}	ND^b	47 ± 4	39 ± 8
	10^{-7}	ND	5	4 ± 1.7
Expt. 2	10^{-5}	615 ± 41	464 ± 30	477 ± 21

^{a} Mean value $\pm$ standard deviation or mean of two values.
^{b} ND, Not detectable.

culture medium for 1 hour. Enzyme immunoassay and USERIA can easily determine approximately 25-fmole adducts in 5 μg DNA in cells exposed to 10^{-7} M ($\pm$)-BPDE I, whereas RIA is not sensitive enough to measure accurately the amounts of adducts in samples exposed to either 10^{-6} or 10^{-7} M ($\pm$)-BPDE I. Nevertheless, the results of the three assays are similar (Table IV).

B. DETERMINATION OF AAF–DNA ADDUCTS

The carcinogen, AAF, and its activated derivatives, N-Ac-AAF and hydroxy AAF, bind covalently to guanosine in DNA producing G-8-AAF and dG-8-AAF as the two major adducts (Miller *et al.*, 1966). Antibodies against these adducts were prepared by immunization of rabbit with G-8-AAF-coupled proteins; the hapten, G-8-AAF, was first oxidized by NaIO$_4$, reduced by NaBH$_4$, and then coupled to BSA. Using the rabbit antiserum, a standard curve for RIA was constructed by competing the [^{3}H]dG-8-AAF with unlabeled G-8-AAF or dG-8-AAF, both of which competed equally well (Poirier *et al.*, 1977). Approximately 2 pmole of G-8-AAF gave 50% inhibition; dG, N-Ac-AAF, and AAF produced a slight inhibition. At concentrations up to 100 μg, dT, dA, and dC were totally ineffective.

For EIAs (Hsu *et al.*, 1980), polyvinyl U microtiter plates were coated with 0.1 ml per well of a DNA solution (DNA either with or without AAF metabolite modification) dissolved in 50 mM carbonate buffer, pH 9.6, for 16 hours at 37°C in a humidified chamber; the DNA containing dG-8-AAF is stable and does not undergo deacetylation at pH 9.6 for at least 24 hours. The wells with bound DNA were washed five times with PBS–Tween. To prevent nonspecific binding of antibody to the plates, each DNA-coated well was exposed to 0.2 ml of 1% horse serum (Grand Island Biological Co.) in PBS–Tween for 1 hour at 37°C and then washed twice with PBS–Tween. Standard curves for the competition assays were determined by mixing serial dilutions of dG-8-AAF with dilutions of the rabbit antiserum (USERIA, 600,000-fold dilution; EIA, 60,000-fold dilution) and adding 0.1 ml of the mixtures to each well containing a standard amount of bound AAF–DNA. After 1-hour incubation at 37°C, the plates were washed five times with PBS–Tween and then incubated with 0.1 ml per well of goat anti-rabbit IgG alkaline phosphatase conjugate (1 : 400 dilution) for 1 hour. The plates were washed five times with PBS–Tween and then twice with 0.1 M diethanolamine buffer, pH 9.6, before adding 0.1 ml per well of enzyme substrates (USERIA, 100 pmole [^{3}H]AMP per well; EIA, 0.1 mg p-nitrophenyl phosphate per well; Sigma Chemical Co., St. Louis, MO) diluted in the diethanolamine buffer. The activity of alkaline phosphatase bound to the solid phase by the above reactions was determined either by measuring radioactive adenosine (USERIA) (Harris *et al.*, 1979) or by spectrophotometrically assaying p-nitrophenol at 405 nm (EIA) (Engvall and Perlmann, 1972). Experiments were performed in triplicate and the results of the triplicate samples varied less than 20%.

The standard curves for the results of the competition assays by RIA, ELISA, and USERIA are shown in Fig. 11. The amounts of dG-8-AAF at which a 50% inhibition was observed were 250 fmole for RIA, 40 fmole for ELISA, and 4 fmole for USERIA. In addition to a 60-fold increase in sensitivity for USERIA as compared to RIA, the optimal amount of rabbit antiserum used in the assay was 60- to 600-fold less than that used in RIA (i.e., the optimal serum dilutions were 1000-fold for RIA, 60,000-fold for ELISA, and 600,000-fold for USERIA).

The competition assay can be used to determine small quantities of dG-8-AAF in DNA. 2-Acetylaminofluorine-modified calf thymus DNA was hydrolyzed by S_1 nuclease (Sigma Chemical Co.) (Hsu *et al.*, 1980) and dG-8-AAF adducts were determined as 35, 29, and 32 pmole per μg DNA by RIA, USERIA, and ELISA, respectively. S_1 nuclease-hydrolyzed AAF–DNA yielded competition curves similar to those shown for authentic dG-8-AAF in Fig. 11 for all three assays. Previous results have indicated that RIA reliably quantitates the level of AAF binding determined by radiochemical techniques (Poirier *et al.*, 1977; Poirier *et al.*, 1979). The close correlation of results with RIA, EIA, and USERIA indicates that quantitation of these more sensitive assays is also valid.

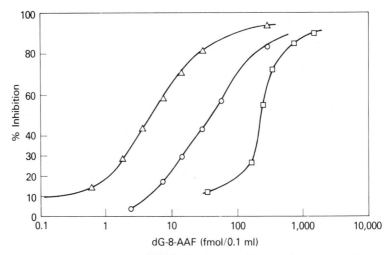

FIG. 11. Percentage inhibition curves for detection by competitive assays of dG-8-AAF in AAF–DNA by RIA (□), ELISA (○), and USERIA (△). For USERIA, the microtiter plates were coated with 0.4 ng of AAF–DNA per well. The reaction mixture contained rabbit antiserum (600,000-fold dilution) with serial dilutions of dG-8-AAF (0–290 fmole in 0.1 ml). [³H]AMP concentration was 1 μM. For ELISA, the plates were coated with 4 ng of AAF–DNA per well. The reaction mixture contained rabbit antiserum (60,000-fold dilution) with serial dilution of dG-8-AAF (0–2900 fmole in 0.1 ml). The detailed methodologies of RIA, USERIA, and ELISA are described in the text.

When the immunoassays were used to measure dG-8-AAF in rat hepatocytes exposed to 10^{-5} M AAF for 5 hours, they yielded binding values of 12, 13, and 17 fmole of dG-8-AAF as determined by USERIA, EIA, and RIA, respectively, in repeated experiments (Hsu *et al.*, 1980). An important advantage of these assays to such studies is that they require less than 10 μg of DNA for multiple assays, whereas techniques using radiolabeled carcinogens usually require much larger quantities of starting material.

Using a second approach, AAF bound to DNA can also be detected with a noncompetitive immunological assay by adsorbing the carcinogen-modified DNA in wells of the microtiter plates and directly measuring the carcinogen–DNA adducts (Hsu *et al.*, 1980). To determine the sensitivity of this noncompetitive assay, wells were coated with single-stranded calf thymus DNA, 10 ng/well, containing serial dilutions of AAF-modified DNA in 50 mM carbonate buffer, pH 9.6. After incubation for 16 hours at 37°C, each well in the microtiter plate was (1) washed five times with PBS–Tween, (2) incubated with 0.2 ml per well of 1% horse serum for 1 hour, (3) washed five times with PBS–Tween, (4) incubated with 0.1 ml

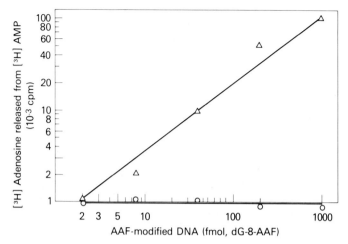

Fɪɢ. 12. Dose–response curve of noncompetitive USERIA. The plates were coated with 10 ng calf thymus DNA per well containing 0, 2, 8, 40, 200, and 1000 fmole of dG-8-AAF adducts. The methodology for USERIA is described in the text. Experimental values (△) were determined from wells coated with various amounts of AAF-modified DNA; control values (○) were determined from wells coated with 10 ng calf thymus DNA only.

per well of diluted rabbit antiserum for 1 hour, and (5) incubated with 0.1 ml per well of goat anti-rabbit IgG alkaline phosphatase conjugate, as described above. As shown in Fig. 12, alkaline phosphatase activity, as measured by the release of [³H]adenosine from [³H]AMP, increased linearly with increasing concentrations of AAF-modified DNA. As little as 2 fmole of dG-8-AAF can be detected in a total of 10 ng of DNA (Hsu *et al.*, 1980).

V. Measurement of Biologically Active Molecules and Viruses

A. Gᴇɴᴇʀᴀʟ Cᴏɴꜱɪᴅᴇʀᴀᴛɪᴏɴꜱ

As discussed in Section II, the sensitivity and specificity of EIA systems are dependent to a great extent on the properties of the immunoreactants utilized in the assay (Yolken, 1980; Pesce *et al.*, 1978; Ekins, 1980). This is particularly a consideration in the measurement of viruses, bacterial toxins, and other biologically active macromolecules since these antigens can be difficult to obtain in large quantities in pure form. It is thus important that care be taken in the preparation of antisera to these macromolecules to ensure a minimum of nonspecific reactivity with extraneous antigens. We have found that the most critical determinant of the specificity of the antisera is the absence of contaminating antigens in the preparation used to immunize the animal. In the case of viruses the main source of extraneous antigens is nonviral proteins derived from the tissue culture or animal cells used to propagate the virus (Rubenstein, 1978; Dienstag *et al.*, 1976; Fisher, 1980). This is particularly a problem in the case of enveloped viruses such as herpes simplex and herpes zoster, since whole virions can contain some proteins of host origin which are incorporated into the virion in the process of viral release (Hampar and Martea, 1973). Antisera made to these virions might contain antibodies to human proteins, thus leading to a false-positive reaction when a specimen with these proteins is tested. In the case of viral antigens obtained from whole animals, an additional source of contaminating material is immunoglobulin. Such immunoglobulins might be part of the natural host response of the animal to viral infection. When viral proteins complexed with antibodies are used as an immunogen, antibodies to immunoglobulins are produced as well as antibodies to the viral antigen. The use of such antibodies in an immunoassay system will lead to false-positive reactions in the case of specimens containing cross-reactive antibodies. This is particularly a problem in the case of viruses obtained from human sources, such as Norwalk virus, hepatitis A and B viruses, and rotavirus, since the antibodies will be directed with a high degree of reactivity toward immunoglobulins in human clinical specimens (Yolken, 1980; Dienstag *et al.*, 1976). In the case of bacterial toxins, the main source of potential cross-reactivity is with some bacterial products which are not themselves active. Antibodies directed against such proteins will cross-react with non-toxin-producing strains of bacteria, thus leading to false-positive results.

With these considerations, it is important that the antigen utilized to immunize the animal be purified to the greatest degree possible. In the case of viral antigens, purification by means of repeated density sedimentations is usually sufficient. However, in the case of enveloped viruses, such treatment might not adequately separate viral from mammalian proteins. It thus might be necessary to disrupt the viruses and isolate specific viral proteins. In addition, care should be taken to utilize animals which do not have detectable antibodies to antigens which might be present in humans.

Once an antiserum is obtained it should be tested to ensure its specificity. If adequate specificity is not obtained then the investigator can attempt to purify it by means of immunological techniques such as affinity chromatography. One limitation of this technique is that sufficient quantities of antigen are often not available to allow for the production of adequate volumes of antibodies. However, in many cases, sufficient concentrations of cross-reacting antigens such as uninfected tissue culture fluid or cells can be utilized to absorb the nonspecific activity.

Due to the problems of the production of specific antisera, especially in the case of the more sensitive assay systems, there has been an interest in utilizing systems *in vitro* for the production of antibody. One such system is the "hybridoma" system developed by Kohler and Milstein (1975). This system involves the fusion of effector cells derived from an immunized animal with an antibody-producing cell line and the selection of clones which produce antibodies with the desired specificity. One limitation of some monoclonal antibodies is that their affinity constants are often not as high as those of polyclonal antibodies. As shown in Table I, the use of antibodies with less favorable affinity constants might partially offset the decrease in nonspecific activity which could be gained from them. However, the availability of monoclonal antibodies with affinity constants similar to those of most polyclonal antibodies (10^8–10^9) should markedly improve the specificity of EIA systems, especially in the case of the ultrasensitive systems utilizing fluorescent and radioactive substrates.

B. PROTOCOL FOR THE PERFORMANCE OF THE ASSAY SYSTEMS FOR BIOLOGICALLY ACTIVE MOLECULES AND VIRUSES

1. Optimal Concentration of Reagents

The optimal concentration of reagents utilized should be determined by titration. That is, dilutions of all reagents should be tested and the relative sensitivity and specificity of the systems should be determined with a test antigen. In our experience, EIA reagents used in the following ranges gave satisfactory results:

1. Serum used to coat plates (Ab_1):   1:10,000– 1:100,000
2. IgG fraction used to coat plates: 0.5–2 μg/ml
3. Unlabeled second antibody: 1:1000– 1:4000
4. Enzyme-labeled conjugates: 1:200– 1:2000
5. Antigen used to coat plates for binding-antibody test: 1:20– 1:1000
6. Staphylococcal Protein A: 2–10 μg/ml
7. Enzyme–antienzyme complex: 1:200– 1:1000

Note that all reactants are used in a quantity of 100 μl/well.

2. *Example of a Protocol for Measurement of Virus*

Detailed protocols for the measurement of rotavirus have been published (Yolken, 1980). Antigen assays are described.

a. *Direct Assay for Antigen*

1. Coat alternate rows of wells of the microtiter plate with a dilution of goat anti-rotavirus serum (or IgG) and an equal dilution of goat serum (or IgG) which does not contain measurable antibody to rotavirus.
2. Incubate the plate at least overnight at 4°C. If the plate is not used the next day, it should be covered with Parafilm and stored at 4°C until use.
3. Wash the plate five times with PBS–Tween.
4. Add 50 μl of *N*-acetylcysteine (adjusted to pH 7) to each of the wells. Add an equal amount of specimen to two wells coated with goat anti-rotavirus serum and two wells coated with normal goat serum. Include a weakly positive control and four negative controls in each test.
5. Incubate the plate for 2 hours at 37°C or overnight at 4°C.
6. Wash the plate five times with PBS–Tween.
7. Add to the wells enzyme-labeled anti-rotavirus serum (either goat or guinea pig) diluted in PBS–Tween containing 2% fetal calf serum (PBS–Tween–FCS).
8. Incubate the plate for 1 hour at 37°C.
9. Wash the plate five times with PBS–Tween.
10. Add appropriate substrate. Incubate the plate at 37°C or room temperature until the weakly positive control has a visible color equivalent to an optical density of approximately 0.1. Calculate a rotavirus specific activity by subtracting the mean activity of the specimen in wells coated with the rotavirus-negative serum from the mean activity of the wells coated with the anti-rotavirus serum. To ensure accurate quantitation, specimens giving readings of greater than 1.2 optical density units should be diluted 1 : 10 and retested. Calculate the mean and standard deviation of the rotavirus specific activity of the negative controls. A specimen is considered positive if its mean activity is greater than 2 standard deviations above the mean of the negative controls. Alternatively, a specimen can be considered positive if its activity is greater than that of the weakly positive control.

If qualitative visual determinations are used, a specimen is considered positive if its color in the goat anti-rotavirus wells is greater than its color in the normal goat wells and greater than the color of the weakly positive control in the goat anti-rotavirus wells.

b. Indirect Antigen Assay

1. Coat the plate and add the specimens as described in steps 1–6 of "Direct Assay for Antigen."
2. Add unlabeled guinea pig anti-rotavirus serum diluted in PBS–Tween–FCS.
3. Incubate the plate for 1 hour at 37°C.
4. Wash the plate five times with PBS–Tween.
5. Dilute enzyme-labeled anti-guinea pig immunoglobulin, prepared in either goat or rabbit, in PBS–Tween and add it to the wells.
6. Incubate the plate for 1 hour at 37°C.
7. Wash the plate five times with PBS–Tween.
8. Add substrate and interpret the results as described in step 10 under "Direct Assay for Antigen."

VI. Perspectives

Enzyme immunoassays are an important addition to the many methods currently used in cancer research. The primary advantages of EIAs are their sensitivity, rapidness, and inexpensiveness. Although solid-phase immunoassays such as EIA are easy to perform, one has to be aware of the principles and practical aspects of these assays. In addition, optimal assay conditions for each antigen–antibody combination have to be determined by direct experimentation. The information provided in this chapter should be a useful guide.

Enzyme immunoassays will supplement and, in some cases, replace RIAs for the measurement of chemical carcinogens, carcinogen–DNA adducts, oncofetal proteins, ectopic hormones, viruses, drugs, etc. Enzyme immunoassays will be improved by the availability of solid phases that have larger surface areas and more uniform absorptive characteristics. Equipment for semiautomation of the various technical manipulations and endpoint measurements is already available: complete automation will no doubt be the next step.

The ultimate limit in the sensitivity of EIAs such as USERIA will depend on the specificity and the affinity of the antibodies. As high-affinity monoclonal antibodies become available, the current level of sensitivity will be surpassed.

REFERENCES

Avrameas, S., and Ternyck, T. (1971). *Immunochemistry* **8**, 1175–1181.

Baum, E. J. (1978). *In* "Polycyclic Hydrocarbons and Cancer" (H. V. Gelboin and P. O. P. Ts'o, eds.), pp. 45–70. Academic Press, New York.

Berg, R. A., Yolken, R. H., Rennard, S. I., Dolin, R., Murphy, B. R., and Straus, S. E. (1980). *Lancet* **1**, 851–853.

Bullock, S., and Walls, K. (1977). *J. Infect. Dis.* **136**, 5279–5288.

Cantarero, L. A., Butler, J. E., and Osborne, J. W. (1980). *Anal. Biochem.* **105**, 375–382.

Davies, D. A. L. (1973). *In* "Handbook of Experimental Immunology" (D. M. Weir, ed.), pp. 4.1–4.14. Blackwell, Oxford.

Dienstag, J. L., Schulman, A. N., Gerety, R. J., Hoffnagle, J. H., Lorenz, D. E., Purcell, R. H., and Barker, L. F. (1976). *J. Immunol.* **11**, 876–881.

Ekins, R. (1980). *Nature (London)* **284**, 14–15.

Engvall, E. (1978). *Scand. J. Immunol.* **8**, 25–31.

Engvall, E., and Perlmann, P. (1972). *J. Immunol.* **109**, 129–135.

Erlanger, B. F., and Beiser, S. M. (1964). *Proc. Natl. Acad. Sci. U.S.A.* **52**, 68–74.

Fisher, D. (1980). *In* "Manual of Clinical Immunology" (E. H. Lennette, ed.), 3rd Ed., pp. 339–342. American Society of Microbiology, Washington, DC.

Haining, J. L., and Legan, J. S. (1972). *Anal. Biochem.* **45**, 469–472.

Hampar, B., and Martes, L. M. (1973). *In* "The Herpesviruses" (A. S. Kaplan, ed.), pp. 114–128. Academic Press, New York.

Haugen, A., Groopman, J. D., Hsu, I.-C., Goodrich, G. R., Wogan, G. N., and Harris, C. C. (1981). *Proc. Natl. Acad. Sci. U.S.A.* **78**, 4124–4127.

Harris, C. C., Autrup, H., Connor, R., Barrett, L. A., McDowell, E. M., and Trump, B. F. (1976). *Science* **194**, 1067–1069.

Harris, C. C., Yolken, R. H., Krokan, H., and Hsu, I.-C. (1979). *Proc. Natl. Acad. Sci. U.S.A.* **76**, 5336–5339.

Hsu, I.-C., Stoner, G. D., Autrup, H., Trump, B. F., Selkirk, J. K., and Harris, C. C. (1978). *Proc. Natl. Acad. Sci. U.S.A.* **75**, 2003–2007.

Hsu, I.-C., Poirer, M. C., Yuspa, S. H., Yolken, R. H., and Harris, C. C. (1980). *Carcinogenesis* **1**, 455–458.

Hsu, I.-C., Poirier, M. C., Yuspa, S. H., Grunberger, D., Weinstein, I. B., Yolken, R. H., and Harris, C. C. (1981). *Cancer Res.* **41**, 1091–1095.

Hunter, W. M. (1973). *In* "Handbook of Experimental Immunology" (D. M. Weir, ed.), pp. 1–17. Blackwell, Oxford.

Jeffrey, A. M., Weinstein, I. B., Jennette, K. W., Grzeskowiak, K., Nakanishi, K., Harvey, G. W., Autrup, H., and Harris, C. C. (1977). *Nature (London)* **269**, 348–350.

Kato, K., Umeda, U., Suzuki, F., Hayashi, D., and Koseka, A. (1979). *FEBS Lett.* **102**, 253–256.

Kohler, G., and Milstein, C. (1975). *Nature (London)* **256**, 495–498.

Kriek, E. (1972). *Cancer Res.* **32**, 2042–2048.

Kriek, E., Miller, J. A., Juhl, U., and Miller, E. C. (1967). *Biochemistry* **6**, 177–182.

Lehtonen, O. P., and Viljanen, M. K. (1980). *J. Immunol. Methods* **34**, 61–70.

Miller, E. C., Juhl, U., and Miller, J. A. (1966). *Science* **153**, 1125–1127.

Muller, R., and Rajewsky, M. F. (1980). *Cancer Res.* **40**, 887–896.

Ngo, T. T., and Lenhoff, H. M. (1980). *FEBS Lett.* **116**, 285–288.

Pesce, A. J., Modesto, R. R., Ford, D. J., Sethi, K., Clyne, D. N., and Pollak, V. E. (1976). *In* "Immunoenzymatic Techniques" (G. Feldmann, ed.), pp. 7–18. North-Holland Publ., Amsterdam.

Pesce, A., Ford, D., Gaizutis, M., and Pollak, V. (1977). *Biochim. Biophys. Acta* **492**, 399–407.

Pesce, A. J., Ford, D. J., and Gaizutis, A. (1978). *Scand. J. Immunol.* **8**, 1–7.

Plescia, O. J., Brown, W., and Palczuk, N. C. (1964). *Proc. Natl. Acad. Sci. U.S.A.* **52**, 279–285.

Poirier, M. C. (1980). *In* "DNA Repair: A Laboratory Manual of Research Procedures" (E. C. Freidberg and P. C. Hanawalt, eds.), pp. 143–153. Dekker, New York.

Poirier, M. C., Yuspa, S. H., Weinstein, I. B., and Blobstein, S. (1977). *Nature (London)* **270**, 186–188.

Poirier, M. C., Dubin, M. A., and Yuspa, S. H. (1979). *Cancer Res.* **39**, 1377–1381.

Poirier, M. C., Santella, R., Weinstein, I. B., Grunberger, D., and Yuspa, S. H. (1980). *Cancer Res.* **40**, 412–416.

Rubenstein, K. E. (1978). *Scand. J. Immunol.* **8**, 57–62.

Salonen, E. M., Vaheri, A., Suni, J., and Wager, O. (1980). *J. Infect. Dis.* **142**, 250–255.

Shalev, A., Greenberg, A. H., and McAlpine, P. (1980). *J. Immunol. Methods* **38**, 125–139.

Sims, P., Grover, P. L., Swaisland, A., Pal, K., and Hewer, A. (1974). *Nature (London)* **252**, 326–328.

Voller, A., Bidwell, D., and Bartlett, A. (1980). *In* "Manual of Clinical Immunology" (E. H. Lennette, ed.), 3rd Ed., pp. 359–371. American Society of Microbiology, Washington, DC.

Winchester, R. (1980). *In* "New and Useful Techniques in Rapid Viral Diagnosis Meeting" National Institutes of Health, Bethesda, Maryland.

Wisdom, E. B. (1976). *Clin. Chem.* **22**, 1243–1258.

Yolken, R. H. (1980). *Yale J. Biol. Med.* **53**, 85–92.

Yolken, R. H., and Stopa, P. J. (1979a). *J. Clin. Microbiol.* **10**, 317–321.

Yolken, R. H., and Stopa, P. J. (1979b). *J. Clin. Microbiol.* **10**, 703–707.

Yolken, R. H., and Stopa, P. J. (1980). *J. Clin. Microbiol.* **11**, 546–551.

Yolken, R. H., Stopa, P. J., and Harris, C. C. (1980). *In* "Manual of Clinical Immunology" (E. H. Lennette, ed.), 3rd Ed., pp. 692–699. American Society of Microbiology, Washington, DC.

Yuspa, S. H., and Harris, C. C. (1974). *Exp. Cell Res.* **86**, 95–105.

Zidoni, E., and Kramer, M. L. (1974). *Arch. Biochem. Biophys.* **161**, 658–661.

CHAPTER VII

METHODS FOR THE DETERMINATION OF DEOXYRIBONUCLEOSIDE TRIPHOSPHATE CONCENTRATIONS*

DAREL HUNTING AND J. FRANK HENDERSON

* The preparation of this chapter and the original work reported were supported by the National Cancer Institute and Medical Research Council of Canada.

245

I. Introduction

Deoxyribonucleoside triphosphates are substrates for DNA synthesis and hence are essential for cell multiplication as well as for DNA repair. Thus their concentrations in cells are of interest in relation to the regulation of DNA synthesis and repair and to the action of a number of cancer chemotherapeutic agents that affect nucleotide metabolism. In addition, altered concentrations of deoxyribonucleoside triphosphates have been implicated in certain human immunodeficiency diseases and in the toxicity of certain deoxyribonucleosides.

Deoxyribonucleoside triphosphates are present in cells at very low concentrations and are not readily separated from the corresponding ribonucleotides; hence they were not detected in early studies of nucleotide metabolism and nucleotide concentrations in cells. Their existence had been demonstrated by the mid-1950s, however, and thereafter a number of approaches to their assay in cell extracts were undertaken. In all, six general methods have been developed: microbiological assay, isolation by conventional chromatography and detection by spectrophotometry, isotope dilution in intact cells, labeling with radioactive orthophosphate, high-performance liquid chromatography, and enzymatically using DNA polymerase. Several appreciably different variants of each general method exist.

This article describes the principal methods for the measurement of deoxyribonucleoside triphosphates, and evaluates them critically. Its purpose is (1) to provide an assessment of the factors that are important in each method, so that published deoxyribonucleoside triphosphate measurements can be critically evaluated; (2) to help investigators choose the method best suited to their needs; and (3) to indicate where further improvements may be necessary or desirable.

For each of the six major types of deoxyribonucleoside triphosphate assays, the general principle and historical development of the method will be presented and its advantages and disadvantages considered. As an introduction, however, problems encountered in extracting these nucleotides from cells will be discussed.

II. Extraction of Deoxyribonucleoside Triphosphates

Deoxyribonucleoside triphosphate values in the literature are probably influenced as much by the method of extraction as by the method of assay. Cell extraction methods in general have been reviewed by Hauschka (1973) and will not be discussed here in detail. However, some points that are relevant to the problem at hand include the following:

1. The washing of cells prior to extraction is not only unnecessary but unwise. As pointed out by Hauschka (1973), washing can result in the hydrolysis of nucleoside tri-, di-, and monophosphates. Tyrsted (1975) thoroughly studied the effects of washing on the deoxyribonucleotide triphosphate content of cells and found that a single wash with ice-cold medium or isotonic sodium chloride resulted in a 43–80% loss of deoxyribonucleoside triphosphates. This was confirmed by Kinahan et al. (1979) and by Walters et al. (1974), who also found that washing the cells caused deoxyribonucleotide breakdown, though exact values were not given.

2. Perchloric acid (PCA) extraction usually gives the highest yield of nucleotides (review: Hauschka, 1973).

3. The optimal PCA concentration for extraction is 0.4 M (Bagnara and Finch, 1972).

4. Trichloroacetic acid (TCA) (5–10%) will extract cellular nucleotides, but the yields are not as reproducible as with PCA, possibly because TCA does not efficiently extract nucleotides bound to intracellular polycations (review: Hauschka, 1973).

5. Sixty percent methanol or 70% ethanol has been used to extract nucleotides from cells with the advantage of being readily lyophilized (review: Hauschka, 1973). North et al. (1980) have reported that several enzymes that interfere with the enzymatic assay of deoxynucleoside triphosphates are present in 60% methanol extracts of cultured HeLa cells. These activities included a nuclease, a nucleoside diphosphate kinase, and deoxynucleoside monophosphate kinases which can phosphorylate dAMP, dGMP, and dCMP. They suggest that methanol extraction of cells will give artificially high values for the deoxyribonucleoside triphosphates when assayed enzymatically because of degradation of the DNA template and phosphorylation of the degradation products to deoxyribonucleoside triphosphates by the contaminating enzymes. Although their findings will not be reviewed here in detail, there were some inconsistencies in the results. For example, they did not observe any exonuclease activity during the assay of standards, but did find this activity during the assay of the methanol extracts, despite the fact that the Escherichia coli DNA polymerase I, which was used in their assay, contains both $5' \rightarrow 3'$ and $3' \rightarrow 5'$ exonuclease activities as part of the same enzyme. Furthermore, the small amount of deoxynucleoside monophosphate kinase activity that they observed is inadequate to explain the 500% increase in the apparent amount of deoxyribonucleoside triphosphates in methanol extracts as compared to PCA extracts.

Nevertheless, methanol extraction of cells will have to be carefully reexamined to determine if it introduces errors into the enzymatic assay. In fact, contaminating enzymes such as phosphatases can result in errors, regardless of the assay method used.

6. If cell extracts are lyophilized and redissolved in a known volume, then the recovery of the nucleotides through the overall process should be measured. If cells are extracted with a known volume of extraction medium and a portion of this extract is used for analysis, then dilution of the extract by cellular water and by medium around the cells should be determined.

7. Even if the best extraction method and the greatest care are used, it is still important to assess the quality of the final extract. While this is not an exact parameter, we have found that the nucleoside triphosphate to diphosphate ratio is a sensitive indicator of nucleotide breakdown in the cells (D. Hunting and J. F. Henderson, unpublished). We therefore routinely measure the ATP/ADP ratio, as determined by high-performance liquid chromatography (HPLC), and consider a value of 10 or more for cultured cells to be an indication of satisfactory extraction and sample-handling technique. Excessive manipulation of cells, such as washing prior to extraction, an inappropriate extraction medium, failure to keep the extract cold, or neutralizing it within 1 hour may significantly lower the ATP/ADP ratio.

A few examples may be given to indicate how ATP/ADP ratios may vary. In two extracts made using cold 0.4 M PCA, these ratios were 11.0 and 13.5. In another extract, using 60% methanol at 30°C for 10 minutes followed by storage overnight at -20°C, it was 12.6. However, when the extraction was made using 60% methanol at -20°C overnight, the ratios for two samples were 5.8 and 3.9.

To show the different extraction procedures that have been used, Table I compares various procedures used to prepare cell extracts for enzymatic assays. The majority of methods do not involve washing cells, but there are a few exceptions, one of which includes three washings. Since Tyrsted (1975) reported a value of 60% for the average amount of deoxyribonucleoside triphosphate breakdown from a single wash, three washes could result in a recovery of only 6% of the original deoxyribonucleoside triphosphates present in the cell. The degree of breakdown during cell washing probably varies from cell type to cell type, but one should regard nucleotide values obtained from washed cells with some caution.

Most of the extraction media were used at optimum concentrations. The majority of procedures did not include the measurement either of recovery or of dilution. Rarely were attempts made to minimize dilution by wiping media from the inside of the centrifuge tube before extraction. Finally, the quality of the extracts was rarely assessed.

TABLE I

METHODS USED TO EXTRACT DEOXYRIBONUCLEOSIDE TRIPHOSPHATES

Cells washed before extraction	Extraction medium	Dilution or recovery measured	Quality of extract assessed	Reference
No	60% MeOH	Recovery	No	Skoog (1970)
No	PCA	No	No	Lindberg and Skoog (1970)
No	60% MeOH	Recovery	No	Skoog et al. (1973)
No	1.0 M PCA	No	Yes	Kinahan et al. (1979)
No	60% EtOH	Recovery	Yes	Tyrsted (1975)
No	60% MeOH	Recovery	Yes	Munch-Petersen et al. (1973)
1×	66% EtOH	Recovery	Yes	Kyburg et al. (1979)
2×	0.5 M PCA	No	No	Tattersall and Harrap (1973)
No	0.5 M PCA	No	No	Walters et al. (1973)
1×	60% MeOH	No	No	Tattersall et al. (1975b)
No	0.5 M PCA	No	No	de Saint Vincent and Buttin (1979)
No	2.0 M PCA	No	No	Solter and Handschumacher (1969)
No	0.5 M PCA	No	No	Lowe and Grindey (1976)
No	0.4 M PCA	Dilution	Yes	Lowe et al. (1977)
1×	0.5 M PCA	No	No	Fridland (1974)
No	2.0 M PCA	No	No	Cohen et al. (1978)
2×	0.5 M PCA	No	No	Bray and Brent (1972)
1×	60% MeOH	No	No	Tattersall et al. (1975a)
3×	5% TCA	No	No	Adams et al. (1971)
No	0.5 M PCA	No	No	Baumunk and Friedman (1971)
No	5% TCA	No	No	Wittes and Kidwell (1975)
No	0.4 M PCA	No	No	Goetz and Carell (1978)
No	60% MeOH	No	No	Mitchell et al. (1978)
No	0.4 M PCA	Dilution	Yes	D. Hunting and J. F. Henderson (1981)

III. Microbiological Assay

The microbiological assay for deoxyribonucleotides was introduced in 1957 and subsequent modifications resulted in an accurate assay of high specificity, but of relatively low sensitivity. Although the last reported use of the microbiological assay was more than 10 years ago, it will be considered in this chapter because it still is a valid technique which played an important role in the early studies of cellular deoxyribonucleotide pools, and because some of the results obtained with this method have not been repeated using other assay methods and are still being cited (review: Henderson *et al.*, 1980). Therefore this assay will be discussed in the context of all of the presently used assay methods in terms of its accuracy, sensitivity, reproducibility, and problems or possible pitfalls.

A. GENERAL PRINCIPLE

The microbiological assay is based on the principle that certain organisms, such as *Lactobacillus acidophilus,* require exogenous deoxyribonucleosides or deoxyribonucleoside monophosphates for growth. Standard curves can be constructed by plotting cell number or, more commonly, turbidity at approximately 650 nm, after 24–36 hours of incubation at 37°C, against the amount of deoxyribonucleoside standard in each culture. The standard curves are linear up to approximately 2 nmole/tube but then flatten off as maximum growth stimulation is approached. Deoxyribonucleoside di- and triphosphate concentrations can be determined by converting these compounds to the deoxyribonucleosides with phosphatases. Some specificity can be obtained by hydrolyzing the purine deoxyribonucleosides under mild acidic conditions; thus, values for the total purine and the total pyrimidine deoxyribonucleoside content can be obtained. Further specificity can be achieved by chromatographing the cell extracts to separate the individual deoxyribonucleosides and then assaying each one separately.

B. DEVELOPMENT OF THE ASSAY

The origins of the microbiological determination of deoxyribonucleotides lie in an assay for DNA which was developed by Hoff-Jorgensen (1952). This assay was based on the fact that DNA would support the growth of the deoxyribonucleoside-requiring bacterium *L. acidophilus* R26 after hydrolysis of the DNA to monophosphates with DNase. Five years later, Hoff-Jorgensen (1957) published an assay for deoxyribonucleoside monophosphates based on his 1952 method for DNA, and he also demonstrated that hydrolysis of deoxyribonucleoside monophosphates to deoxyribonucleosides with phosphatase did not change the results. The phosphatase was not used routinely, nor did he determine the ability of the assay to measure deoxyribonucleoside di- and triphosphate concentrations. Separate values for purine and pyrimidine deoxyribonucleoside monophosphates were determined by first measuring the total deoxyribonucleoside monophosphate content, and then hydrolyzing the purine derivatives under mild acidic conditions and assaying again for the pyrimidine deoxyribonucleoside monophosphate content.

In contrast to Hoff-Jorgensen's results, Siedler *et al.* (1957) found that the sensitivity of this assay varied with different deoxyribonucleoside monophosphates, and that the sensitivity to monophosphates was much less than to deoxyribonucleosides. They suggested that the assay would be improved by treating all samples with phosphatase. Schneider and Potter (1957) studied the method further and reported that *L. acidophilus* R26 could grow on medium supplemented with deoxyribonucleosides or deoxyribonucleoside monophosphates, but not on diphosphates or triphosphates. They also found that the procedure of Hoff-Jorgensen, which required autoclaving the medium and extracts prior to the addition of the bacterial inoculum, resulted in the hydrolysis of nucleoside di- and triphosphates, so that the bacteria could grow in media supplemented with these compounds; previous measurement of the deoxyribonucleoside and deoxyribonucleoside monophosphate content of tissue extracts (Schneider, 1955) was probably too high because of deoxynucleoside di- and triphosphate breakdown during autoclaving. Schneider and Potter (1957) recommended that filtration should be substituted for autoclaving and that the deoxynucleoside di- and triphosphate content of tissue extracts could be determined by enzymatic hydrolysis of these compounds before performing the assay. Siedler and Schweigert (1959) soon clarified the question of whether or not deoxyribonucleoside monophosphates were used as readily as deoxyribonucleosides by *L. acidophilus* when they reported that ribonucleotides, if present in the assay medium, inhibited the utilization of deoxyribonucleoside monophosphates but not of deoxyribonucleosides. This explained why different laboratories had reached different conclusions regarding the utilization of deoxyribonucleoside monophosphates. Schneider (1962) confirmed these results and decided that the best routine assay procedure was to hydrolyze all the ribo- and deoxyribonucleoside phosphates with phosphatase to remove interference by ribonucleotides and allow the assay of all the deoxyribonucleoside derivatives in extracts.

Larsson (1963) subsequently demonstrated that either *L. acidophilus* R26 or *Lactobacillus leichmannii* could be used in the assay, although when *L. leichmannii* was used it was necessary to remove all vitamin B_{12} from the medium and extracts since this organism can be grown on medium supplemented with either vitamin B_{12} or deoxyribonucleosides.

Finally, Brown and Handschumacher (1966) used the fully developed assay to measure deoxyribonucleotide pools in *Streptococcus fecalis*. Their procedure also included a further refinement in that they chromatographically separated all the deoxyribonucleoside triphosphates, then hydrolyzed each with phosphatase and assayed them separately.

In conclusion, this method is specific for deoxyribose compounds, and the specificity can be increased by chromatographically separating the compounds before assaying them. This method allows the measurement of amounts of deoxyribonucleotides greater than 0.5 nmole, with a standard error of approximately 5% (Schneider and Potter, 1957). The main problem with this technique is that it is quite insensitive compared to more recently developed techniques (e.g., the enzymatic assay is as much as 1000 times more sensitive). It is also very laborious, especially if the amount of each deoxyribonucleoside triphosphate, rather than the sum total, is to be determined.

IV. Chromatographic–Spectrophotometric Assay

The first reported use of chromatographic isolation followed by ultraviolet (UV) measurement to determine quantitatively deoxynucleoside triphosphate concentrations in cell extracts was in 1955 (Potter, 1955; Potter and Schlesinger, 1955), the same year the microbiological assay was introduced. Although the chromatographic method has not been used frequently, it has provided valuable information on topics such as adenosine toxicity and thymineless death (Klenow, 1962; Munch-Petersen and Neuhard, 1964; Kummer and Kraml, 1977). Its most recent use was in 1977 in a study of thymidine triphosphate concentrations in malignant tumors (Kummer and Kraml, 1977). The main drawbacks of this method are that it is laborious and relatively insensitive.

A. GENERAL PRINCIPLE

The chromatographic assay is based mainly on two principles.

1. Separation

Deoxyribonucleotides can be isolated from cell extracts using anion-exchange column chromatography. However, complete purification of the deoxyribonucleoside triphosphates requires further chromatography on paper. Although one-step purification of the deoxyribonucleotides from cell extracts is possible using two-dimensional thin-layer chromatography, its usefulness is limited because not enough deoxyribonucleotide can be isolated to permit accurate measurement. However, there are two published procedures in which this method has proved useful (Kummer and Kraml, 1977; Bucher and Oakman, 1969).

2. Quantitative Measurement

Three methods which have been used to determine the amount of each deoxyribonucleotide after chromatographic separation are measurement of UV absorbance, the luciferase assay, and bioassay, with the measurement of UV absorbance being the most common method used. The bioassay has been discussed separately and will be mentioned only briefly here. The luciferase assay has been used only in one study (Klenow, 1962), and all four deoxyribonucleoside triphosphates could be assayed by this method.

B. DEVELOPMENT OF THE ASSAY

Potter (1955) and Potter and Schlesinger (1955) reported the quantitative measurement of pyrimidine deoxynucleotides in calf thymus extracts in 1955 and gave a complete description of the method in 1957 (Potter *et al.*, 1957). The basic procedure was as follows: Neutralized, concentrated tissue extracts were chromatographed on an anion-exchange column and the nucleotides were eluted using a gradient. Fractions were collected and the UV absorbance was determined. Preliminary identification of the fractions was based on the A_{275}/A_{260} ratio. The deoxyribonucleotides did not separate well from the ribonucleotides, and a second column chromatographic procedure followed by paper chromatography was necessary to isolate pure dTTP and dCTP. The amounts isolated were determined by UV absorbance, with identification of the compounds based on deoxyribose and phosphorus content and on spectral data. No purine deoxyribonucleotides could be isolated by this technique, and data on accuracy and sensitivity were not reported.

LePage (1957) used a similar procedure to determine the dATP concentration of rat tumor extracts. ATP and dATP were separated from the other nucleotides by anion-exchange chromatography and, after desalting on a charcoal–Celite column, dATP was separated from ATP by three sequential runs on paper chromatograms. The amount of pure dATP isolated was 2 μmole, and the recovery determined by using a dATP standard was 50–67%.

Klenow (1962) used a substantially different procedure to measure dATP concentrations in extracts of Ehrlich ascites tumor cells. He simply chromatographed the cell extracts on Whatman No. 40 filter paper, eluted the dATP, and determined its absorbance. Its identity was confirmed from spectral data and by using the diphenylamine reaction. One disadvantage of this method was that the chromatography step required 75 hours, which could have resulted in dATP hydrolysis. He did not report values for dATP recovery.

Klenow (1962) also introduced an ingenious modification to the assay by using luciferase as well as UV measurements to measure the amount of deoxyribonucleoside triphosphate that had been purified by paper chromatography. Values for the sensitivity and accuracy of the determinations were not given. Although the luciferase assay is a convenient method of determining deoxyribonucleoside triphosphates after chromatography, no other reports of its use for this purpose could be found. The luciferase assay was originally used to determine dATP in extracts that had been treated with periodate to oxidize ATP (Klenow, 1962; Coddington and Bagger-Sorensen, 1963). However, since all the deoxyribonucleoside triphosphates can be measured by the luciferase assay, it is probable that this technique measured the total deoxyribonucleoside triphosphate concentration and not just that of dATP.

Potter and Nygaard (1963) used the chromatography–UV measurement procedure of Potter *et al.* (1957) to measure dTTP concentrations in extracts of rat spleen and thymus. However, they found that the UV measurements were too insensitive to measure dTTP in thymus extract; they therefore used the microbiological assay instead. Although they did not report values for sensitivity, the lowest amount of dTTP determined was 19 nmole.

The assay was improved by Bucher and Oakman (1969), who introduced both two-dimensional thin-layer chromatography and isotope dilution. The thin-layer chromatographic method, based on the procedure of Randerath and Randerath (1967), involved one-dimensional thin-layer chromatography on poly(ethylene)imine (PEI)-cellulose plates. Although a single sample was streaked across the origin of three plates, the plates were heavily overloaded and the dTTP that was isolated had to be purified by rechromatographing on PEI-cellulose using a two-dimensional system. The dTTP was then eluted and measured spectrophotometrically.

The isotope-dilution technique involved the addition of [^{14}C]dTTP of a known specific activity to the PCA before extracting the tissue. After isolating the dTTP as described above, the endogenous dTTP content was calculated from the reduction of the specific activity of [^{14}C]dTTP. This assay method was simpler than previous chromatographic–spectrophotometric procedures, and the use of the isotope-dilution technique automatically corrected for loss of dTTP by incomplete recovery of breakdown during the isolation procedure. In principle, this method should have been quite accurate; however, no values for accuracy were reported.

The most recent use of the chromatographic–spectrophotometric assay was by Kummer and Kraml (1977). The method utilized two-dimensional thin-layer chromatography, as described above, followed by determination of dTTP by UV absorbance. A minimum sensitivity can be determined from the fact that 400 pmole of dTTP was detected in an extract of 10^7 cells. Thus if all the extract was chromatographed, the sensitivity of the assay would be less than 400 pmole.

In conclusion, although the chromatographic–spectrophotometric assay is quite laborious, it has the advantages of being direct and accurate, especially if the recovery is measured or if the isotope-dilution technique is used.

V. Isotope Dilution in Intact Cells

The method of measuring intracellular nucleotide pool sizes by applying the isotope-dilution principle to intact cells by developed by Forsdyke (1968). Deoxyribonucleoside triphosphate pool size measurements using this method have been made in only two laboratories, that of Forsdyke himself (Forsdyke, 1968, 1971; Sjöstrom and Forsdyke, 1974; Scott and Forsdyke, 1976, 1978) and that of R. L. P. Adams (1969). It must be clearly understood that although the isotope-dilution principle is valid in itself, the assumptions involved in applying it to the measurement of intracellular nucleotide pools have not been properly tested. Few changes have been made in Forsdyke's original procedure, although it has been applied to different types of problems. For this reason, the development of the method will not be discussed separately.

A. GENERAL PRINCIPLE

The isotope dilution assay of Forsdyke is based on the isotope-dilution principle and probably also on the enzymatic isotope-dilution method developed by Newsholme and Taylor (1968), Brooker and Appleman (1968), and Gander (1970). The assumptions and reasonings of this method will first be stated as clearly as possible, and then critically evaluated.

1. If cells are incubated *in vitro* with a radioactive deoxyribonucleoside precursor of DNA, then the rate of incorporation of radioactivity into DNA will be proportional to the specific activity of the precursor and to the V_{max} of the rate-limiting step in the pathway.
2. It is assumed that the specific activity of the deoxyribonucleoside precursor will be reduced by any compounds (nucleosides and nucleotides), either extracellular or intracellular, which enter the pathway of metabolism and incorporation of the precursor prior to the rate-limiting step; therefore, the total pool of these compounds will be measured through isotope dilution. The total amount of these compounds normally present in the cells and medium is called the "intrinsic pool," while the total amount of these compounds which might be added to the medium experimentally is called the "extrinsic pool."

3. It is also assumed that compounds which enter the pathway after the rate-limiting step will not reduce the specific activity of the external deoxyribonucleoside precursor and therefore will not be detected by the isotope-dilution assay.

4. Operationally, if a constant quantity of radioactive precursor is added to the medium, along with varying quantities of the same, nonradioactive precursor, then a plot of the reciprocal of the radioactivity incorporated into DNA (abscissa) against the total concentration of added precursor (extrinsic pool) will be linear. The slope of this plot is taken to be a measure of the V_{max} of the rate-limiting step, while the negative intercept at the ordinate is taken to be a measure of the intrinsic pool (which, as stated above, may include both intracellular and extracellular compounds).

5. A change in the position of the rate-limiting step in the pathway, as induced, for example, by treatment with drugs, will change the number of compounds which reduce the specific activity of the radioactive deoxyribonucleoside precursor, and therefore will change the size of the intrinsic pool.

B. ANALYSIS OF THE METHOD

Two especially important assumptions involved in the use of the isotope-dilution method for the measurement of intracellular nucleotide pools remain untested.

1. It is assumed that both intracellular deoxyribonucleotide pools and extracellular nonradioactive deoxyribonucleoside precursors reduce the incorporation of added radioactive deoxyribonucleoside precursor into DNA by exactly the same mechanism (i.e., it is assumed that intracellular deoxyribonucleotides can reduce the specific activity of the extracellular deoxyribonucleoside via a rapid chemical equilibrium). Therefore, if a radioactive deoxyribonucleoside were incubated with cells and then isolated from the medium, its specific activity should have decreased by an amount dependent on the size of the intrinsic pool which, depending on the position of the rate-limiting step in the pathway, could include intracellular nucleotides as well as nucleosides. There is no evidence that this assumption is valid. Furthermore, it is likely that this point has caused some confusion since generally when one refers to the dilution of, for example, radioactive thymidine by intracellular thymidine nucleotides, it is implied that the dilution occurs only within the cells and only after the radioactive thymidine has been converted to nucleotides.

2. It is assumed that intracellular nucleotide pools and synthetic pathways which enter the pathway under study distal to the rate-limiting step have no effect on the incorporation of the extracellular radioactive precursor into DNA. Thus, for example, in a situation in which the phosphorylation of thymidine is the rate-limiting step for the incorporation of radioactive thymidine into DNA, it is assumed that the rate of incorporation of radioactivity into DNA is independent both of the size of the thymidine nucleotide pool and of the rate of thymidylate synthesis *de novo*. This is contrary to what one would intuitively predict, and it is therefore difficult to accept this assumption without any supporting experimental evidence.

Sjöstrom and Forsdyke (1974) have reported that at thymidine concentrations less than 5 μM, the rate-limiting step for the incorporation of radioactive thymidine into DNA in cultured thymus cells was thymidine kinase. Therefore, according to the isotope-dilution theory of Forsdyke, the specific activity of the extracellular thymidine would have been diluted only by the intracellular thymidine pool and by any thymidine normally present in the medium. As well, the assay would have measured only the size of these thymidine pools. However, at thymidine concentrations above 5 μM, Sjöstrom and Forsdyke concluded that the most likely rate-limiting step was DNA polymerase. Therefore, the specific activity of the extracellular thymidine would have been diluted by the intracellular dTTP, dTDP, dTMP, and thymidine pools as well as by the synthesis *de novo* of thymidylate. Theoretically, the assay would then have measured the size of the total intracellular thymidine nucleotide and nucleoside pools.

When Adams (1969) used the method of Forsdyke to measure dTTP pools in cultured mouse fibroblast cells, he indicated his understanding of the assumptions by stating that the method "assumes that exogenous (thymidine) and endogenous dTTP are in direct equilibrium," but he did not justify or test this assumption.

In conclusion, the measurement of deoxyribonucleotide pools by the isotope-dilution assay is based on two untested—but testable—assumptions. Until these assumptions are proven, this method cannot be presumed to be valid for the measurement of deoxyribonucleotide concentrations in cells.

VI. Radioactive Orthophosphate Assay

The first use of the $^{32}P_i$ method to measure deoxyribonucleotide pool sizes was by Neuhard and Munch-Petersen (1966). This method has not been used frequently and its use is declining, probably as a result of the increased use of more direct methods utilizing enzymatic or HPLC assays. The main assets of the $^{32}P_i$ method are that it is quite sensitive, conceptually and methodologically simple, and requires few assumptions. The main problems with this method are the long incubation times required for $^{32}P_i$ to equilibrate completely with the intracellular acid-soluble phosphate compounds, and the difficulty in chromatographicallly separating the deoxyribonucleotides cleanly from other labeled compounds. It seems unlikely that further significant improvements can be made on this method.

A. General Principle

The basic premise of this method is that if the pool of phosphate compounds in cells is equilibrated with external $^{32}P_i$ of known specific activity, then measurement of the amount of radioactivity in a given phosphate compound, such as dATP, will allow the calculation of the pool size of that compound.

The general procedure is that cells are labeled with $^{32}P_i$ of known specific activity until equilibrium is reached; that is, until the specific activity of each phosphate in each acid-soluble phosphate compound equals the specific activity of the added $^{32}P_i$. Attainment of equilibrium is variously taken as the time at which the total acid-soluble radioactivity becomes constant, the time at which the rate of incorporation of label into DNA becomes linear, or the time at which the amount of radioactivity in the compounds of interest becomes constant. The equilibration time should be determined for each treatment condition [i.e., for each drug, or for stationary- or log-phase cells, since equilibrium times can vary greatly from one condition to another (Weber and Edlin, 1971)]. The cells are then extracted, and generally the extracts are treated with sodium periodate to oxidize the ribonucleotides, which are difficult to separate from the deoxyribonucleotides. The extracts are chromatographed and the amount of radioactivity in each deoxyribonucleotide is determined. These data, plus the value for the specific activity of the $^{32}P_i$, allow the calculation of each pool size. Generally, only the triphosphates, the largest of the deoxyribonucleotide pool, can be determined accurately.

B. Development of the Assay

The measurement of ribonucleotide pools by the $^{32}P_i$ method is relatively simple, but measurement of the very much smaller deoxyribonucleotide pools has been more difficult, mainly due to the inability to separate the deoxyribonucleotides totally from the heavily labeled ribonucleotides and from $^{32}P_i$. By 1965 procedures developed by Randerath and Randerath (1964a,b) and by Neuhard et al. (1965) allowed the separation of all eight ribo- and deoxyribonucleoside triphosphates using a two-dimensional chromatographic system on PEI-cellulose thin-layer plates. The first-dimension solvent was 2 M LiCl:2 N acetic acid (1:1 v/v) and the second-dimension solvent was 3 M ammonium acetate in 5% boric acid, pH 7. Neuhard and Munch-Petersen (1966) and Neuhard (1966) used this chromatographic system in conjunction with $^{32}P_i$ labeling to determine the size of the four deoxyribonucleoside triphosphate pools in E. coli 15T$^-$A$^-$U$^-$.

Colby and Edlin (1970) subsequently improved the chromatographic method of Neuhard et al. (1965) in two ways: (1) Two concentrations of each solvent in each dimension were used, creating a concentration gradient and improving separations. (2) The cells were washed once with cold 0.15 M NaCl–0.1 M Tris, pH 7.4, to remove excess $^{32}P_i$ before extraction and thereby reduce the streaking of $^{32}P_i$. However, the washing procedure probably also caused nucleotide breakdown so that the net advantage of this step is questionable. Colby and Edlin (1970) also studied the kinetics of $^{32}P_i$ labeling of both the ribo- and deoxyribonucleoside triphosphate pools in growing, Rous sarcoma virus (RSV)-transformed, and growth-inhibited chick fibroblast cells. They found substantial differences in $^{32}P_i$-labeling kinetics among these cells, although the nucleotide pool sizes were similar. Although these were preliminary experiments, they demonstrated the need to determine the $^{32}P_i$ equilibration conditions under different growth conditions. Colby and Edlin (1970) also cautioned that their determinations of the deoxyribonucleoside triphosphates were quite variable due to $^{32}P_i$ streaking.

Weber and Edlin (1971) confirmed the observation of Colby and Edlin regarding differences in the rate of $^{32}P_i$ uptake by growing and density-inhibited cells. They used a preliminary separation of inorganic and organic phosphates to reduce the extent of $^{32}P_i$ streaking during chromatography.

Probably the most significant improvements in the assay were introduced by Yegian (1974). He used periodate to oxidize the ribofuranosyl ring of the ribonucleotides, and thereby prevented the overlap of heavily labeled ribonucleotides with the deoxyribonucleotides during chromatography; this increased the accuracy of the determinations. This use of periodate oxidation to remove interference by ribonucleotides was not a new idea; in fact, Klenow (1962) had used it to permit him to measure dATP concentrations using luciferase.

Yegian (1974) also introduced a new chromatographic system that separated the four deoxyribonucleoside triphosphates much better than before and eliminated interference from $^{32}P_i$ and the oxidized ribonucleotides. The main innovation was that samples were spotted in the middle of the plate and the $^{32}P_i$ was washed into the wick, which was then cut off. The plate was then rerun with a different solvent in the opposite direction to separate the nucleotides. Finally, Yegian (1974) also checked the purity of each lot of $^{32}P_i$, using only lots that had less than 0.02% impurity. This precaution was not mentioned by previous researchers. In a review of this method, Hauschka (1973) noted that $^{32}P_i$ is often contaminated with polyphosphates and phosphosilicates, and these complicate the chromatographic purification of the nucleotides.

Bersier and Braun (1974) made additional changes in the method. They first measured directly the specific activity of the four ribonucleoside triphosphate pools by labeling large numbers of cells with $^{32}P_i$ for various times, extracting the cells, and isolating the ribonucleoside triphosphates by ion-exchange column chromatography. They found that in *Physarum polycephalum* the ribonucleotide pools reached their maximum specific activity after 30 minutes of labeling; unfortunately they did not compare the specific activity of the ribonucleotide pools with that of the $^{32}P_i$ in the medium. This comparison would have been a test of the main assumption made by others that when the amount of label in a nucleotide pool becomes constant, the specific activity of each phosphate of the acid-soluble compounds equals the specific activity of the $^{32}P_i$ in the medium. Bersier and Braun (1974) then used the specific activities determined for the ribonucleotides plus the amount of label in each deoxyribonucleoside triphosphate to calculate the deoxyribonucleoside triphosphate pool sizes. One other improvement they introduced was to measure nucleoside triphosphate recovery during extraction by adding tritiated nucleoside triphosphates to the extraction medium just before extracting the cells. They found that a considerable loss (60–70%) of the triphosphates had occurrred, due mainly to triphosphate breakdown; the results were corrected for this loss during recovery.

Although improvements in the assay were being made, they were not always used. Thus Nexo (1975) published a study of deoxyribonucleoside triphosphate concentrations in *Tetrahymena pyriformis* using exactly the same procedures that Neuhard and Munch-Petersen (1966) had developed 9 years earlier.

Finally, Reynolds and Finch (1977) made still further improvements. They found that the chromatographic method developed by Yegian (1974) did not completely remove all the oxidized ribonucleotides; some of these remained at the origin following washing, and radioactive orthophosphate was released during the chromatography, contaminating the deoxyribonucleotide spots. Reynolds and Finch (1977) overcame this by using the chromatographic system of Neuhard *et al.* (1965) for periodate-treated extracts. Streaking of orthophosphate occurred in the first dimension, but in the second dimension the overlapping orthophosphate ran ahead of the nucleotides, while any remaining orthophosphate that continued to leach from the origin ran parallel to, but away from, the nucleotides.

No values have been published regarding the accuracy, reproducibility, or sensitivity of the $^{32}P_i$ deoxyribonucleoside triphosphate assay. However, in a few cases enough information has been given so that an estimate of the maximum sensitivity under those conditions can be made.

Bersier and Braun (1974) found the equilibrium-specific activity of the ribonucleotide pools in *Physarum* to be 13.5 counts per minute (cpm) per pmole; since the $^{32}P_i$ had equilibrated the deoxyribonucleotide pools should have had the same specific activity. This value gives an indication of the sensitivity, but a value for the background radioactivity of the chromatograms would be necessary to complete the picture. Neuhard and Munch-Petersen (1966) reported the specific activity of the $^{32}P_i$ used to be $1-3$ $\mu Ci/\mu mole$, and theoretically this should have given equilibrium-specific activities in the *E. coli* deoxyribonucleoside triphosphates of between 6.6 and 20 disintegrations per minute (dpm) per pmole. Again, no value for the background radioactivity on the chromatogram was reported, so the actual sensitivity cannot be determined. The use of higher specific activities would increase the sensitivity, but would also increase radiation damage to the cells. This is an important limitation on the sensitivity of this method.

C. DISCUSSION

The $^{32}P_i$-deoxyribonucleotide assay has been in use for 14 years, undergoing constant evolution during this time. It is not possible to refer to a standard $^{32}P_i$ assay because almost every user of the assay has added some improvements. However, it is possible to examine all the variations and pick the best features of each. General features that should be included in a standard assay are as follows:

1. Purity checks of each batch of $^{32}P_i$, followed by purification if there is significant contamination by polyphosphates or polysilicates which cochromatograph with nucleotides.

2. Use of the highest $^{32}P_i$ specific activity which does not cause significant radiation damage, and of the lowest phosphate concentration in the medium which will still give normal growth rates.

3. Measurement of the $^{32}P_i$ equilibration times for each treatment condition; attainment of equilibrium could reasonably be taken as the point at which the amount of radioactivity in the deoxyribonucleotide pools becomes constant.

4. Extraction of cells, with no prior washing, and neutralization on ice to minimize nucleotide breakdown. The extraction medium should contain a tritiated deoxyribonucleoside triphosphate for determination of overall recovery.

5. Oxidation of ribose compounds using sodium periodate in order to improve chromatographic separation.

6. Use of a two-dimensional chromatography system such as that developed by Neuhard et al. (1966) or Colby and Edlin's (1970) modification of their system.

Although an assay incorporating these features would be the optimum $^{32}P_i$ deoxyribonucleoside triphosphate assay, it would still have the drawback of being more laborious than the enzymatic or HPLC assays.

VII. High-Performance Liquid Chromatography

The use of HPLC to measure deoxyribonucleoside triphosphates in cell extracts is a recent extension of the use of this technique to measure ribonucleotide concentrations. The HPLC method is direct, involves few assumptions, and allows the simultaneous measurement of all four deoxyribonucleoside triphosphates. It is less sensitive than the enzymatic assay, but offers approximately the same sensitivity as the $^{32}P_i$ assay. The HPLC assay is slower than the enzymatic assay when many samples must be processed, but it is better suited for a few samples or for infrequent measurements. Since the HPLC assays in use are quite varied, there is a need to assess each one, to compare them to other methods, particularly the enzymatic assay, and to determine what further improvements should be made.

A. GENERAL PRINCIPLE

The HPLC assay relies mainly on three principles.

1. Separation

Deoxyribonucleotides can be rapidly separated using anion-exchange columns and high-performance chromatography apparatus. Separation from ribonucleotides is facilitated by periodate oxidation of the ribonucleotides to change their mobilities.

2. Detection

Deoxyribonucleotides can be detected by measuring their UV absorbance. The ease and sensitivity of detection depend on the detector and the separation method. Solvents with relatively high refractive indexes or high UV absorbances reduce the sensitivity of deoxyribonucleotide detection. As well, gradient separations generally result in a changing baseline due to changes in the refractive index or absorbance of the solvents. Finally, the sharpness of the peak will affect the accuracy of detection.

The amplification of the detector signal can usually be varied and a common measure of the detector sensitivity is the number of absorbance units required for full-scale deflection of the recorder pen. For example, the Varian Aerograph LCS 1000 detector has a maximum sensitivity setting of 0.02 optical density (OD) units full scale, which may be equivalent to between 2000 and 3000 pmole of dATP. Most new models, such as the Spectra-Physics 8000 HPLC detector and the Waters Associates HPLC detector, have a maximum sensitivity setting of 0.005 OD units full scale, which may be equivalent to between 500 and 750 pmole of dATP. Although it is useful to know the detector sensitivity settings, these values can be misleading because the detectors are limited not only by how much the signal can be amplified, but also by the signal-to-noise ratio. Therefore, if this ratio is low, or if the separation method results in a shifting baseline, high sensitivity settings are of little value.

3. Quantitation

The amount of compound in a peak is proportional to its area on the recorder tracing. Other parameters, such as peak height, can be used for quantitative measurements, but except for very sharp, symmetrical peaks, they are not as sensitive or as accurate as measuring peak area. Peak areas are usually measured either by planimetry, which is accurate but tedious, or by automatic electronic integration. Although automatic integration is very convenient, it requires careful programming to ensure accuracy and reproducibility

B. DEVELOPMENT OF THE METHOD

The first published use of HPLC for the determination of deoxyribonucleoside triphosphate concentrations was in 1978 (Ullman *et al.*, 1978;

Gudas *et al.*, 1978). These reports were both from the same laboratory and the same method was used in each case. The separations were done isocratically on a Whatman Partisil SAX column (a strong anion-exchange resin), using 0.45 M potassium phosphate buffer, pH 3.6. The peaks were monitored at both 254 and 280 nm, but the detector sensitivity settings were not reported. The only deoxyribonucleotides determined were dATP and dGTP. Adenosine triphosphate and dATP were not separated at the baseline, which was unstable, thus making accurate integration of the peaks difficult; the method of integration was not given. Although dATP and dGTP values were also determined by the enzymatic method, the results obtained by the two methods were not compared.

The next obvious step was to get rid of interfering ribonucleotides using periodate oxidation. In 1979, this step was introduced by three laboratories (Ullman *et al.*, 1979; Ritter and Bruce, 1979; Garrett and Santi, 1979), though two different procedures were used. Ritter and Bruce (1979) used the following procedure to oxidize the ribonucleotides: 200 μl of 2 N formic acid and 200 μl of sodium periodate solution (0.07 gm/ml) were added with mixing to 200 μl of cold neutralized PCA extract. After 45 minutes at 4°C in the dark, 200 μl of ethylene glycol was added to reduce unused periodate. After 15 minutes, 50 μl of concentrated ammonium hydroxide was added and 5 minutes later the pH was adjusted to 7.5. Although variable degrees of ribonucleotide oxidation were obtained with this procedure, they were satisfied with this method because as long as the ribonucleotide and deoxyribonucleotide concentrations were similar, all could be separated. Separation was achievd using two 250 × 4.6-mm Whatman Partisil 10 SAX anion-exchange columns in series at 40°C, with a linear gradient from 0.2 M NH$_4$H$_2$PO$_4$, pH 3.2, to 0.6 M NH$_4$H$_2$PO$_4$, pH 4.4, at a flow rate of 1.0 ml/minute for 2 hours. The peaks were monitored at 254 nm, which is optimal for dATP but not for dCTP (λ_{max} = 280). The detector sensitivity was quite low (0.05 OD units full scale) and the peak areas were measured by planimetry.

This procedure has been tested in our laboratory using both standards and cell extracts with added tritiated ribo- or deoxyribonucleoside triphosphates; it was found that the ribonucleotides were completely oxidized, and that the deoxyribonucleotides were completely stable (J.K. Lowe and J.F. Henderson, unpublished). Ritter and Bruce (1979) had concluded that the ribonucleotides were not always completely oxidized by this procedure and showed a chromatogram of a periodate-treated cell extract in which there was a peak with the same retention time as UTP. Lowe and Henderson (unpublished) also noted this peak in periodate-treated cell extracts but not in treated standards. They concluded that the peak was not UTP since tritiated UTP added to a cell extract was completely oxidized, whereas this peak remained. The identity of this peak has not been established, nor is it known if it is produced during periodate treatment or if it normally cochromatographs with UTP. Ritter and Bruce (1979) used two Partisil 10 SAX columns in series with a 2-hour linear gradient with column washing between runs, whereas Lowe and Henderson (unpublished) were able to obtain equally good resolution using a single Partisil 10 SAX column eluted isocratically with 0.25 M KH$_2$PO$_4$, 0.5 M KCl, pH 4.5, in about 40 minutes; no column washing was required between runs.

The major problem with this oxidation procedure is the production of a very large and tailing peak of ribonucleotide oxidation products on whose shoulder the dCTP and dTTP peaks appear. This makes electronic integration virtually impossible and limits the accuracy of planimetric integration because of the difficulty in choosing a baseline.

Garrett and Santi (1979) solved the problem of the large tailing peak of ribonucleotide oxidation products by reacting them with methylamine to eliminate the phosphate groups and cleave the N-glycosidic bond. The resulting bases elute well before the deoxyribonucleoside triphosphates. The actual procedure of Garrett and Santi was as follows: to 1.0 ml of neutralized cell extract was added 40 μl 0.5 M NaIO$_4$, followed within several minutes by 50 μl of 4 M methylamine which had been slowly brought to pH 7.5 with H$_3$PO$_4$. After 30 minutes at 37°C, 10 μl of 1 M rhamnose was added to reduce any remaining periodate. The oxidized samples were chromatographed on a Whatman Partisil 10 SAX anion-exchange column (4.6 × 250 mm) and eluted isocratically with 0.4 M ammonium phosphate, pH 3.25:acetonitrile (10:1) at 30°C. The peaks were monitored at 254 nm at 0.013 OD units full scale. Peaks of less than 500 pmole could not be reliably integrated with an automatic electronic integrator and were quantitated by comparing the height with that of standard peaks (rather than by planimetry, which would have probably been more accurate because the peaks were asymmetric). They reported a lower limit of sensitivity of 30 pmole. Values for accuracy and reproducibility were not given.

Lowe and Henderson (unpublished) used this method both for deoxyribonucleoside triphosphate standards and for neutralized cell extracts. After periodate and methylamine treatment the cells were chromatographed on a Whatman Partisil 10 SAX anion-exchange column and eluted isocratically with either 0.4 M ammonium phosphate, pH 3.25:acetonitrile (10:1) or 0.25 M KH$_2$PO$_4$, 0.5 M KCl, pH 4.5; equivalent results were obtained with both solvents. The peaks were detected at 254 nm, at a sensitivity of 0.02 or 0.005 OD units full scale, and were measured by planimetry rather than electronically because of an unstable baseline. In agreement with Garrett and Santi (1979), Lowe and Henderson (unpublished) found that the methylamine treatment greatly reduced the tailing of the initial peak, making the dTTP and dCTP peak measurements easier than in cell extracts oxidized by the method of Ritter and Bruce (1979). Although peaks containing as few as 30 pmole were visible, it was impossible to obtain consistent values for the areas because the position of the baseline could not be accurately determined. Although Garrett and Santi (1979) reported that 30 pmole of deoxyribonucleotide could be measured by this method, Lowe and Henderson (unpublished) found this value to be about 100–200 pmole. This difference may simply reflect the different machines used by the two groups. Garrett and Santi used a Hewlett-Packard HPLC, whereas Lowe and Henderson used both a Varian and a Waters Associates HPLC.

The most recent changes to the method have been made by Maybaum et al. (1980). Their method involves the separation and collection of each ribo- and corresponding deoxyribonucleotide using an anion-exchange column. Each pair of nucleotides is converted to the corresponding nucleoside by acid phosphatase and then separated and collected using a preparative reversed-phase column. When higher sensitivity is required, the fractions are rerun on an analytical reversed-phase or cation-exchange column. Thus they are able to measure the eight major ribo- and deoxyribonucleotides, although the assay will be described and discussed only in the context of the deoxyribonucleotide measurements. The published procedure is restricted to pyrimidines, but an unpublished modification of the procedure has been developed for purines.

The actual procedure used by Maybaum et al. (1980) was as follows: Neutralized cell or tissue extracts were chromatographed on an analytical anion-exchange column. Monophosphates were eluted isocratically followed by a linear gradient to elute the di- and triphosphates. Ribonucleotides were not separated from the corresponding deoxyribonucleotides, so each pair was collected, lyophilized, and treated with acid phosphatase to convert the nucleotides to nucleosides. Each pair of ribo- and deoxyribonucleosides was run on a preparative reversed-phase column, because the high salt content would saturate an analytical column. Uracil and cytosine nucleosides were eluted with methanol: H_2O and thymidine was eluted with acetonitrile: H_2O. Detection was at 254 and 280 nm with the lower limit of sensitivity at 100 pmole and a net recovery of 80%. In order for this method to be of practical use in measurement deoxyribonucleotides in cell extracts, much lower sensitivity was required. Therefore, each deoxyribonucleoside was collected, dried, and redissolved. Deoxyuridine and deoxythymidine were rechromatographed on a reversed-phase column and eluted with 10 mM NaH_2PO_4, pH 3.0: acetonitrile and

10 mM sodium acetate, pH 7.4 : acetonitrile, respectively, while deoxycytidine was rechromatographed on a cation-exchange column and eluted isocratically. With detection at 254 and 280 nm, the lower limit of sensitivity was 10 pmole and the net recovery of the entire procedure was 66%. The standard deviation, based on three determinations for each deoxyribonucleotide, ranged from 3 to 15%.

Although this procedure can provide a considerable amount of information from one sample, it is very tedious and time consuming, with only a threefold more sensitive measurement of the deoxyribonucleoside triphosphates over that obtained by Garrett and Santi (1979).

C. Discussion

High-performance liquid chromatography has been used to assay deoxyribonucleoside triphosphates for only 4 years, but it is quite useful within certain limitations of sensitivity, speed, and cost. Although Maybaum *et al.* were able to measure amounts of deoxynucleotides as low as 10 pmole, an almost prohibitive amount of work was required (Maybaum *et al.*, 1980). Their method would not be practical for analyzing more than a few samples.

There are two main ways the sensitivity of the HPLC method could be enhanced: (1) with the development of new columns with higher theoretical plates and (2) with the development of new detectors with a higher signal-to-noise ratio than is presently available.

Given the limitations of the present equipment, the HPLC assay is still useful if a large number of cells can be extracted or if the deoxyribonucleotide pool to be measured is artificially elevated. For example, the dATP pool in red blood cells incubated with deoxyadenosine plus 2'-deoxycoformycin is sufficiently elevated to allow it to be easily measured using HPLC (C. M. Smith and J. F. Henderson, unpublished).

VIII. Enzymatic Assay

The enzymatic assay of deoxyribonucleoside triphosphates was originally developed by Solter and Handschumacher (1969). Many subsequent improvements and modifications have resulted in a plethora of assays. Presently there are more than 20 different variations of this method in the literature, many of which have not been thoroughly evaluated, and some of which certainly are not optimal. As a result, it is difficult to compare data obtained using different variations of the method without having an assessment of the reliability of the different methods; and as well, researchers wishing to use the enzymatic assay are faced with a difficult choice. Finally, there are improvements which would benefit even the best of the present assays. The purpose of this section is to describe the development of the enzymatic assay, to present both the advantages and the drawbacks of each variation of the assay, and, finally, to present the method used in our laboratory, in which we have attempted to incorporate the best features of previous assays as well as further improvements.

A. General Principle

The enzymatic assay is based on the fact that DNA polymerase I will accurately catalyze the incorporation of four deoxyribonucleoside triphosphates into DNA, which serves both as the template and the primer for the reaction. If three of these triphosphates are present in excess and one of the three is radioactive, then at the completion of the polymerization reaction the amount of radioactivity in DNA will be proportional to the amount of the fourth, limiting triphosphate that was originally present. One of the important improvements to the original assay was the later substitution of synthetic alternating copolymers for the DNA.

An important requirement of the assay is that in order for the optimum incubation time of the reaction to be independent of the amount of limiting deoxyribonucleotide present, the kinetics of the polymerization reaction must be first order with respect to the limiting deoxyribonucleoside. Thus, maximum incorporation will be reached at the same time, regardless of the amount of deoxyribonucleotide being assayed.

B. Development of the Assay

The first enzymatic assay for deoxynucleoside triphosphates used undenatured calf thymus DNA as the primer-template and *E. coli* DNA polymerase I as the polymerization enzyme; deoxynucleoside triphosphate pools in extracts of bacterial and mammalian cells were measured (Solter and Handschumacher, 1969). Time courses demonstrated that the reaction was first order with respect to the limiting substrate and also that the product was degraded with time as a result of $3' \rightarrow 5'$ exonuclease activity, an inherent property of the *E. coli* DNA polymerase I. The assay was quite insensitive by modern standards, with a lower limit of 100 pmole/tube, although the authors pointed out that the sensitivity could be increased by increasing the specific activity of the labeled deoxyribonucleotides. By assaying the extracts in the presence and absence of standards, Solter and Handschumacher (1969) demonstrated that cell extracts did not affect the accuracy of the assay.

Skoog (1970) and Lindberg and Skoog (1970) introduced a significant improvement in the assay by using poly[d(I-C)] as the primer-template for the dGTP and dCTP assays, and poly[d(A-T)] for the dATP and dTTP assays. The synthetic alternating copolymers offered several advantages over DNA in that they were readily soluble, resulted in a faster polymerization rate, and, because of their alternating deoxynucleotide sequence, incorporated labeled and unlabeled nucleotide in exactly equal amounts and required only two substrates for the reaction. By also using nucleotides with higher specific activities than did Solter and Handschumacher (1969), Lindberg and Skoog (1970) reported a lower limit of sensitivity of 0.2 pmole. Unlike Solter and Handschumacher (1969), Lindberg and Skoog (1970) tested for and found phosphatase activity in the DNA polymerase I preparation; they were able to inhibit this by pretreating the polymerase with mercuric ion.

The next significant improvement was added by Munch-Petersen *et al.* (1973), who recognized that the specific activities of the labeled deoxyribonucleotides were being diluted by the same unlabeled deoxyribonucleotides in the cell extract. For example, an increase in the amount of dATP in the cell extracts would lower the apparent concentration of dTTP by diluting the specific activity of the [³H]dATP in the assay. To correct the data for this effect, they constructed appropriate simultaneous equations.

Between 1973 and 1980, few if any improvements were made on the assay. Our own recent improvements involve the use of a 3' → 5' exonuclease inhibitor to increase the stability of the product polymer. The other improvement is the result of the discovery that background incorporation can occur in the presence of the labeled deoxyribonucleotide alone, presumably as the result of terminal addition of the labeled nucleotide onto the primer-template. When the specific activity of the label is increased in order to increase the sensitivity and accuracy of the assay, the background incorporation increases proportionally. Thus achievement of greater sensitivity and accuracy requires that the background incorporation be corrected for the dilution of the specific activity of the radioactive precursor by unlabeled nucleotide in the cell extract.

One final improvement, which probably would not increase accuracy or sensitivity but which would make the assay less tedious, would be the use of a DNA polymerase with no associated 3' → 5' exonuclease activity, such as calf thymus DNA polymerase. This would eliminate the need for an exonuclease inhibitor, which is not completely effective, and would also eliminate the need for precise sampling times. Our attempts to use a commercial calf thymus DNA polymerase preparation in this assay were unsuccessful because the preparation was contaminated with both phosphatase and exonuclease activities.

C. Important Variables in Individual Methods

More than 20 variant DNA polymerase assays for deoxyribonucleoside triphosphates have been published. The important differences among them will be described in the following section and in Tables II–V.

1. DNA Polymerase

Three types of DNA polymerase have been used in the enzymatic assay: *E. coli* polymerase I, *Micrococcus luteus* polymerase I, and the large fragment of *E. coli* polymerase I (Table II). The *E. coli* and *M. luteus* polymerases are very similar and have the same types of activities, while the large fragment of *E. coli* polymerase I contains 5′ → 3′ polymerase and 3′ → 5′ exonuclease, but not 5′ → 3′ exonuclease, activity (Kornberg, 1974).

The main problem with DNA polymerase preparations is that they often contain contaminating phosphatase activity which at the very least reduces the sensitivity of the assay by dephosphorylating the substrates, thus making them unavailable for DNA synthesis. We have found phosphatase activity in DNA polymerase preparations from several sources, but have been able to obtain phosphatase-free preparations from Boehringer-Mannheim Inc. (D. Hunting and J. F. Henderson, 1981; see Appendix, Section X,B). Although it is useful to know the specific activity of the enzyme preparation, it is more important to test for the presence of phosphatase, even in preparations of high specific activity. Table II shows that even a polymerase preparation of high specific activity contained significant amounts of phosphatase activity. Unfortunately, phosphatase activity was only assayed in 3 of the 24 variations of the assay.

2. Reaction Conditions

The polymerases used in this assay all contain 3′ → 5′ exonuclease activity; therefore, when the polymerization reaction has gone to completion, degradation of the product begins, releasing labeled deoxyribonucleotides. The presence of this exonuclease activity makes it essential to optimize the incubation time. We use an exonuclease inhibitor (dAMP) to stabilize the product polymer and reduce the error caused by small changes in sampling times, the rate of polymerization, or the 3′ → 5′ exonucleation. Even in the presence of an exonuclease inhibitor some exonucleation occurs, so optimization of the sampling time is still important. The actual value for the sampling time is probably not too important;

TABLE II
DNA POLYMERASE PREPARATIONS USED

Type of polymerase	Specific activity (units/mg protein)	Phos-phatase detected	Reference
E. coli Pol I	8,900	Yes	Skoog (1970)
E. coli Pol I	18,000	ND[a]	Lindberg and Skoog (1970)
E. coli Pol I	NR[b]	ND	Skoog *et al.* (1973)
M. luteus Pol	1336	Yes	Kinahan *et al.* (1979)
E. coli Pol I, large fragment	NR	ND	Tyrsted (1975)
E. coli Pol I, large fragment	NR	ND	Munch-Petersen *et al.* (1973)
M. luteus Pol	600	ND	Kyburg *et al.* (1979)
M. luteus Pol	NR	ND	Tattersall and Harrap (1973)
M. luteus Pol	NR	ND	Walters *et al.* (1973)
M. luteus Pol	NR	ND	Tattersall *et al.* (1975a)
E. coli Pol I, large fragment	NR	ND	de Saint Vincent and Buttin (1979)
E. coli Pol I, large fragment	7,050	ND	Solter and Handschumacher (1969)
E. coli Pol I, large fragment	NR	ND	Lowe and Grindey (1976)
M. luteus Pol	NR	ND	Lowe *et al.* (1977)
M. luteus Pol	420	ND	Fridland (1974)
E. coli Pol I	NR	ND	Cohen *et al.* (1978)
E. coli Pol I	59,000	ND	Bray and Brent (1972)
M. luteus Pol	NR	ND	Tattersall *et al.* (1975b)
E. coli Pol I	22	ND	Adams *et al.* (1971)
M. luteus Pol	10,000	ND	Baumunk and Friedman (1971)
E. coli Pol I	4,600	ND	Wittes and Kidwell (1975)
M. luteus Pol	NR	ND	Goetz and Carell (1978)
M. luteus Pol	NR	ND	Mitchell *et al.* (1978)
E. coli Pol I	3,600	No	D. Hunting and J. F. Henderson (1981)

[a] ND, Not determined.

[b] NR, Not reported.

however, excessively long incubations at 37°C may result in triphosphate breakdown and should be avoided.

The amount of primer-template used per tube is important for two reasons. There should be sufficient primer-template to make the polymerization reaction independent of its concentration, but since background incorporation is proportional to the amount of primer-template, excessive amounts should not be used. Unfortunately, it is difficult to compare the amounts of primer-template used in the various assays because different units were used. In addition, the properties of primer-templates from different sources vary. For example, we have found that poly[d(I-C)] purchased from the Sigma Chemical Co. had much less primer-template activity per A_{260} unit than did a similar polymer obtained from the Miles Chemical Co. (D. Hunting and J. F. Henderson, unpublished). Information concerning the relative sizes of the polymers was not available. As well, in some assays the DNA primer-template was pretreated by denaturation or treatment with DNase I to increase the activity (Bray and Brent, 1972; Fridland, 1974).

As discussed earlier, the synthetic polymers are better suited to the enzymatic assay than is DNA. If DNA is used it would be wise to ensure that the labeled nucleotide is complementary to the nucleotide being assayed, so that one can be sure they will be incorporated in equal amounts.

Table III compares the reaction conditions used in the various enzymatic assays. Sampling time was optimized in only 50% of the assays. Some of the sampling times were quite long (e.g., 120 minutes, 360 minutes), but most were between 30 and 60 minutes. In a few assays the amount of primer-template used seems to have been excessive, thereby increasing the background incorporation. We have found 0.02 A_{260} units of either poly[d(A-T)] or poly[d(I-C)] to be sufficient in our system. In many cases in which DNA was the primer-template, the labeled nucleotide and the nucleotide being assayed were not complementary; often the same labeled nucleotide was used to determine the concentrations of the other three nucleotides, so that the labeled and unknown nucleotides were complementary in only one of the assays.

3. Controls

There are a number of controls which need to be performed on the assay before using it routinely. First, it is important to measure the purity of the nonradioactive nucleotides which are used as standards in the assay in order that the true concentration of the deoxyribonucleotides can be determined, rather than just relative values. We have found, for example, that the deoxyribonucleoside triphosphates purchased from the Sigma Chemical Co. and shipped at ambient temperatures contained about 2–10 molar % of the mono- and diphosphates, as determined by HPLC. Triphosphates shipped on dry ice contained only about 2 molar % of the mono- and diphosphates upon arrival, but even storage at $-20°C$ over a desiccant for a few months resulted in as much as 15% hydrolysis of the triphosphates; dGTP was the least stable but substantial hydrolysis of all the triphosphates occurred. Maximum stability was achieved by preparing stock solutions of the triphosphates in buffer followed by storage at $-20°C$. These solutions were stable for at least several months.

TABLE III

REACTION CONDITIONS

Sampling time optimized	Sampling time (minutes)	Primer-template/tube		DNA (μg)	Label and unknown complementary	Reference
		poly[d(A-T)]	poly[d(I-C)]			
Yes	40	—	0.6 nmole		Yes	Skoog (1970)
Yes	35	4 nmole	—		Yes	Lindberg and Skoog (1970)
Yes	35–40	4 nmole	0.6 nmole		Yes	Skoog et al. (1973)
Yes	25	0.1 μg	0.1 μg		Yes	Kinahan et al. (1979)
Yes	30–40 or 80–120	—	0.2–0.8 nmole		Yes	Tyrsted (1975)
Yes	30–40	10 nmole	—		Yes	Munch-Petersen et al. (1973)
No	60	4–23 A_{260} U	—		Yes	Kyburg et al. (1979)
No	30	0.01 A_{260} U	—	NR[a]	No	Tattersall and Harrap (1973)
Yes	60	5 nmole	5.0 nmole		Yes	Walters et al. (1973)
No	35	0.05 A_{260} U	—	5	No	Tattersall et al. (1975a)
No	40	—	0.6 nmole		Yes	de Saint Vincent and Buttin (1979)
Yes	60	—	—	10	Not always	Solter and Handschumacher (1969)
Yes	25	—	—	10	Not always	Lowe and Grindey (1976)
Yes	120	—	—	10	Not always	Lowe et al. (1977)
No	45	—	—	1.5	Not always	Fridland (1974)
No	60	—	—	10	Yes	Cohen et al. (1978)
No	45	—	—	12	Not always	Bray and Brent (1972)
No	60	—	—	5	Not always	Tattersall et al. (1975b)
No	30	—	—	10	Not always	Adams et al. (1971)
No	360	—	—	7.5	No	Baumunk and Friedman (1971)
No	90	—	—	7.5	No	Wittes and Kidwell (1975)
Yes	90	—	—	5	Not always	Goetz and Carell (1978)
No	NR	—	—	10	Not always	Mitchell et al. (1978)
Yes	10–20 or 40–60	0.02 A_{260} U	0.02 A_{260} U	—	Yes	D. Hunting and J. F. Henderson (1981)

[a] NR, Not reported.

In addition, if the data are to be corrected for dilution of the specific activity of the radioactive nucleotide by the extract, then the purity and specific activity of the radioactive deoxyribonucleotides must be known. We have found that in tritiated deoxyribonucleoside triphosphate preparations supplied by ICN and by Schwarz Mann Inc., 6–14% of the radioactivity in the nucleotides was present as mono- and diphosphates, as determined by thin-layer chromatography. As well, substantial amounts (up to 50%) of the radioactivity in some preparations were present on arrival as tritiated water. Therefore, it is important to determine the amount of hydrolysis of the radioactive triphosphate and the amount of exchange of the tritium that has occurred.

Finally, the effect of the cell extract on the assay must be determined for each different type of extract and each type of experimental condition used. This can be done in three ways: (1) by addition of deoxyribonucleoside triphosphate standards to the cell extracts to determine if the final amount measured is equal to the sum of the amounts in the standard and cell extract; (2) by determining if the values obtained from the assay are proportional to the amount of cell extract assayed; and (3) by performing time courses to determine if the assays containing standards, control cell extracts, and extracts of drug-tested cells reach the maximum incorporation at the same time.

These controls on the effect of the extract on the assay are very important. As mentioned in the discussion of extraction methods, North et al. (1980) have reported that methanol extracts of cells gave artificially high deoxyribonucleoside triphosphate values. They also reported that PCA extracts of cells interfered slightly with the assay procedure, although this is not consistent with our results (D. Hunting and J. F. Henderson, 1981) or the results of many other researchers. As well, Tyrsted (1975) has reported that 60% methanol extracts of unwashed cells interfered with the enzymatic assay of dCTP.

Table IV presents the results of a comparison of the controls performed on the different assays. In most cases, the purity of neither the labeled nor unlabeled nucleotides was determined, making it impossible to correct the results for dilution of the labeled nucleotide by the extract. This correction was made in only 5 of the 24 assays, even though the importance of this correction was demonstrated by Munch-Petersen et al. (1973). In a few cases, however, this correction would not have been too important because a large excess of radioisotope was used and little dilution would have been caused by the sample.

Our own assay procedure is the only one which includes a correction for the effects of dilution of the specific activity of the labeled nucleotide on background incorporation. This correction is required only when ra-

TABLE IV
CONTROLS PERFORMED

Purity of unlabeled nucleotides measured	Purity of radioactive nucleotides measured	Effect of cell extract on assay measured	Reference
Yes	Yes	Yes	Skoog (1970)
Yes	Yes	Yes	Lindberg and Skoog (1970)
Yes	Yes	Yes	Skoog et al. (1973)
No	No	Yes	Kinahan et al. (1979)
No	No	Yes	Tyrsted (1975)
No	No	Yes	Munch-Petersen et al. (1973)
No	No	No	Kyburg et al. (1979)
No	No	No	Tattersall and Harrap (1973)
Yes	Yes	Yes	Walters et al. (1973)
No	No	Yes	Tattersall et al. (1975a)
No	No	No	de Saint Vincent and Buttin (1979)
No	No	Yes	Solter and Handschumacher (1969)
No	No	Yes	Lowe and Grindey (1976)
No	No	No	Lowe et al. (1977)
No	No	Yes	Fridland (1974)
No	No	Yes	Cohen et al. (1978)
Yes	No	Yes	Bray and Brent (1972)
No	No	No	Tattersall et al. (1975b)
No	No	No	Adams et al. (1971)
No	No	Yes	Baumunk and Friedman (1971)
Yes	Yes	Yes	Wittes and Kidwell (1975)
No	No	Yes	Goetz and Carell (1978)
No	No	No	Mitchell et al. (1978)
Yes	Yes	Yes	D. Hunting and J. F. Henderson, (1981)

dioactive nucleotides of high specific activity are used or when small amounts of nucleotides are measured. Only 7 of the 24 methods did not include a check on the effect of the cell extract on the assay.

4. Sensitivity, Reproducibility, Accuracy, and Range

These parameters are all important, but in fact only reproducibility and accuracy are measures of the quality of a particular method. Often, the sensitivity and range used are simply determined by the type of samples that are to be analyzed. Table V compares the sensitivity, reproducibility, and range of the various assays. Accuracy values were available for only one of the assay.

TABLE V

SENSITIVITY, REPRODUCIBILITY, AND RANGE

Sensitivity $\left(\dfrac{\text{cpm incorporated}}{\text{pmole substrate}}\right)$	Reproducibility	Range (pmole)	Reference
150–900	NR[a]	0.2–4	Skoog (1970)
700–1000	NR	0.5–7	Lindberg and Skoog (1970)
NR	NR	NR	Skoog et al. (1973)
700–1200	SD = 0.1%	0.2–40	Kinahan et al. (1979)
300–600	NR	0–6	Tyrsted (1975)
350	NR	1–10	Munch-Petersen et al. (1973)
1600	NR	0.1–5	Kyburg et al. (1979)
NR	NR	1–100	Tattersall and Harrap (1973)
NR	SEM < ±7%	NR	Walters et al. (1973)
NR	COV = 1.2%	0–50	Tattersall et al. (1975a)
NR	NR	NR	de Saint Vincent and Buttin (1979)
1–3	NR	100–1000	Solter and Handschumacher (1969)
NR	NR	1–20	Lowe and Grindey (1976)
NR	NR	2–50	Lowe et al. (1977)
NR	NR	0–100	Fridland (1974)
NR	NR	NR	Cohen et al. (1978)
NR	NR	5–100	Bray and Brent (1972)
NR	NR	NR	Tattersall et al. (1975b)
NR	NR	5–500	Adams et al. (1971)
NR	NR	0–100	Baumunk and Friedman (1971)
4	NR	0–200	Wittes and Kidwell (1975)
NR	NR	NR	Goetz and Carell (1978)
NR	NR	NR	Mitchell et al. (1978)
500–5000	SD = 2.5–8.5%	0.5–200	D. Hunting and J. F. Henderson (1981)

[a] NR, not reported.

The sensitivity is expressed as the number of counts per minute incorporated into the polymer for each picomole of limiting substrate. In most cases these values were calculated from standard curves presented in the literature. Values for sensitivity in picomoles per tube were generally not available. It is obvious that the enzymatic assay is capable of very high sensitivity since the radioactive deoxyribonucleoside triphosphates are available at very high specific activities, such as 20 Ci/mmole. Although values for reproducibility are rarely presented, those given are good. It is also apparent that the enzymatic assay can be used over a very wide range (about 10,000-fold) of concentrations.

D. CONCLUSIONS

Although in principle the enzymatic assay of deoxyribonucleoside triphosphate concentrations is capable of very good sensitivity, accuracy, and reproducibility, in practice it is often not used to its full potential. Several improvements, such as the use of synthetic copolymers, tests for phosphatase activity in the DNA polymerase preparation, and correction of the results for the dilution of the radioactive precursor by nonradioactive precursor in the sample, are still not incorporated into all the versions of the assay. Furthermore, several versions of the assay have not been thoroughly tested to determine if they measure the actual deoxyribonucleoside triphosphate concentrations in cell extracts. It is hoped that this article will alert researchers to the possible pitfalls in this method as well as to its potential.

IX. Conclusions

There are three useful methods for measuring deoxyribonucleoside triphosphate concentrations in cells at the present time: the $^{32}P_i$, HPLC, and enzymatic assays. The microbiological and chromatographic methods are too insensitive to be useful unless large amounts of biological material are available. Table VI gives the approximate maximum sensitivity that has been achieved with each method, as well as the main limitations on the sensitivity of each method. All of the methods can be reliable and accurate when used properly. The HPLC assay has the advantage of requiring less setup time than the enzymatic or $^{32}P_i$ assays, which require more control experiments. Therefore, if few or infrequent measurements are to be made, the HPLC method may be best suited. The enzymatic method has the advantages of being about 100-fold more sensitive than the $^{32}P_i$ or HPLC assays, as well as faster when large numbers of samples are involved. The $^{32}P_i$ assay has no apparent advantages over the HPLC or enzymatic assays, since it is slower than both and less sensitive than the latter. The final choice of methods is probably between the HPLC and enzymatic assays, and this choice will depend on the particular requirements of the researcher and the equipment that is available.

Finally, when comparing intracellular deoxyribonucleotide concentra-

TABLE VI

SENSITIVITIES OF DIFFERENT DEOXYRIBONUCLEOSIDE TRIPHOSPHATE ASSAY METHODS

Assay method	Maximum sensitivity achieved (pmole/assay)	Factors limiting sensitivity	References
Microbiological	500	Growth response of organism to deoxyribonucleosides; volume required for determination of growth rate	Hoff-Jorgensen (1957)
Chromatography with UV measurement	<400[a]	Sensitivity of UV measurement; background absorbance	Kummer and Kraml (1977)
Radioactive orthophosphate ($^{32}P_i$)	10[b]	Sensitivity of organism to radiation; background radioactivity on chromatogram	Neuhard and Munch-Petersen (1966)
HPLC with UV detection	10	Sensitivity of UV detection; background absorbance	Maybaum et al. (1980)
Enzymatic	0.1	Specific activity of deoxyribonucleoside triphosphates; washing background due to incomplete removal of unincorporated radioactive triphosphates	Skoog (1970); Kinahan et al. (1979); Kyburg et al. (1979)

[a] This value is based on the fact that Kummer and Kraml extracted 1×10^7 cells containing 400 pmole of dTTP. However, since they did not report the amount of extract that was chromatographed, the value given is a minimum estimate of the sensitivity of the method.

[b] This value is based on an intracellular deoxyribonucleoside triphosphate specific activity of 20 dpm/pmole and the assumption that 200 dpm can be accurately determined.

tions given in the literature, one must assess not only the general assay method, but also the particular variant method used.

X. Appendix: Improved Enzymatic Assay

The measurement of intracellular deoxyribonucleoside triphosphates by the enzymatic method, as used in our laboratory, is described here. This procedure incorporates the best features of other assay procedures, as well as improvements of our own, as discussed above.

A. Cell Extraction

Preparation of extracts for nucleotide pool size measurements was as follows: $0.25-4.0 \times 10^7$ cells were centrifuged at 1000 g for 2 minutes at 4°C. The medium was aspirated and the tube recentrifuged at 1000 g for 5 seconds to remove medium from the centrifuge tube wall. The pellet was extracted on ice with 0.4 M PCA containing [³H]adenosine for determination of dilution. After 30 minutes the extract was centrifuged and the supernatant was removed and neutralized by extraction with 0.5 M alamine 336 (tricapryl tertiaryamine) in Freon-TF (trichlorotrifluoroethane) (Khym, 1975). Supernatants were stored at -20°C. Analysis by HPLC of samples stored for several weeks showed no nucleotide breakdown.

B. Purity of Reagents

The purities of the nonradioactive deoxyribonucleoside triphosphates were 90–98 molar %, as determined by HPLC. The final concentration of each deoxyribonucleoside triphosphate was corrected for the presence of the impurities which were deoxyribonucleoside mono- and diphosphates. The standard nucleotide solutions were stable for several months at -20°C.

The radioactive deoxyribonucleoside triphosphates were supplied and stored in 50% ethanol. The ethanol and tritiated water were removed by lyophilization followed by dissolution in 100 mM HEPES, pH 7.4. The radiochemical purity was 86–94%, as determined by chromatography followed by sample oxidation and liquid scintillation counting. The solution was stable for several months at -20°C.

DNA polymerase I (*E. coli*) was supplied and stored in 50% glycerol, pH 7.0. A working solution was prepared by diluting the stock solution with 50 mM Tris–HCl, pH 7.8, containing 12 mg/ml bovine serum albumin. This solution was stored not longer than 1 month. Each new batch was checked for phosphatase activity by incubating the enzyme with all the components of the assay except the copolymer. The formation of deoxyribonucleoside mono- and diphosphates indicated the presence of phosphatase activity. All the enzyme preparations used in the assay were phosphatase free.

C. Reaction Conditions

The following components were common to both the dATP and dTTP assay in a final volume of 180 μl: 0.02 A_{260} units poly[d(A-T)], 1.8 μmole

MgCl$_2$, 1.8 μmole dAMP, 18 μmole HEPES buffer, pH 7.4, and 0.75 Richardson units of DNA polymerase I (Richardson *et al.*, 1964). As well, the dATP assay contained 100 pmole (0.5 μCi) [^{3}H]dTTP, and 0–75 pmole dATP standard, while the dTTP assay contained 100 pmole (0.5 μCi) [^{3}H]dATP and 0–75 pmole dTTP standard.

The following components were common to both the dGTP and the dCTP assays in a final volume of 180 μl: 0.02 A_{260} units poly[d(I-C)], 1.8 μmole MgCl$_2$, 1.8 μmole dAMP, and 18 μmole HEPES buffer, pH 7.4. As well, the dGTP assay contained 100 pmole (2.2 μCi) [^{3}H]dCTP, 0–10 pmole dGTP standard, and 1.9 units DNA polymerase I. The dCTP assay contained 240 pmole (0.5 μCi) [^{3}H]dGTP, 0–200 pmole dCTP standard, and 3.0 units DNA polymerase I.

The dAMP was used to inhibit the 3' $\rightarrow$ 5' exonuclease activity of the DNA polymerase I (Byrnes *et al.*, 1977).

The reaction was started by the addition of the DNA polymerase I, followed by incubation at 37°C. At each time point aliquots were removed and spotted on squares of Whatman 3MM filter paper which had been wetted with 200 μl of 2% sodium pyrophosphate. The squares were washed (3 $\times$ 15 minutes) with a solution of 5% TCA and 1% sodium pyrophosphate (20 ml/square), then rinsed once with 95% ethanol and finally washed (1 $\times$ 15 minutes) with 95% ethanol. The dried filters were counted in toluene scintillation cocktail (4 gm PPO and 0.1 gm POPOP per liter of toluene).

Results were corrected for the washing background and for the effects of the dilution of the specific activity of the labeled deoxyribonucleotide by the sample on both the sample incorporation and the background incorporation.

The final value for the deoxynucleoside triphosphate concentration, which was independent of the amount of extract used in the assay, was within the limits of the standard curves. As well, addition of standards to cell extracts was used to demonstrate that the assay was not affected by the cell extracts. Finally, time courses were performed with standards, cell extracts of control cells, and cell extracts of drug-treated cells to ensure that the maximum incorporation was reached at the same time under all conditions.

D. CORRECTION OF THE DATA FOR THE ISOTOPIC DILUTION CAUSED BY THE SAMPLE

The samples being assayed usually contain nonradioactive deoxyribonucleoside triphosphate which will dilute the specific activity of the radioactive nucleotide used in the assay. As a result, both the background incorporation and the sample incorporation will be lowered in proportion to the amount of isotopic dilution that has occurred.

The following derivation provides the equations to correct the incorporation data for the isotopic dilution caused by the sample.

Definitions

dNTP1, dNTP2	Deoxyribonucleoside triphosphate 1 and 2 which are incorporated into the alternating copolymer
P1	Picomoles of radioactive dNTP2 per tube in the dNTP1 assay
P2	Picomoles of radioactive dNTP1 per tube in the dNTP2 assay
d1, d2	Dilution of the radioactive nucleotide caused by the sample in the dNTP1 and dNTP2 assay, respectively
C1, C2	Actual radioactivity incorporated into the polymer in the dNTP1 and dNTP2 assays, respectively
Y1, Y2	Dilution-corrected radioactivity incorporated into the polymer
m1, m2	Slope of the standard curve in each assay
X1, X2	Picomoles of dNTP1 and dNTP2, respectively, in the sample of standard per tube
b1, b2	Background incorporation in the assays (i.e., the y intercepts of the standard curves)
V1, V2	Volumes of sample used in each of the assays

Since the standard curves are linear the following relationships can be defined:

$$Y1 = m1X1 + b1, \qquad Y2 = m2X2 + b2$$

But the dilution-corrected cpm (Y) is equal to the actual radioactivity incorporated (C) divided by the isotopic dilution caused by the sample (d).

$$Y1 = C1/d1, \qquad Y2 = C2/d2$$

The isotopic dilution, when corrected for the volume of sample used in each tube, can be expressed as:

$$d1 = \frac{P1}{P1 + (X2V1/V2)} = \frac{P1V2}{P1V2 + X2V1}$$

$$d2 = \frac{P2}{P2 + (X1V2/V1)} = \frac{P2V1}{P2V1 + X1V2}$$

These equations can be solved for X1 and X2:

$$X1 = \frac{C1P1P2m2V2 + C1C2P2V1 - P2C1b2V1 - b1P1P2m2V2}{V2(P1P2m1m2 - C1C2)}$$

$$X2 = \frac{C2P1P2m1V1 + C1C2P1V2 - P1C2b1V2 - b2P1P2m1V1}{V1(P1P2m1m2 - C1C2)}$$

We have incorporated these equations into a computer program, written in APL, which also includes linear regression analysis. The program determines the slopes and y intercepts of the standard curves and then uses this information in the solution of the equations for X1 and X2.

REFERENCES

Adams, R. L. P. (1969). *Exp. Cell Res.* **56**, 55–58.
Adams, R. L. P., Berryman, S., and Thompson, A. (1971). *Biochim. Biophys. Acta* **240**, 455–462.
Bagnara, A. S., and Finch, L. R. (1972). *Anal. Biochem.* **45**, 24–34.
Baumunk, C. N., and Friedman, D. L. (1971). *Cancer Res.* **31**, 1930–1935.
Bersier, D., and Braun, R. (1974). *Biochim. Biophys. Acta* **340**, 463–471.
Bray, G., and Brent, T. P. (1972). *Biochim. Biophys. Acta* **269**, 184–191.
Brooker, G., and Appleman, M. M. (1968). *Biochemistry* **7**, 4182–4184.
Brown, N. C., and Handschumacher, R. E. (1966). *J. Biol. Chem.* **241**, 3083–3089.
Bucher, N. L. R., and Oakman, N. J. (1969). *Biochim. Biophys. Acta* **186**, 13–20.
Byrnes, J. J., Downey, K. M., Que, B. G., Lee, Y. W., Black, V. L., and So, A. G. (1977). *Biochemistry* **16**, 3740–3746.
Coddington, A., and Bagger-Sorensen, M. (1963). *Biochim. Biophys. Acta* **72**, 598–607.
Cohen, A., Hirshhorn, R., Horowitz, S. D., Rubinstein, A., Polmar, S. H., Hong, R., and Martin, D. W., Jr. (1978). *Proc. Natl. Acad. Sci. U.S.A* **75**, 472–476.
Colby, C., and Edlin, G. (1970). *Biochemistry* **9**, 917–920.
de Saint Vincent, B. R., and Buttin, G. (1979). *Somatic Cell Genet.* **5**, 67–82.
Forsdyke, D. R. (1968). *Biochem. J.* **107**, 197–105.
Forsdyke, D. R. (1971). *Biochem. J.* **125**, 721–732.
Fridland, A. (1974). *Cancer Res.* **34**, 1883–1888.
Gander, J. E. (1970). *Biochim. Biophys. Acta* **201**, 179–184.
Garrett, C., and Santi, D. V. (1979). *Anal. Biochem.* **99**, 268–273.
Goetz, G. H., and Carell, E. F. (1978). *Biochem. J.* **170**, 631–636.
Gudas, L. J., Ullman, B., Cohen, A., and Martin, D. W., Jr. (1978). *Cell* **14**, 531–538.
Hauschka, P. V. (1973). *Methods Cell Biol.* **2**, 361–462.
Henderson, J. F., Scott, F. W., and Lowe, J. K. (1980). *Pharmacol. Ther.* **8**, 573–604.
Hoff-Jorgensen, E. (1952). *Biochem. J.* **50**, 400–403.
Hoff-Jorgensen, E. (1957). *In* "Methods in Enzymology" (S. P. Colowick and N. O. Kaplan, eds.), Vol. III, pp. 781–785. Academic Press, New York.
Hunting, D., and Henderson, J. F. (1981). *Can. J. Biochem.* **59**, 723–727.
Khym, J. X. (1975). *Clin. Chem.* **21**, 1245–1252.
Kinahan, J. J., Otten, M., and Grindey, G. B. (1979). *Cancer Res.* **39**, 3531–3539.
Klenow, H. (1962). *Biochim. Biophys. Acta* **61**, 885–896.
Kornberg, A. (1974). "DNA Synthesis," p. 70. Freeman, San Francisco, California.
Kummer, P., and Kraml, F. (1977). *Z. Krebsforsch.* **88**, 129–143.
Kyburg, S., Schaer, J., and Schindler, R. (1979). *Biochem. Pharmacol.* **28**, 1885–1891.
Larsson, A. (1963). *J. Biol. Chem.* **238**, 3414–3419.

LePage, G. A. (1957). *J. Biol. Chem.* **226**, 135–137.
Lindberg, U., and Skoog, L. (1970). *Anal. Biochem.* **34**, 152–160.
Lowe, J. K., and Grindey, G. B. (1976). *Mol. Pharmacol.* **12**, 177–184.
Lowe, J. K., Brox, L., and Henderson, J. F. (1977). *Cancer Res.* **37**, 736–743.
Maybaum, J., Klein, F. K., and Sadee, W. (1980). *J. Chromatogr.* **188**, 149–158.
Mitchell, B. S., Mejias, E., Daddona, P. E., and Kelley, W. N. (1978). *Proc. Natl. Acad. Sci. U.S.A.* **75**, 5011–5014.
Munch-Petersen, A., and Neuhard, J. (1964).*Biochim. Biophys. Acta* **80**, 542–551.
Munch-Petersen, B., Tyrsted, G., and Dupont, B. (1973). *Exp. Cell Res.* **79**, 249–256.
Neuhard, J. (1966). *Biochim. Biophys. Acta* **129**, 104–115.
Neuhard, J., and Munch-Petersen, A. (1966). *Biochim. Biophys. Acta* **114**, 61–71.
Neuhard, J., Randerath, E., and Randerath, K. (1965). *J. Chromatogr.* **13**, 211–222.
Newsholme, E. A., and Taylor, K. (1968). *Biochim. Biophys. Acta* **158**, 11–24.
Nexo, B. A. (1975). *Biochim. Biophys. Acta* **378**, 12–17.
North, T. W., Bestwick, R. K., and Mathews, C. K. (1980). *J. Biol. Chem.* **255**, 6640–6645.
Potter, R. L. (1955). *Fed. Proc. Fed. Am. Soc. Exp. Biol.* **14**, 263–264.
Potter, R. L., and Nygaard, O. F. (1963). *J. Biol. Chem.* **238**, 2150–2155.
Potter, R. L. and Schlesinger, S. (1955). *J. Am. Chem. Soc.* **77**, 6714–6715.
Potter, R. L., Schlesinger, S., Buettner-Janusch, V., and Thompson, L. (1957). *J. Biol. Chem.* **226**, 381–394.
Randerath, K., and Randerath, E. (1964a). *J. Chromatogr.* **16**, 111–125.
Randerath, K., and Randerath, E. (1964b). *J. Chromatogr.* **16**, 126–129.
Randerath, K., and Randerath, E. (1967). *In* "Methods in Enzymology" (L. Grossman and K. Moldave, eds.), Vol. 12, Part A, pp. 323–347. Academic Press, New York.
Reynolds, E. C., and Finch, L. R. (1977). *Anal. Biochem.* **82**, 591–595.
Richardson, C. C., Schildkraut, C. L., Aposhian, H. V., and Kornberg, A. (1964). *J. Biol. Chem.* **239**, 222–231.
Ritter, E. J., and Bruce, L. M. (1979). *Biochem. Med.* **21**, 16–21.
Schneider, W. C. (1955). *J. Biol. Chem.* **216**, 287–301.
Schneider, W. C. (1962). *J. Biol. Chem.* **237**, 1405–1409.
Schneider, W. C., and Potter, R. L. (1957). *Proc. Soc. Exp. Biol. Med.* **94**, 798–800.
Scott, F. W., and Forsdyke, D. R. (1976). *Can. J. Biochem.* **54**, 238–248.
Scott, F. W., and Forsdyke, D. R. (1978). *Biochem. J.* **170**, 545–549.
Siedler, A. J., and Schweigert, B. S. (1959). *J. Bacteriol.* **77**, 514–515.
Siedler, A. J., Nayder, F. A., and Schweigert, B. A. (1957). *J. Bacteriol.* **73**, 670–675.
Sjöstrom, D. A., and Forsdyke, D. R. (1974). *Biochem. J.* **128**, 253–262.
Skoog, L. (1970). *Eur. J. Biochem.* **17**, 202–208.
Skoog, L., Nordenskjold, B. A., and Bjursell, K. G. (1973). *Eur. J. Biochem.* **33**, 428–432.
Solter, A. W., and Handschumacher, R. E. (1969). *Biochim. Biophys. Acta* **174**, 585–590.
Tattersall, M. H. N., and Harrap, K. R. (1973). *Cancer Res.* **33**, 3086–3090.
Tattersall, M. H. N., Ganeshaguru, K., and Hoffbrand, A. V. (1975a). *Biochem. Pharmacol.* **24**, 1495–1498.
Tattersall, M. H. N., Lavoie, A., Ganeshaguru, K., Tripp, E., and Hoffbrand, A. V. (1975b). *Eur. J. Clin. Invest.* **5**, 191–202.
Tyrsted, G. (1975). *Exp. Cell Res.,* **91**, 429–440.
Ullman, B., Gudas, L. J., Cohen, A., and Martin, D. W., Jr. (1978). *Cell* **14**, 365–375.
Ullman, B. Gudas, L. J., Clift, S. M., and Martin, D. W., Jr. (1979). *Proc. Natl. Acad. Sci. U.S.A.* **76**, 1074–1078.

Walters, R. A., Tobey, R. A., and Ratliff, R. L. (1973). *Biochim. Biophys. Acta* **319,** 336–347.

Walters, R. A., Gurley, L. R., Tobey, R. A., and Ratliff, R. L. (1974). *Radiat. Res.* **60,** 173–201.

Weber, M. J., and Edlin, G. (1971). *J. Biol. Chem.* **246,** 1828–1833.

Wittes, R. E., and Kidwell, W. R. (1975). *J. Mol. Biol.* **78,** 473–486.

Yegian, C. D. (1974). *Anal. Biochem.* **58,** 231–237.

MONOCLONAL ANTIBODIES AND THE TUMOR CELL SURFACE

CHAPTER VIII

MONOCLONAL ANTIBODY DEVELOPMENT IN THE STUDY OF COLORECTAL CARCINOMA-ASSOCIATED ANTIGENS

ZENON STEPLEWSKI AND HILARY KOPROWSKI

I. Introduction

The subject of human tumor immunology has expanded dramatically in the last decade. Although it was realized for a long time that malignant animal cells expressed specific cell surface molecules, tumor-associated transplantation antigens (TATA) recognized by the host as nonself (Gross, 1943; Klein *et al.*, 1960; Old and Boyse, 1964; Hellstrom and Hellstrom, 1969), the detection of human tumor antigens proved to be elusive. There are two main reasons for the search for biochemical markers that are unique to human tumor cells. First, the unregulated, malignant growth of tumor cells, their invasiveness, and their high growth rates suggest that these cells do not perceive the modulation by the organism's control mechanisms that influence and regulate the behavior of normal cells. Thus the tumor cells must be different from the normal cells from which they are presumably derived. Second, the hypothesis that tumors may again become susceptible to control or suppression by the activity of the autolo-

285

286 ZENON STEPLEWSKI AND HILARY KOPROWSKI

gous immune system predicts the existence of biochemical (antigenic) differences between tumor cells and normal cells of the same lineage. This hypothesis is supported by the observation that some tumors, in fact, do regress spontaneously (Bodurtha *et al.*, 1967).

The presence of infiltrating lymphocytes in the primary tumor bed (Edelson *et al.*, 1975) and the induction of hypersensitivity responses with tumor extracts in cancer patients (Bluming *et al.*, 1972) support the notion that patients can respond immunologically against their own tumors. The serological evidence also indicates that patients respond with antibodies that bind to autologous tumors (Gupta *et al.*, 1974; Irie *et al.*, 1979; Sidell *et al.*, 1980) and frequently to other tumors of similar histological type (Embleton *et al.*, 1980). The ability of patients to respond immunologically to their own and to allogeneic tumors thus seems to be well established (Morton *et al.*, 1968; Lewis *et al.*, 1969; Cornain *et al.*, 1975; Carey *et al.*, 1976; Garret *et al.*, 1977), yet tumor-specific responses have not been clearly demonstrated, nor have the antigens been identified. The analysis of human tumor-associated antigens by xenoantisera (Bray, 1978; Galloway *et al.*, 1981; Liao *et al.*, 1979; Mutzner *et al.*, 1980; Smith and O'Neill, 1971; Von Kleist and Burtin, 1969; Martin and Martin, 1970; Gold and Freedman, 1965) is complicated by the great number of normal antigens immunogenic for animals. Extensive absorption procedures on normal human tissues and serum quite often remove minor specific antibodies that are nonetheless important.

Introduction of hybridoma technology has revolutionized the analysis of cell surface antigens (Köhler and Milstein, 1975, 1976). For the first time it is possible to have pure, monoclonal antibodies that react specifically with a single antigenic epitope. Original attempts to detect antigens specific for human leukemia cells by hybridoma technology (Levy *et al.*, 1978) resulted in establishment of a panel of monoclonal antibodies reactive with different subsets of lymphocytes and their tumors. Specific monoclonal antibodies were produced against antigens present on cortical thymocytes and leukemia cells of patients with thymic acute lymphoblastic leukemia (ALL) (Levy *et al.*, 1979; Bradstock *et al.*, 1980). A large set of antigens present on different subsets of T cells has already been characterized (Reinhertz *et al.*, 1979; Hansen *et al.*, 1980; Royston *et al.*, 1980), some of which have potentially important diagnostic and therapeutic value. Similarly, a number of B-cell-specific antigens have been detected by monoclonal antibodies (Hansen *et al.*, 1980; Beckman *et al.*, 1980; Nadler *et al.*, 1980; Ritz *et al.*, 1980). These antigens are expressed differently on normal and malignant cells. Analyses of these antigens by the use of monoclonal antibodies have shown that, although they do not have the characteristics of tumor-specific antigens, it is possible to predict which particular stage of lymphoid development the malignant cell represents.

Antibodies that react with human melanomas were first described by Koprowski et al. (1978). Reactivities of some of these antibodies were later studied in detail, and antigens detected by these monoclonal antibodies were found to be glycoproteins, expressed not only by tumor cells in tissue culture, but also by melanoma cells freshly isolated from patients (Steplewski et al., 1979; M. Herlyn et al., 1980; Steplewski, 1980). One such antibody, designated Nu4B, was established from splenocytes of a mouse immunized with a melanoma somatic cell hybrid which contained only three human chromosomes (14, 17, and 21) and which retained the tumorigenic phenotype of the parental melanoma cell line. The Nu4B antigen was found on all tested melanoma cell lines (Koprowski et al., 1978; M. Herlyn et al., 1980) and all melanomas freshly isolated from patients (Steplewski et al., 1979). The antigen is also expressed by some astrocytoma cell lines and seems to represent a reexpression of antigen of neural tube origin (Steplewski, 1980). The antigen was not expressed by nonmalignant pigmented cells from nevi (Steplewski et al., 1979) or Spitz tumors. The target antigen of Nu4B antibody has a tetramolecular structure composed of three disulfide-linked polypeptide chains with molecular weights of 116,000, 29,000, and 26,000 noncovalently associated with a fourth polypeptide chain of molecular weight 95,000 (Mitchell et al., 1980, 1981). Another antibody was found to detect DR antigen (Mitchell et al., 1980; M. Herlyn et al., 1980). Antimelanoma antibody 19–19 reacts with most melanoma and some astrocytoma cells (Koprowski et al., 1978; M. Herlyn et al., 1980; Steplewski, 1980), but the antigen is distinct from that of Nu4B antibody, with a major component of molecular weight 260,000 (Steplweski et al., 1982; Mitchell et al., 1982).

Another report (Yeh et al., 1979) described an antibody which reacted with the antigen expressed strongly on the immunizing cell line and weakly with two allogeneic melanoma and one breast carcinoma cell line. Two other distinct melanoma antigens have been detected by monoclonal antibodies. The same antigens were also immunoprecipitated by xenoantisera (Reisfeld et al., 1980; Imai et al., 1980). The antigens have molecular weights of 240,000 and 94,000. Antigens with similar molecular weights were described by Brown et al. (1980). Their antigen has a molecular weight of 97,000. Another group of antigens described by this group (Woodbury et al., 1980) includes antigens with molecular weights of 33,000 and 50,000, 23,000, 27,000, 40,000, 200,000, and 27,000, 80,000, and 110,000. Dippold et al. (1980) described six monoclonal antibodies detecting antigens of the 95,000 group and antibodies reacting with glycoproteins of molecular weight 150,000, as well as a group in the 50,000–

70,000 range. Again, some of these antibodies are melanoma specific and some cross-react with other tumors, including astrocytomas. We have described a group of antimelanoma antibodies that detect antigens with molecular weights of 60,000, 196,000, and 28,000 (Steplewski et al., 1981). Monoclonal antibodies directed against other tumors included antineuroblastoma (Kennett and Gilbert, 1979) and anticolorectal carcinoma (M. Herlyn et al., 1979; Koprowski et al., 1979) antibodies. Antigens detected by anticolorectal carcinoma antibodies include carcinoembryonic antigen (CEA) and a monosialoganglioside (Magnani et al., 1981). The monosialoganglioside is present in sera of patients with colon, gastric, and pancreatic carcinomas (Koprowski et al., 1981), and its presence is not correlated with or related to CEA. The antigen is not present in serum of patients with other tumors or inflammatory diseases, or in normal subjects of different age, sex, and smoking habits.

It is clear at present that the availability of monoclonal antibodies has circumvented one major problem that hampered the characterization of cell surface antigens, the heterogeneity of antibodies present in antisera. The second problem—the low avidity of some antibodies—has been overcome through two circumstances: the large amounts of antibody present in hybridoma milieu and the selection procedure, which tends to eliminate clones that secrete only small amounts of low-affinity antibody.

II. Hybridoma Technology

In recent years two major facts have contributed to the explosive development of the analysis of tumor-associated antigens. It is well established that some tumors express on their surfaces antigens not present on the normal cells of the same lineage. At the same time, hybridoma technology (Köhler and Milstein, 1975) produces monoclonal antibodies. Using hybridoma technology it is now possible to produce large amounts of homogeneous monoclonal antibodies, each directed against a single antigenic epitope. In conjunction with immunochemical methods it is possible to define precisely the chemical structures of each antigen as defined by monoclonal antibodies. The fusion of a panel of immune splenocytes with drug-resistant hypoxanthine–aminopterin–thymidine (HAT)-sensitive myeloma cells results in a large number of clones. Each clone secretes a single type of antibody against a single antigenic determinant. These hybridoma clones grow continuously in tissue culture and form ascitic tumors when injected into syngeneic mice. A high titer of homogeneous antibodies theoretically could be produced in unlimited quantity. The general protocol used to produce anti-human tumor monoclonal antibodies is described below. Methods of immunization, analysis of detected antigens, and approaches to the analysis of antibody functions vary depending on the goals of each experiment.

A. IMMUNIZATION

Immunization protocols are designed according to the requirements of each experiment and depend on the type of antigen used. Animals are immunized with live cells from tumor tissue culture, cells freshly isolated from cancer patients, membrane or purified antigen preparations from tumor cells, or serum-free supernatants (SFS) from tumor cells grown in tissue culture.

1. Immunization with Tumor Cells Grown in Culture

Mice are immunized for primary or secondary responses with tissue culture-derived tumor cells. Tumor cells grown in suspension are collected and washed three times in phosphate-buffered saline (PBS) before injection. Cells grown in monolayers are trypsinized 1 day before, until all are detached, and are replenished with fresh (or used) medium. On the next day, a short trypsinization is used to detach all cells. The tumor cells are then collected, washed three times in PBS, and kept at room temperature in the last wash for 3–4 hours. For primary immunization 1×10^6– 1×10^7 cells in 0.3 ml PBS are injected intravenously (iv) into a mouse. Five days later splenocytes are collected for fusion with mouse myeloma cells. For secondary response, mice are injected subcutaneously (sc) and/or intraperitoneally (ip) with $1–2 \times 10^7$ cells in 0.5 ml of PBS. These injections could be performed once or repeated at 2- to 3-week intervals. About 3–4 weeks after the last injection, a booster iv injection is given with 1×10^6 similarly prepared tumor cells. Three to four days later, splenocytes are prepared for fusion (M. Herlyn et al., 1979; Koprowski et al., 1978, 1979).

2. Immunization with Tumor Cell Membranes

Tumor cells collected from tissue culture by a rubber policeman or cells isolated from freshly obtained tumors are washed three times in PBS and resuspended at a concentration of 5×10^7 cells/ml in PBS containing 2 mM phenylmethylsulfonyl fluoride (PMSF). Cells are disrupted by nitrogen cavitation or with a Potter/Elvejhem homogenizer at 4°C and nuclei and debris are removed by centrifugation at 600 g. Membranes contained in the supernatant are pelleted at 100,000 g, resuspended in 1 ml of PBS containing 2 mM PMSF, and stored at -70°C.

Mice are immunized with 1×10^7 tumor cells injected sc and ip, as before, and 3–4 weeks later boostered with an iv injection of 0.2 ml cell membrane preparation. Three days later splenocytes are prepared for fusion. In another protocol, mice are injected sc with 0.3 ml of cell membrane preparation, suspended in incomplete Freund's adjuvant, and ip injected. Three to four weeks later, 0.2 ml of the membrane preparation is iv injected, the mice are sacrificed 3 days later, and splenocytes are purified for fusion.

3. Immunization by Serum-Free Spent Medium

Most of the tumor cell lines survive and divide for up to 8 days in serum-free medium (SFM) (MEM or RPMI 1640) supplemented with 1% nonessential amino acids, 5 μg/ml insulin, and 5 μg/ml transferrin (Chang et al., 1980; Steplewski et al., 1981). Supplemented SFM (SSFM) from 8-day-old cultures contains large quantities of antigens shed by tumor cells (Steplewski et al., 1981); it is an excellent source of immunogenic molecules (unpublished data). Ten-times concentrated, cell-free SSFM is used for immunization in exactly the same way as the membrane preparation. The protease inhibitor, PMSF, should be included.

B. HYBRIDOMA PRODUCTION

1. Myeloma Cell Lines

The most often used HGPRT-deficient myeloma cell lines are P3x63/Ag8 (Köhler and Milstein, 1975), which secretes γ1 immunoglobulin, its nonsecreting derivative, 653 (Kearney et al., 1979), nonsecreting Sp 2/0-Ag 14 (Shulman et al., 1978), and P3/NS1-AG4-1 (Köhler et al., 1976).* The cells are grown in MEM with high glucose (4.5 μg/liter) or in RPMI 1640 medium with high glucose (4.5 μg/liter). The medium contains 10% donor horse serum or 20% FCS (both heat inactivated). Addition of 15 μg/ml of 8-azaguanine ensures that no revertants of drug resistance will appear. Cells are maintained at a density of $10^5–10^6$/ml and are divided every 2–3 days to maintain high (>90%) viability. One day before fusion the myelomas are split 1:2 to obtain optimal fusion conditions.

---

* These are available from American Type Culture Collection, 12301 Parklawn Drive, Rockville, MD 20852, or from the Institute for Medical Research, NIGMS Cell Repository, Copewood and Davis Streets, Camden, NJ 08103.

2. Immune Splenocytes

At days 5 (primary response) or 3–4 (secondary response), the spleens are removed and placed in tissue culture medium containing 10% FCS in 60-mm Petri dishes. Single-cell suspension is obtained by teasing the spleen with tweezers or through perfusion of the spleen by injecting medium several times into the spleen with a 26-gauge needle at several sites until all the splenocytes are removed (Kennett, 1980). The usual recovery is about 10^8 cells/spleen. Spleen cells are collected in the centrifuge tube, underlayered with 2 ml of FCS, and gently centrifuged (~ 600 g for 5 minutes) to remove debris. The supernatant is discarded and the pellet is suspended in 5 ml of 0.17 M NH_4Cl to lyse erythrocytes. After 3 minutes at room temperature, 5–19 ml of medium containing 20% FCS is added, and the mixture is underlayered again with 2 ml of FCS. After centrifugation (~ 600 g for 5 minutes), the pellet is resuspended in serum-free medium.

3. Cell Fusion

Ten percent of the splenocytes are set aside and kept on wet ice to serve as feeder layer for fused cells. Splenocytes ($1–9 \times 10^7$) are mixed with $5 \times 10^7 – 5 \times 10^8$ myeloma cells centrifuged (600 g for 10 minutes), and washed three times in SFM (RPMI 1640). After the third wash, the supernatant is removed by suction and the cell pellet is loosened by tapping the tube. Polyethyelene glycol (PEG) 1000 or 1500 40–50% in SFM prewarmed to 37°C is added. The PEG tends to lower the pH, and the pH should be adjusted to approximately 8.0 with sodium bicarbonate. After 1 minute, 1 ml of SFM (37°C) is added, and then after each minute, 1.5, 2.0, and 2.5 ml of SFM (37°C) are added. Two minutes after the last SFM, 5 ml of medium containing 20% FCS (37°C) is added. The whole mixture is then gently centrifuged (400 g, 6 minutes, room temperature). Diluted PEG is removed by suction. The fused cells are resuspended in HAT medium containing 20% FCS and the previously set-aside 10% of the original splenocytes are added. One spleen fusion with feeder layer splenocytes is usually resuspended in 150 ml of HAT medium (Szybalski et al., 1962; Littlefield, 1964) and distributed into three 24-well tissue culture plates (Linbro FB-16-24 TC). The next day the medium is changed (two-thirds) with fresh HAT medium containing 20% FCS. Within 10 to 15 days, single colonies of hybridomas appear microscopically. As soon as colonies become visible macroscopically (15–25 days), they are carefully collected with Pasteur pipets and each is placed separately in wells of new 24-well Linbro plates. Colonies are observed daily and supernatants are tested as soon as a colony grows to confluency (change of medium color to yellow).

C. Screening and Cloning

1. Screening

In the analysis of hybridoma-secreted antibodies for their binding specificities to tumor cells, supernatants are collected from wells containing single colonies. The binding of the antibody is usually detected in radioimmunoassay (RIA). When colon carcinoma cells grown in culture are used for immunization of mice, the screening procedure should include targets as presented in Table I.

Binding of the antibodies could be detected by RIA, mixed hemadsorption assay (MHA), enzyme-linked immunoassay (ELISA), or by any immunoadherence assay. We are using RIA, as described below.

a. Radioimmunoassay. Tumor cells are detached from the growth surface by trypsin–versene the day before. The next day cells are collected after very short trypsinization, washed three times in RIA buffer (PBS with 2% IgG-free horse serum), and then suspended at a concentration of 1×10^7 cells/ml. Aliquots of cell suspension (50 μl) are distributed into the wells of 96-well Linbro plates and 50 μg volumes of dilution of monoclonal antibody-containing supernatant are added. The plates are incubated with shaking for 1 hour at room temperature. The cells are washed three times in RIA buffer by sequential resuspension, centrifugation, and removal of supernatant. The cells are then incubated for 1 hour with ^{125}I-labeled rabbit anti-mouse $F(ab')_2$ antiserum (30,000–100,000 cpm/well) with shaking, and then washed three more times before the content of each well is counted in a gamma spectrometer.

b. Mixed Hemadsorption Assay (MHA). The method developed by Espmark and Fagreus (1962) and modified by Cary *et al.* (1976) is very suitable for the analysis of cells grown in monolayers. Tumor cells are

TABLE I

SELECTION OF TARGETS FOR SPECIFICITY SCREENING OF
ANTICOLON CARCINOMA ANTIBODIES

Target preparation	Number of different cell lines				
	Colon carcinoma	Other than immunizer	Other GI tumors	Other tumors	Normal cells
Live cells	Immunizer	1	2^a	1	3^b
SSF medium	Immunizer	1	2^a	1	3

[a] Usually pancreatic and gastric carcinoma.

[b] One fibroblast cell line and one each from freshly isolated peripheral blood erythrocytes and leukocytes.

prepared 1 day before the assay by the seeding of 1×10^3 cells/well (Falcon 30.40 microtest II plate). Attached cells are washed 24 hours later with MHA buffer (Veronal-buffered 0.87% NaCl, pH 7.5, containing 0.1% glucose, 0.1% gelatine, 0.15 mM CaCl$_2$, 0.5 mM MgCl$_2$, 5.7 mM KCl, 3.1 mM Veronal, and 1.8 mM sodium Veronal). Dilutions of hybridoma supernatant are added to the wells and incubated for 60 minutes at room temperature. Unbound antibody is removed, the plates are washed with MHA buffer, and 100 μl (0.2% v:v) of indicator system (sensitized sheep erythrocytes with mouse antiserum against sheep erythrocytes and goat anti-mouse IgG—Cappel Laboratories, Cochranville, Pennsylvania) in PBS is added. Plates are incubated for 60 minutes at room temperature, and then agitated gently, washed, and examined by phase-contrast microscopy. A cell is considered positive when 25% or more of its perimeter is covered by indicator erythrocytes (M. Herlyn et al., 1979). Original screening of colonies usually results in rejection of those that do not produce antibodies binding in the assay and those producing antibodies that bind to all targets. Remaining colonies with a selective pattern of binding specificities are cloned and further analysis of antibodies is performed on supernatants from clones of secondary clones.

2. Cloning of Hybridoma Colonies

a. Cloning by Limiting Dilutions in Fluid Phase. Cloning is performed in the presence of feeder layer (mouse macrophages, rat or mouse thymocytes) or in the presence of 20% conditioned medium (usually a 48-hour-old supernatant from a parental myeloma cell line grown in the absence of 8-azaguanine and in medium containing 20% FCS). Aseptically collected macrophages or thymocytes (from 5- to 6-week-old animals) are prepared as single-cell suspensions and irradiated (1500–1600 rads of gamma irradiation). Feeder layer cells are adjusted to 10^6–10^7/ml, and 0.1 ml of this suspension in medium containing 20% FCS is placed into each well of the 96-well tissue culture plates (Linbro FB96TC). Suspensions of hybridoma cells are adjusted to contain 200, 20, and 10 cells/ml. To each of the 96 wells 0.1 ml of hybridoma suspension is added. For each of the dilutions one plate is prepared.

If conditioned medium is used, similar concentrations of hybridoma cells are prepared in MEM or RPMI 1640 medium containing 20% FCS and 20% conditioned medium. One plate is set up for each dilution of hybridoma cells. After about 10–12 days, macroscopically visible single colonies are selected and their supernatants are tested for binding. If positive, the clones are expanded into 24-well Linbro plates.

b. Cloning in Semisolid Agarose. Normal human, rabbit, or mouse fibroblasts are plated in 60-mm Petri dishes and irradiated 24 hours later

(1500–1600 rads). A layer of 2 ml of 0.5% agarose (Seakem agarose, Marine Colloids, Rockland, Maine) is applied and incubated with the fibroblasts at 37°C in a CO_2 incubator for 24 hours. The next day 0.25% agarose is prepared and mixed with two concentrations of hybridoma cells (approximately 200 and 1000/plate). The agarose is permitted to solidify at room temperature and then placed in a CO_2 incubator. At about 10–15 days visible colonies of cloned cells appear and are transferred into 24-well Linbro plates. Agarose batches are screened and the best batch is selected. Agarose is suspended at 2.5% concentration in 0.15 M NaCl and sterilized by boiling for 30–45 minutes. After cooling to 56°C, dilutions are made in prewarmed 2 × Dulbecco's MEM supplemented with 30% FCS.

D. SELECTION OF TUMOR-SPECIFIC MONOCLONAL ANTIBODIES

Hybridoma clones found to secrete antibodies that bind to a desired target tumor cell are further characterized by screening a large panel of cells of different origins for the expression of antigen detected by such a monoclonal antibody. For example, after a single iv injection of SW 1083 human colon carcinoma cell line (Leibovitz et al., 1976) into BALB/c mouse, and fusion of splenocytes 5 days later with P3x63/Ag8 myeloma cells, clone 1083-17-1A (17-1A) was found to secrete a γ2a antibody that was colon carcinoma-specific as defined under tissue culture conditions (M. Herlyn et al., 1979). Figure 1 represents the binding specificity, as detected by radioimmunoassay, of antibody 17-1A to live cells. All nine colorectal carcinoma cell lines bound antibody 17-1A, but breast carcinoma, three lung carcinomas, 10 melanomas, 2 astrocytomas, and a panel of other tumor and normal cell lines did not express the antigen against which the antibody is directed. We found (Steplewski et al., 1981) that this antigen is confined to the surface of tumor cells and is not shed into tissue culture supernatant. From another immunization (secondary response) with SW 1116 colon carcinoma cells (Leibovitz et al., 1976) and fusion of splenocytes with the 653 variant of P3x63/Ag8 mouse myeloma cells (Kearney et al., 1979), 50 of 76 colonies isolated secreted antibodies that bound to various kinds of human cells. Nineteen of these 50 had specificity for human tumors (Koprowski et al., 1979). In this panel of 19 antibodies, one antibody of the IgM isotype, 1116 NS-3d (3d), bound only to colon carcinoma cells (Fig. 2) and immunoprecipitated from tumor cells and from commercial CEA preparations (Mitchell, 1980) a single CEA molecule with a molecular weight of 180,000. Hybridoma 3d was subcloned and subclones were found which secreted IgG1 isotype with binding specificity to 180,000 CEA retained (unpublished data). Two mono-

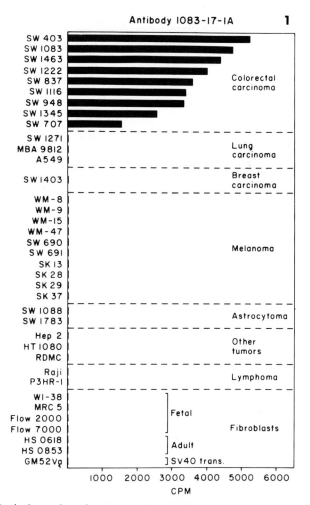

FIG. 1. Anticolorectal carcinoma monoclonal antibody 1083-17-1A binding to live cells maintained in tissue culture. Radioimmunoassay detects binding of mouse monoclonal antibody to live cells by using rabbit anti-mouse F(ab′)₂ radioiodinated IgG. Bars represent counts per minute of bound antibody minus cpm of control P3x63/Ag8 immunoglobulin (usually 150–200 cpm).

clonal antibodies in this group, 1116 Ns-19 (19; Fig. 3) and 1116 NS-52a (52a; Fig. 4), reacted with the majority of colon carcinoma cells, but not with other tumors (except for a low reactivity with SK 37 melanoma) or normal cells tested. Later it was found that freshly isolated lymphocytes and erythrocytes also did not bind antibodies 19 and 52a. Two antibodies, 1116 NS-38a (38a; Fig. 5) and 1116 NS-38c (38c; Fig. 6), both of IgM class, bound only to colon carcinoma cells. Similarly, antibody 1116 NS-10 (10;

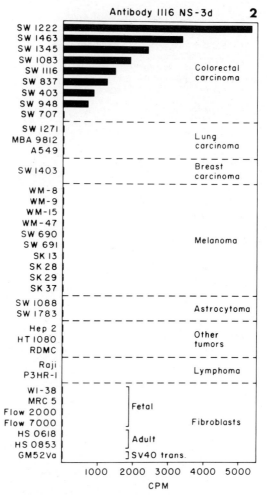

Fig. 2. Binding to live cells of an anti-CEA monoclonal antibody 1116 NS-3d secreted by a hybridoma established from splenocytes of mice immunized with SW 1116 colorectal carcinoma cell line. For detailed description, see legend to Fig. 1.

Fig. 7) bound to colon carcinoma and, in a panel of other tumors, only to melanoma cells SK 37.

Freshly isolated tumor cells could also be used to elicit antitumor monoclonal antibodies. In one experiment mice were immunized with freshly isolated colon carcinoma cells and 3 weeks later boostered with membrane preparation from the same cell pool, 3 days prior to spleen collection and fusion. Three antibodies selected from this experiment are

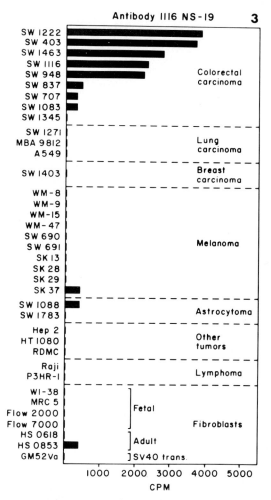

FIGS. 3 and 4. Monoclonal antibodies 1116 NS-19 and 1116 NS-52a. Specificity of binding of these monoclonal antibodies is directed against gastrointestinal carcinoma antigen (GICA), defined as a monosialoganglioside. For details see legend to Fig. 1.

presented in Fig. 8. All three antibodies bound to the majority of colorectal carcinoma cells (except SW 1116 and SW 1345), but not to a large panel of other tumor and normal cells.

In similar experiments, after immunization of mice with freshly isolated gastric carcinoma cells, three tumor-associated antibodies were selected. Antibody WGHS-9-1 (9-1) bound to all cells of the gastrointestinal (GI) tract, including pancreatic carcinoma CAPAN-2 (Fig. 9). A quite similar

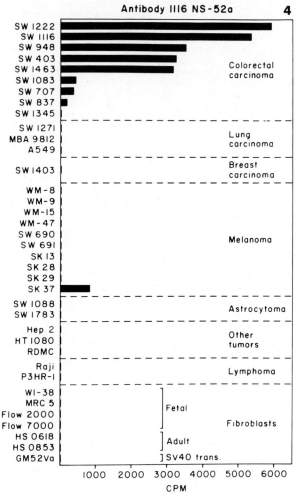

FIG. 4.   See legend on p. 297.

binding pattern is represented by antibody WGHS-22-2 (22-2), although with different levels of binding to different GI tract tumors (Fig. 10). The third antibody, WGHS-29-1 (29-1; Fig. 11), had a different binding pattern. It bound to all colorectal carcinomas, to a gastric carcinoma, but also to bronchogenic carcinoma MBA 9812 and to lymphocytes of normal subjects.

The panel of cells used for selection of monoclonal antibodies directed against GI tumor-associated antigens should always include normal pe-

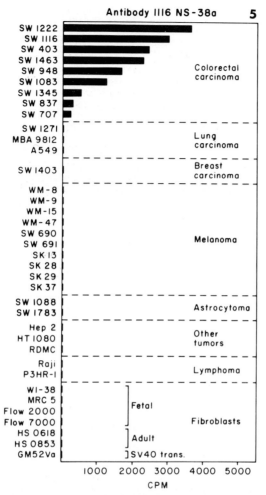

FIGS. 5–7. Monoclonal antibodies 1116 NS-38a, 1116 NS-38c, and 1116 NS-10. Binding specificities as defined in RIA on live cells. The antigen detected by these antibodies was defined as blood group Le^b substance. For details see legend to Fig. 1.

ripheral blood cells, including erythrocytes. As shown in Table II, four different antibodies selected after immunization of mice with freshly isolated colon carcinoma cells from liver metastasis had very good association with tumor cells, except that erythrocytes and lymphocytes, from two other individuals bound all four antibodies.

The isotypes of selected monoclonal antibodies with specificities for tumor-associated antigens are tested in Ouchterlony immunodiffusion

TABLE II

BINDING OF WC-ZYG HYBRIDOMA ANTIBODIES AS DETECTED IN RIA

Target cells		Hybridoma-secreted antibodies WC-ZYG-NS-			
Origin	Cell	13	14	66	11
Colorectal carcinoma	SW 620	2250	2480	270	2140
	SW 1116	570	580	5060	680
	SW 1222	2850	2170	3900	1970
Mammary carcinoma	SW 1403	690	650	2020	840
Lung carcinoma	MBA-9812	1630	1240	150	1430
	SW 1271	0	0	0	0
Melanoma	WM 28-7	0	0	0	0
	WM 28-9	0	0	0	0
	WM 46	0	0	0	0
	WM 47-3	0	0	0	0
Fibroblasts	Flow 7000	0	0	NT[a]	0
Lymphocytes	WC-ZYG	0	0	0	0
Erythrocytes	WC-ZYG	2490	260	1650	5090
	ZS	NT	270	280	1544
	PRBC	1870	2150	1690	1640

[a] NT, Not tested.

(Koprowski *et al.*, 1979). Diffusion is carried out in 1% agarose in 0.02 *M* Tris–HCl buffer, pH 8.0, and 0.1 *M* NaCl. Monospecific antisera purchased from commercial sources (Bionetics, Bethesda, Maryland, and others) should be tested prior to use with a panel of myeloma proteins. The same antisera can be used in radioimmunoassay for the classification of immunoglobulins.

III. Monoclonal Antibody-Defined Antigens

Well-characterized monoclonal antibodies of high avidity may be produced in large quantities in tissue culture or in ascitic fluid of suitable mice. This permits studies of monoclonal antibody-defined antigens on the tumor cell surfaces (Koprowski *et al.*, 1979; Mitchell *et al.*, 1980, 1981, 1982). For immunoprecipitation of antigens, cell surfaces are labeled biosynthetically or by radioiodination (Koprowski *et al.*, 1979).

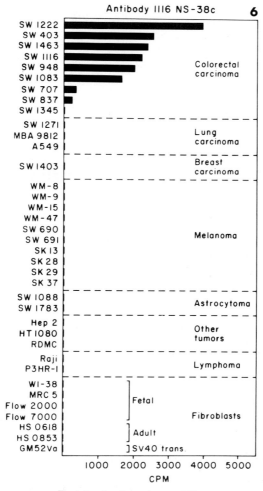

FIG. 6. See legend on p. 299.

A. IMMUNOPRECIPITATION OF PROTEIN ANTIGENS

1. Biosynthetic Labeling of Tumor Cells

Cells are grown for 48 hours in methionine-free medium (GIBCO, Grand Island, New York) containing 50 μCi of [^{75}Se]selenomethionine (Amersham/Searle, Arlington Heights, Illinois). Cell monolayers are then washed three times in PBS and solubilized by incubation for 15 minutes at

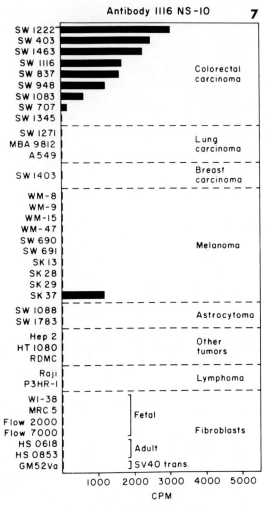

FIG. 7. See legend on p. 299.

4°C in 1 ml of NET buffer [0.15 M NaCl, 0.05 M Tris, 5 mM ethylenedi-
aminetetraacetic acid (EDTA), 0.2 mM PMSF, pH 7.0] containing 0.5%
Nonidet P-40 (NP-40) (Shell Chemical Co., London, England). The solubilized material is centrifuged at 100,000 g for 30 minutes and absorbed
serially with two 0.5-ml volumes of packed *Staphylococcus aureus*
Cowan I (SaCI) previously washed with NET buffer containing 0.05%
NP-40 and 1 mg/ml bovine serum albumin (BSA). SaCI-cleared preparations could be stored at −70°C.

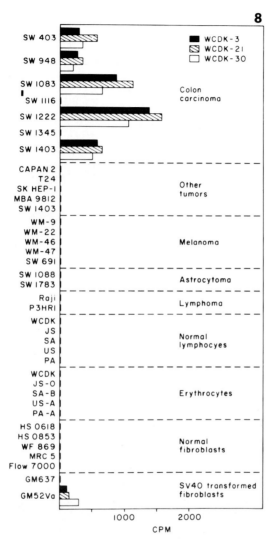

FIG. 8. Binding specificity of three monoclonal antibodies secreted by hybridomas established after immunization of mice with freshly isolated colorectal carcinoma cells from patient DK. For details see legend to Fig. 1.

2. Radioiodination of Tumor Cells

Cell surfaces are radiolabeled with ^{125}I by the lactoperoxidase method (Marchalonis *et al.*, 1971). Adherent monolayer tumor cells are labeled *in situ* or after trypsinization. Cells are trypsinized, washed twice with PBS,

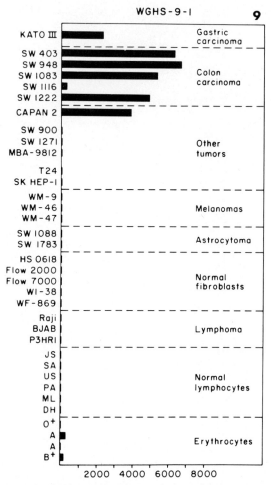

Figs. 9–11. Binding specificities of three monoclonal antibodies secreted by hybridomas established by fusion of splenocytes from mouse immunized with freshly isolated tumor cells from patient HS with gastric carcinoma. For details see legend to Fig. 1.

and iodinated for 15 minutes after successive addition of lactoperoxidase, glucose oxidase, ^{125}I, and glucose. The radioiodinated cells are washed three times in PBS and solubilized as described for biosynthetically labeled cells. Cell lysates are cleaved and processed as described above.

3. Immunoprecipitation

Radiolabeled cell surface antigens are precipitated from NP-40-solubilized cells by hybridoma antibodies. Aliquots of SaCI-cleaved lysates are

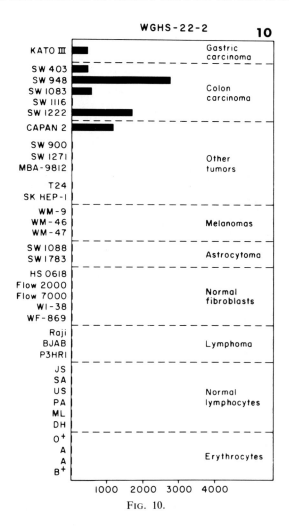

FIG. 10.

mixed with 200 μl of hybridoma tissue culture supernatant and incubated at 4°C for 15 minutes. Immune complexes are adsorbed onto rabbit or goat anti-mouse IgG-coated SaCI (10 μl packed SaCI) and incubated for 15 minutes at 4°C. The SaCI pellet is washed three times with 1 ml of 0.1% NP-40 in NET buffer, with careful resuspension of the pellet each time. Antigens are then eluted with 50 μl of sodium dodecyl sulfate sample buffer (Laemmli, 1970; Mitchell *et al.*, 1980).

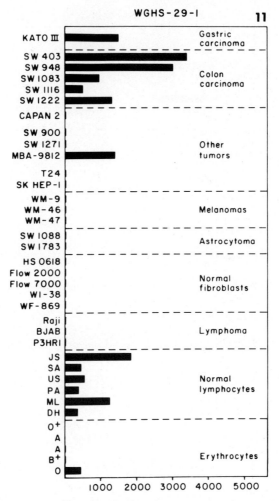

FIG. 11.   See legend on p. 304.

4. Sodium Dodecyl Sulfate–Polyacrylamide Gel Electrophoresis

Sodium dodecyl sulfate–polyacrylamide gel electrophoresis is performed by the method of Laemmli (1970). Prior to electrophoresis, samples are boiled for 1 minute and centrifuged. Electrophoresis is performed with 1.5-mm-thick 10% acrylamide gels with an acrylamide:bisacrylamide ratio of 38:1. Molecular weight standards—myosin, 210,000; phosphorylase a, 92,500; lactoperoxidase, 77,500; bovine serum albumin, 66,000; catalase, 60,000; lactic dehydrogenase, 36,000; and carbonic anhydrase,

29,000—are run on each gel to permit determination of apparent molecular weights. After completion of electrophoresis, gels are stained with 0.02% Coomassie Brilliant Blue R250 in 25% methanol/10% acetic acid. Subsequently, the gels are destained with stain solvent, equilibrated with 5% acetic acid/2% glycerol, and dried. The dried gels are autoradiographed at −70°C by sandwiching a Kodak RP X-Omat film between a DuPont Cronex Lightning-Plus intensifying screen and the dried gel. Quantitation of radioactivity in individual bands is achieved by slicing the acrylamide gel strip into 1-mm fragments that are then assayed in a Packard Autogamma spectrometer.

B. DETECTION OF MONOCLONAL ANTIBODY-DEFINED GLYCOLIPID ANTIGENS

1. Lipid Extraction

The lipid extraction from tumor cells is achieved according to a method described by Magnani *et al.* (1981). Tissue culture cells (1 gm wet weight) are homogenized in 3 ml of water at 4°C. The homogenate is added to 10.8 ml of methanol, to which 5.4 ml of chloroform is added with constant stirring. The mixture is stirred for 30 minutes at room temperature and centrifuged at 15,000 g for 10 minutes. The pellet is rehomogenized in 2 ml of water and extracted as above with 8 ml of a 1:2 chloroform and methanol mixture. The supernatants from both extractions are combined and evaporated under a stream of dry nitrogen and the residues dissolved in 2:1 chloroform and ethanol. This material is used as a target in RIA or for thin-layer chromatography.

2. Detection of Glycolipids by Monoclonal Antibodies

Samples of 1 μl of total lipid extract suitably diluted are spotted 1.5 cm from the bottom of a thin-layer chromatography sheet (Eastman Kodak Co., 100-μm-thick chromatogram, 10 × 10 cm). The sheet is then clamped in a sandwich chamber and developed in a chromatography tank containing chloroform, methanol, and 0.25% KCl (60:35:8). The chromatogram is then air dried and again soaked for 10 minutes at 4°C in 0.01 M sodium phosphate buffer, pH 7.2, containing 0.15 M NaCl, 1% PVP (MW 40,000; Sigma) and 0.1% sodium azide (buffer A). The wet chromatogram is laid horizontally on a smaller, paraffin-covered glass plate. Serum-free hybridoma supernatant (Chang *et al.*, 1980) containing about 10 μg/ml of antibody is diluted 1:4 with buffer A and gently pipetted onto the chromatogram. After incubation in a humid chamber for 6 hours at 4°C, the chromatogram is washed in six successive changes of 0.01 M

sodium phosphate buffer, pH 7.2, containing 0.15 M NaCl (buffer B). The chromatogram is laid again horizontally and layered with ^{125}I-labeled rabbit anti-mouse F(ab')$_2$ immunoglobulin in buffer A (10^6 cpm/ml, about 50 μl/cm^2). After incubation in a humid chamber for 12 hours at 4°C, the chromatogram is washed six times in buffer B, air dried, and exposed to XR-2 X-ray film (Eastman Kodak Co.) for 50 hours (Magnani *et al.*, 1981).

C. COLON CARCINOMA ANTIGENS AS DEFINED BY MONOCLONAL ANTIBODIES

Hybridoma-derived monoclonal anticolorectal carcimona antibodies studied in detail up to date and their corresponding antigens are presented in Table III.

TABLE III

MONOCLONAL ANTICOLORECTAL CARCINOMA ANTIBODIES AND
ANTIGENS DEFINED BY MONOCLONAL ANTIBODIES

Monoclonal antibody			Reactivity with	Monoclonal antibody-defined antigens
Against	Code	Isotype		
Freshly isolated colon carcinoma cells	WGHS-9-1	γ1	Colon, gastric carcinoma	Protein α chain, MW 28,000; β chain, MW 22,000
	WGHS-9-2	γ1	Colon, gastric carcinoma	
	WGHS-29-1	γM	Gastrointestinal, other tumors, granulocytes	Lacto-N-fuco pentaose III
Tissue culture-grown colon carcinoma cells	3d-6	γ1	Colorectal carcinoma	CEA, MW 180,000
	3a	γ1	Colorectal carcinoma and some melanomas	Neutral glycolipids
	33a	γM		Neutral glycolipids
	33b	γM		Neutral glycolipids
	10	γM	Colorectal carcinoma and erythrocytes	Le^b blood group
	38a	γM		Le^b blood group
	43	γ1		Le^b blood group
	19-9	γ1	Gastric, pancreatic carcinoma	Monosialo-ganglioside
	52a	γ1	Colon carcinoma	Monosialo-ganglioside

A bimolecular glycoprotein detected by antibodies 9-1 and 9-2 consists of an α chain of molecular weight 28,000 and a β chain of molecular weight 22,000, and is expressed by colon and gastric carcinomas only. The antigen was not detected in normal gastric and colonic epithelium (R. Dubbs, personal communication). As mentioned above, antibody 3d-6 immunoprecipitates single CEA molecules of molecular weight 180,000. Antibodies 10, 38a, and 43, which were detected only on colon carcinoma cells, were later also found on some erythrocytes. The antigen detected by these antibodies is Le^b blood group substance (Brockhaus et al., 1981). Antibodies 19-9 and 52a are directed against a monosialoganglioside expressed by gastric, pancreatic, and colon carcinomas only. The antigen is also present in meconium (Magnani et al., 1981). The antigen is shed by tumor cells both in vitro (Steplewski et al., 1981a) and in vivo (Koprowski et al., 1981). Antibody WGHS-29-1 is directed to lacto-N-fucopentaose III (Brockhaus et al., 1982; Blaszczyk et al., 1982).

Antibodies 3a, 33a, and 33b are directed against neutral glycolipids present on the surface of colon carcinomas and some melanomas, but not on other tumor or normal cell lines.

IV. Detection of Monoclonal Antibody-Defined Antigens in Serum and Urine

Monoclonal antibodies 19-9 and 52a detect a monosialoganglioside (Magnani et al., 1981) that is expressed by colorectal, gastric, and pancreatic carcinomas (M. Herlyn et al., 1982; Sears et al., 1982) and is present in meconium. This antigen is present on the surface of intact tumor cells in cell membrane extracts and in spent medium of colon carcinoma cells (Steplewski et al., 1981a). Monoclonal antibody 19-9 was selected to devise a binding-inhibition assay for the detection of monosialoganglioside in human sera. Using the binding-inhibition assay for monoclonal antibody 19-9, it was found that patients with colon, gastric, and pancreatic carcinomas have antigen in the serum. The presence of antigen does not correlate with the level of CEA (Koprowski et al., 1981) and it is not present in sera from patients with other tumors or in sera of normal subjects.

A. BINDING-INHIBITION ASSAY

The principle of the binding-inhibition assay is presented in Fig. 12B. Wells of gelatin-coated microtiter plates (left) are filled with aliquots of monoclonal antibody mixed in equal amounts with inhibitor (i.e., human serum); membrane extracts, SSFM from other tumors, or normal human

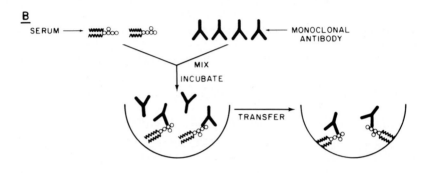

FIG. 12. (A) Binding-inhibition assay of radiolabeled antigen to monoclonal antibody 19-9. Rabbit anti-mouse IgG is attached to a soft plate, followed by monoclonal antibody. The binding of [^{3}H]glucosamine biosynthetically radiolabeled antigen (a monosialoganglioside) is inhibited by different dilutions of patient's serum or urine. (B) Binding-inhibition assay of monoclonal antibody 19-9 to its antigen. Known amount of antibody is incubated with patient's serum or urine and unbound antibody is detected by RIA in a well containing excess of antigen.

serum are used as controls. The mixtures are incubated for 18 hours at 4°C in a humidified chamber and then transferred to wells of plates precoated with either membrane extract or SSFM as the target antigen (right). Following incubation for 18 hours at 4°C in a humidified chamber, the plates are washed with cold Veronal-buffered solution. Binding of monoclonal antibody to the target is then determined as described in the preceding section. In this assay monoclonal antibody is diluted to 50% of maximal binding reactivity as determined by preliminary binding tests. The percentage of specific inhibition of binding of hybridoma antibodies is calculated from the mean value based on a triplicate reading of cpm/antibody aliquot.

$$\% \text{ Inhibition} = 100 - \left[\frac{\text{test cpm} - \text{control cpm}}{\text{maximum cpm} - \text{control cpm}} \right] \times 100$$

Statistical significance of differences in binding is calculated for each experiment by Student's t test.

B. Solid-Phase Binding Assay with Radiolabeled Antigen

Another set of conditions was presently established for the detection of glycolipid antigens. A monosialoganglioside (antibody 19-9) is detected by solid-phase binding inhibition of monoclonal antibody 19-9 to radiolabeled ([^{3}H]glucosamine) antigen. Antigen is found in sera and urine of colon carcinoma patients (Chang *et al.*, 1981). The antigen was found in sera and in urine of most of the colon and pancreatic carcinoma patients only.

1. Preparation of Radiolabeled Soluble Antigen

Human colorectal carcinoma cells (SW 1116) are cultured in 150-cm^2 tissue culture flask with MEM containing 10% FCS. Before confluency, 14 μCi/ml of [^{3}H]glucosamine (38 Ci/mmole; Amersham, England) is added into culture medium, and the cultures are incubated at 37°C for 5 days. The culture supernatant is harvested and centrifuged at 3500 rpm for 15 minutes to remove the cells. This supernatant is used as a soluble [^{3}H]glucosamine-labeled antigen preparation. The [^{3}H]glucosamine-labeled cells are also harvested by rubber policemen and washed three times with PBS. The cells are resuspended in 5 ml of 3 M KCl and frozen and thawed five times with a dry ice/acetone bath. After incubation at 4°C for 2 days, the resulting suspension is centrifuged at 1200 rpm for 10 minutes and the supernatant is recentrifuged at 105,000 g for 90 minutes to remove membranous fragments. The supernatant is then used in an assay as 3 M KCl-extracted [^{3}H]glucosamine-labeled soluble antigen.

2. Preparation of Samples for Binding-Inhibition Assay

Serum samples freshly collected from patients are incubated with 50% methanol overnight at room temperature and then incubated for 30 seconds at 90°C, and the precipitate is centrifuged at 2000 g for 5 minutes. The supernatant is then dried, and the crystals resuspended in agamma horse serum are used for inhibition studies. Urine samples freshly collected from patients are HEPES-buffered to pH 7.0 and centrifuged at 2000 g for 5 minutes to remove precipitates. The supernatant is used for inhibition assay. In this assay only glycolipids are detected.

3. Solid-Phase Radioimmunoassay

Purified rabbit anti-mouse IgG antibody (0.2 mg/100 μl/well) is incubated in polyvinylchloride Linbro U-well plates overnight at room temperature. The plates are then washed three times with RIA buffer (PBS + 10% agamma horse serum + 0.01% sodium azide) and sensitized by addition of hybridoma tissue culture supernatant which contains monoclonal antibodies (100 μl/well). The plates are incubated for 2 hours at room temperature and then washed three times with RIA buffer. ^{3}H-labeled antigen (100 μl/well) is added, and the plates incubated overnight at 4°C. After washing five times with RIA buffer, 100 μl/well of 5% acetic acid + 0.1% NP-40 solution is added to dissolve the labeled antigen–antibody complexes. The eluted material is dissolved in 2 ml of scintillation fluid and the samples counted with a liquid scintillation counter.

4. Solid-Phase Binding-Inhibition Radioimmunoassay

The principle of this assay is shown in Fig. 12A. Plates are prepared as described above and unlabeled antigen source (serum or urine inhibitor; 100 μl/well) is added and the plates again incubated for 2 hours at room temperature. After washing three times with RIA buffer, [^{3}H]glucosamine-labeled antigen (100 μl/well; 60,000 cpm) is added and the plates are incubated overnight at 4°C. After five further washes, the samples are eluted and counted as described above. The binding inhibition is calculated from the equation:

$$\% \text{ Inhibition} = 100 - \left[\frac{\text{sample count } - \text{ nonspecific binding count}}{\text{positive control count } - \text{ nonspecific binding count}} \right] \times 100$$

V. Studies of Biological Functions of Monoclonal Antibodies

We (Koprowski et al., 1978) have described antimelanoma hybridoma mass culture 691-6 which suppressed melanoma tumor growth in nude mice. Experiments performed later with monoclonal anti-CRC antibody 1083-17-1A (17-1A) showed striking inhibition of colon carcinoma tumor growth in nude mice (D. Herlyn et al., 1980). Antibody 17-1A (γ2a) is active in antibody-dependent cell-mediated cytotoxicity (ADCC) in vitro (D. Herlyn et al., 1979) and this cytotoxic effect is restricted to colon carcinoma cells. Since antibody 17-1A is active in ADCC, it is possible that the same mechanism is responsible for tumor inhibition in vivo (D. Herlyn et al., 1979). The participation of complement in the cytotoxicity in vivo has been excluded (Steplewski, unpublished). Antibody 17-1A did not kill tumor cells in vitro in the presence of complement (D. Herlyn et al., 1979). Most of other anti-colorectal carcinoma antibodies of the IgM class were found to mediate complement-dependent cytotoxicity (CDC). The cytotoxicity was detected against human colorectal carcinoma cells grown in tissue culture and against tumor cells freshly isolated from patients. These antibodies were, however, unable to inhibit colon carcinoma tumor growth in nude mice (D. Herlyn and Koprowski, 1981).

VI. Future Applications of Antitumor Monoclonal Antibodies

By selection of monoclonal antibodies of high avidities and antitumor specificities that detect antigens confined to the tumor cell surface and not present in larger quantities in serum of patients, it will be possible to use such antibodies as carriers of radioactive isotopes for nuclear imaging or of toxic substances for therapy. Such efforts to use specificity of monoclonal antibody to target the toxic A chain of diphtheria and ricin toxins have proved successful *in vitro*. Ricin and diphtheria toxin A chains are nontoxic by themselves due to their inability to bind cell surfaces (missing fragment B). These A chains were rendered specifically toxic to colorectal carcinoma cells by conjugating them via disulfide bridges to monoclonal antibodies (Gilliland *et al.*, 1980).

Similarly, selection of high-avidity monoclonal antitumor antibody that detects antigens easily shed into milieu (Steplewski *et al.*, 1981) and present in patients' sera (Koprowski *et al.*, 1981) gives an opportunity to develop highly specific serodiagnostic assays. A range of tumor-associated antigens defined by monoclonal antibodies has already been described, and more will be published. The origins, structure, expression, and reexpression of some of these antigens have to be fully elucidated. Antigens expressed by tumor cells in large numbers may represent only quantitative differences in comparison with their normal lineage. This difference, however, may be sufficient for diagnostic or therapeutic purposes.

Some of the antigens are molecules reexpressed in tumor cells as oncodevelopmental structures. Some inference could be drawn from studies of colon carcinoma-specific antigen 19-9, a monosialoganglioside (Magnani *et al.*, 1981; Koprowski *et al.*, 1981). This antigen occurs on colon, pancreatic, and gastric carcinomas, but is also detectable in meconium. Thus, it is possible that GI tract tumor cells, endodermal in origin, are reexpressing an antigen of embryonal development. Similarly, antimelanoma monoclonal antibody 691I5-Nu4B (Koprowski *et al.*, 1978) detects a glycoprotein tetramolecular antigen (Mitchell *et al.*, 1980, 1981) that is expressed by melanomas, and also by some astrocytomas (M. Herlyn *et al.*, 1980; Steplewski *et al.*, 1982). It was detected on the surfaces of embryonal uveal cells (M. Herlyn *et al.*, in preparation). This antigen may represent a reexpression of neural tube embryonal structure.

The application of hybridoma technology will permit a more detailed analysis and understanding of the tumor-specific or tumor-associated antigens.

ACKNOWLEDGMENTS

The data presented here were derived from experiments in which D. Herlyn, M. Herlyn, M. Blaszczyk, and K. Mitchell also participated. Supported in part by grants CA-10815 and CA-21124 from the National Institutes of Health, Bethesda, Maryland.

REFERENCES

Beckman, I. G. R., Bradley, J., Brooks, D. A., Kupa, A., McNamara, P. J., Thomas, M. E., and Zola, H. (1980). *Clin. Exp. Immunol.* **40,** 593.

Blaszczyk, M., Karlson, K. A., Hansson, G., Larsson, G., Brockhaus, M., Herlyn, M., Steplewski, Z., and Koprowski, H. (1982). *Hybridoma* **2,** 202.

Bluming, A. Z., Vogel, O. L., Ziegler, J. L., and Kiryabwire, J. M. W. (1972). *J. Natl. Cancer Inst.* **48,** 17.

Bodurtha, A., Berkelhammer, J., Kim, Y. H., Laucius, J. F., and Mastrangelo, M. J. (1967). *Cancer* **37,** 735.

Bradstock, K. F., Janossy, G., Pizzolo, G., Hoffbrand, A. V., McMichael, A., Pilch, J. R., Milstein, C., Beverly, P., and Bollum, F. J. (1980). *J. Natl. Cancer Inst.* **65,** 33.

Bray, A. E. (1978). *Surg. Gynecol. Obstet.* **147,** 103.

Brockhaus, M., Magnani, J. L., Blaszczyk, M., Steplewski, Z., Koprowski, H., Karlsson, K-A., Larson, G., and Ginsburg, V. (1981). *J. Biol. Chem.* **256,** 13223.

Brockhaus, M., Magnani, J., Herlyn, M., Blaszczyk, M., and Ginsburg, V. (1982). *Fed. Proc. Fed. Am. Soc. Exp. Biol.* **41,** 897.

Brown, J. P., Wright, P. W., Hart, C. E., Woodbury, R. G., Hellstrom, K. E., and Hellstrom, I. (1980). *J. Biol. Chem.* **255,** 4980.

Carey, T. E., Takahashi, T., Resnick, L. A., Oetgen, H. F., and Old, L. J. (1976). *Proc. Natl. Acad. Sci. U.S.A.* **73,** 3278.

Chang, T. H., Steplewski, Z., and Koprowski, H. (1980). *J. Immunol. Methods* **39,** 369.

Chang, T. H., Steplewski, Z., and Sears, H. F., and Koprowski, H. (1981). *Hybridoma* **1,** 37.

Cornain, S., de Vires, J. E., Collard, J., Vennegoor, C., van Wingerden, I., and Rumke, P. (1975). *Int. J. Cancer* **16,** 981.

Dippold, W. G., Lloyd, K. O., Vi, L. T. C., Ikeda, H., Oettgen, H. F., and Old. L. S. (1980). *Proc. Natl. Acad. Sci. U.S.A.* **77,** 6114.

Edelson, R. L., Hearing, V. J., Dellon, A. L., Frank, M., Edelson, K. K., and Green, I. (1975). *Cancer Immunol. Immunopathol.* **4,** 557.

Embelton, M. J., Price, M. R., and Baldwin, R. W. (1980). *Eur. J. Cancer* **16,** 575.

Espmark, A., and Fagreus, A. (1962). *Acta Pathol. Microbiol. Scand. Suppl.* **154,** 258.

Galloway, D. R., McCabe, R. P., Pellegrino, M. A., Ferrone, S., and Reisfeld, R. A. (1981). *J. Immunol.* **126,** 62.

Garret, T. J., Takahashi, T., Clarkson, B. D., and Old, L. S. (1977). *Proc. Natl. Acad. Sci. U.S.A.* **74,** 4587.

Gilliland, D. G., Steplewski, Z., Collier, R. J., Mitchell, K. F., Chang, T. H., and Koprowski, H. (1980). *Proc. Natl. Acad. Sci. U.S.A.* **77,** 4539.

Gold, P., and Freedman, S. O. (1965). *J. Exp. Med.* **22,** 467.

Gross, L. (1943). *Cancer Res.* **3,** 326.

Gupta, R. K., Silver, H. K. B., Reisfeld, R. A., and Morton, D. L. (1974). *Cancer Res.* **39**, 1683.

Hansen, J. A., Martin, P. J., and Nowinski, R. C. (1980). *Immunogenetics* **10**, 247.

Hellstrom, K. E., and Hellstrom, I. (1969). *Adv. Cancer Res.* **12**, 167.

Herlyn, D., and Koprowski, H. (1981). *Int. J. Cancer* **27**, 769.

Herlyn, D., Herlyn, M., Steplewski, Z., and Koprowski, H. (1979). *Eur. J. Immunol.* **9**, 657.

Herlyn, D., Steplewski, Z., Herlyn, M., and Koprowski, H. (1980). *Cancer Res.* **40**, 717.

Herlyn, M., Steplewski, Z., Herlyn, D., and Koprowski, H. (1979). *Proc. Natl. Acad. Sci. U.S.A.* **76**, 1438.

Herlyn, M., Clark, W. H., Mastrangelo, M. J., Guerry, D., IV., Elder, D. E., LaRossa, D., Hamilton, R., Bondi, E., Tuthill, R., Steplewski, Z., and Koprowski, H. (1980). *Cancer Res.* **40**, 3602.

Herlyn, M., Sears, H. F., Steplewski, Z., and Koprowski, H. (1982) *J. Clin. Immunol.* **2**, 135.

Imai, K., Molinaro, G. A., and Ferrone, S. (1980). *Transplant. Proc.* **12**, 380.

Irie, R. F., Giuliano, A. E., and Morton, D. L. (1979). *J. Natl. Cancer Inst. U.S.* **63**, 367.

Kearney, J. F., Radbruch, A., Liesegang, B., and Rajewski, K. (1979). *J. Immunol.* **123**, 1548.

Kennett, R. H. (1980). *In* "Monoclonal Antibodies" (R. H. Kennett, T. J. McKearn, and K. B. Bechtol, eds.), pp. 365–367. Plenum, New York.

Kennett, R. H., and Gilbert, F. (1979). *Science* **203**, 1120.

Klein, G., Sjogren, H. O., Klein, E., and Hellstrom, K. E. (1960). *Cancer Res.* **20**, 1561.

Köhler, G., and Milstein, C. (1975). *Nature (London)* **257**, 495.

Köhler, G., and Milstein, C. (1976). *Eur. J. Immunol.* **6**, 511.

Köhler, G, Howe, S. C., and Milstein, C. (1976). *Eur. J. Immunol.* **6**, 292.

Koprowski, H., Steplewski, Z., Herlyn, D., and Herlyn, M. (1978). *Proc. Natl. Acad. Sci. U.S.A.* **75**, 3405.

Koprowski, H., Steplewski, Z., Mitchell, K. F., Herlyn, M., Herlyn, D., and Fuhrer, J. P. (1979). *Somatic Cell Genet.* **5**, 957.

Koprowski, H., Herlyn, M., Steplewski, Z., and Sears, H. F. (1981). *Science* **212**, 53.

Laemmli, U. K. (1970). *Nature (London)* **227**, 680.

Leibovitz, A., Stinson, J. C., McCombs, W. B., III, McCoy, C. E., Mazur, C., and Mabry, N. D. (1976). *Cancer Res.* **36**, 4562.

Levy, R., Dilley, J., and Lampson, L. A. (1978). *Curr. Top. Microbiol. Immunol.* **81**, 164.

Levy, R., Dilley, J., Fox, R. I., and Warnke, R. (1979). *Proc. Natl. Acad. Sci. U.S.A.* **12**, 6552.

Lewis, M. G., Ikonopisow, R. L., and Nairn, R. C. (1969). *Br. Med. J.* **3**, 547.

Liao, S. K., Kwong, P. C., Thompson, J. C., and Dent, P. B. (1979). *Cancer Res.* **39**, 183.

Littlefield, J. N. (1964). *Science* **145**, 709.

Magnani, J. L., Brockhaus, M., Smith, D. F., Ginsburg, V., Blaszczyk, M., Mitchell, K. F., Steplewski, Z., and Koprowski, H. (1981). *Science* **212**, 55.

Marchalonis, J. J., Cone, R. E., and Santer, V. (1971). *Biochem. J.* **124**, 921.

Martin, F., and Martin, M. S. (1970). *Int. J. Cancer* **6**, 352.

Mitchell, K. F. (1980). *Cancer Immunol. Immunother.* **10**, 1.

Mitchell, K. F., Fuhrer, J. P., Steplewski, Z., and Koprowski, H. (1980). *Proc. Natl. Acad. Sci. U.S.A.* **77**, 7287.

Mitchell, K. F., Fuhrer, J. P., Steplewski, Z., and Koprowski, H. (1981). *Mol. Immunol.* **18**, 207.

Mitchell, K. F., Steplewski, Z., and Koprowski, H. (1982). *In* "Monoclonal Hybridoma Antibodies: Techniques and Applications" (J. G. Hurrell, ed.), CRC.

Morton, D. L., Malmgren, A. L., and Holmes, E. C. (1968). *Surgery* **64**, 233.

Mutzner, P. A., Stuhlmiller, G. M., and Seigler, H. F. (1980). *J. Surg. Oncol.* **14**, 367.

Nadler, L. M., Stashenko, P., Hardy, R., and Schlossman, S. F. (1980). *J. Immunol.* **125**, 570.

Old, L. J., and Boyse, E. A. (1964). *Annu. Rev. Med.* **15**, 167.

Reinhertz, E. L., Kung, P. C., Goldstein, G., and Schlossman, S. F. (1979). *J. Immunol.* **123**, 1312.

Reisfeld, R. A., Galloway, D. R., Imai, K., Ferrone, S., and Morgan, A. C. (1980). *Fed. Proc. Fed. Am. Soc. Exp. Biol.* **40**, 231.

Ritz, J., Pesando, J. M., Notis-McConanty, J., Lazarus, H., and Schlossman, S. F. (1980). *Nature (London)* **283**, 583.

Royston, I., Majda, J. A., Baird, S. M., Meserve, B. A., and Griffiths, J. C. (1980). *J. Immunol.* **125**, 725.

Sears, H. F., Herlyn, M., DelVilano, B., Steplewski, Z., and Koprowski, H. (1982). *J. Clin. Immunol.* **2**, 141.

Shulman, M., Wilde, C. D., and Köhler, G. (1978). *Nature (London)* **276**, 269.

Sidell, N., Irie, R. F., Nathenson, S. D., and Morton, D. L. (1980). *Cancer Immunol. Immunother.* **9**, 49.

Smith, J. B., and O'Neill, K. T. (1971). *Res. Commun. Chem. Pathol. Pharmacol.* **2**, 1.

Steplewski, Z., Herlyn, M., Herlyn, D., Clark, W. H., and Koprowski, H. (1979). *Eur. J. Immunol.* **9**, 94.

Steplewski, Z. (1980). *Transplant. Proc.* **12**, 384.

Steplewski, Z., Chang, T. H., Herlyn, M., and Koprowski, H. (1981). *Cancer Res.* **41**, 2723.

Steplewski, Z., Mitchell, K. F., and Koprowski, H. (1982). *In* "Melanoma Antigens and Antibodies" (R. Reisfeld, ed.), pp. 365–380. Plenum, New York.

Szybalski, W., Szybalsk, E. H., and Regnie, G. (1962). *Cancer Inst. Monogr.* **7**, 75.

Von Kleist, S., and Burtin, P. (1969). *Cancer Res.* **29**, 1961.

Woodbury, R. G., Brown, J. P., Yeh, M-Y., Hellstrom, I., and Hellstrom, K. E. (1980). *Proc. Natl. Acad. Sci. U.S.A.* **77**, 2183.

Yeh, M-Y., Hellstrom, I., Brown, J. P., Warner, G. A., Hansen, J. A., and Hellstrom, K. E. (1979). *Proc. Natl. Acad. Sci. U.S.A.* **76**, 2927.

CHAPTER IX

HUMAN MELANOMA- AND GLIOMA-ASSOCIATED ANTIGEN(S) IDENTIFIED BY MONOCLONAL ANTIBODIES

STEFAN CARREL, NICOLAS DE TRIBOLET, AND JEAN-PIERRE MACH

I. Introduction

A. MELANOMA-ASSOCIATED ANTIBODIES

Despite the widespread belief that melanoma is an immunogenic tumor in man, the question as to whether patients respond to their tumor by developing humoral and cellular immunity is still highly controversial. The existence of serologically defined tumor-associated antigen(s) on human melanoma cells has been suggested by several studies in which human allogeneic or autologous sera have been used (Morton *et al.*, 1968; Muna *et al.*, 1969; Lewis *et al.*, 1969; Cornain *et al.*, 1975; Gupta and Morton, 1975; Carey *et al.*, 1976; Hersey *et al.*, 1976; Ferrone and Pellegrino, 1977; Shiku *et al.*, 1976, 1977; Liao *et al.*, 1978). Conclusive evidence that the antibodies present in these sera are directed against a melanoma-specific antigen, however, is lacking.

Nevertheless, three operationally distinct systems of antigens have been defined on the surface of melanoma cells (Shiku *et al.*, 1976). Tumor antigens restricted to a single tumor have been referred to as class 1 antigens, antigens present on several melanomas and absent from other tumors or normal tissues have been called class 2 antigens, and antigens not restricted to melanomas and present also on some normal cells have been classified as class 3 antigens. Antibodies that detect class 3 antigens are the ones most commonly found in patients' sera. Major effort has been concentrated on the production of xenoantisera against class 2 antigens, since patients with sera containing such antibodies are extremely rare, if not nonexistent.

Immunization of rabbits, guinea pigs, and monkeys with human melanoma cells has led to the production of several antisera which after absorption reacted preferentially with melanoma cells from primary and long-term cultures (Metzgar *et al.*, 1973; Stuhlmiller and Seigler, 1975; Viza and Phillips, 1975; Fritz *et al.*, 1976; Bystryn, 1977; McCabe *et al.*, 1978; Sorg *et al.*, 1978; Liao *et al.*, 1979; Carrel *et al.*, 1980a). The major drawback of such antisera, however, is the overwhelming amount of contaminating antibodies that must be removed by extensive absorption before any tumor specificity can be demonstrated. Furthermore, the amount of antibodies left after these absorptions is very low and their tumor specificity often remains questionable.

B. MONOCLONAL ANTIBODY TECHNOLOGY AND TUMOR ANTIGENS

The method of Köhler and Milstein (1975) allowing the production of monoclonal antibodies against single antigenic determinants represents a great improvement for the selection of antibodies reacting with tumor-associated antigens. Recently, several investigators have produced monoclonal antibodies against various human tumors, including melanomas (Koprowski *et al.*, 1978; Steplewski *et al.*, 1979; Yeh *et al.*, 1979; Carrel *et al.*, 1980b; Woodbury *et al.*, 1980; Dippold *et al.*, 1980; Morgan *et al.*, 1981; Imai *et al.*, 1981), neuroblastomas (Kennett and Gilbert, 1979), colon carcinomas (Herlyn *et al.*, 1979), gliomas (Schnegg *et al.*, 1981), leiomyosarcomas (Deng *et al.*, 1981), and breast carcinomas (Schlom *et al.*, 1980).

Koprowski *et al.* (1978) reported the production of several hybrids secreting antibodies binding to melanoma cells. Three of them bound to Ia antigens known to be expressed on some melanomas (Winchester *et al.*, 1978; Wilson *et al.*, 1979), while two other antibodies, 19-19 and Nu4B, appeared to detect common structures expressed on melanomas and astrocytomas. Yeh *et al.* (1979) described three monoclonal antibodies which seemed to react with an autologous melanoma antigen, a so-called class 1 antigen. Carrel *et al.* (1980b) described three monoclonal antibodies which had restricted reactivity toward several melanoma cell lines; two of these antibodies also cross-reacted with gliomas. Woodbury *et al.* (1980) reported a hybridoma product that bound to the majority of the melanomas tested and also to several nonmelanoma tumor cells, but not to normal fibroblasts or B cells. The molecular weight of this protein was found to be 97,000 and it has been named p97. Further investigations showed that p97 was also present in small amounts in normal adult tissue as well as in fetal colon and umbilical cord (Brown *et al.*, 1981). Using the same melanoma cell line (SK-Mel-28) for immunization, Dippold *et al.* (1980) obtained eighteen monoclonal antibodies which bound to the immunizing cell line. With these antibodies the authors defined six different antigenic systems. The gp95 antigen seemed to be identical or at least very similar to the p97 described by Brown *et al.* (1981). Four other systems (gp150, M_{19}, R_8, and O_5) appeared to represent class 3 antigens, since they were not restricted to melanomas and astrocytomas. The last antigenic system (R_{24}) was restricted to melanoma and astrocytoma. Interestingly, these antibodies seemed to react not with a glycoprotein, but with a glycolipid.

C. COMMON NEUROECTODERMAL ANTIGENS

It is tempting to assume that the sharing of antigenic determinants by gliomas and melanomas is due to the fact that these two tumors originate from cells embryologically derived from the neural crest. We have previously described (Carrel and Theilkaes, 1973) a rabbit antiserum raised against partially purified melanoma antigen extracted from the urine of melanoma patients. This antiserum reacted with an antigen present in the urine of patients with melanomas and neuroblastomas. More recently, Pfreundschuh *et al.* (1978) reported the presence in the serum of a patient with an astrocytoma of antibodies which cross-reacted with cultured melanomas, neuroblastomas, and sarcomas. Similarly, Coakham *et al.* (1980) found in the serum of another patient with an astrocytoma antibodies which cross-reacted with tumors of neuroectodermal origin, including neuroblastomas, melanomas, and an acoustic neurinoma. By producing monoclonal antibodies against the neuroblastoma cell like IMR-6, Kennett and Gilbert (1979) obtained one hybridoma-secreting antibody which reacted with five other neuroblastomas, one retinoblastoma, and one glioma, as well as with fetal brain tissue. Schnegg *et al.* (1981) immunized mice with glioma cells and obtained, in addition to two monoclonal antibodies reacting exclusively with gliomas, a third antibody which reacted with gliomas, melanomas, and neuroblastomas, but not with the other control cell lines tested. Absorption with homogenates of fetal brain and to a lesser degree of adult brain reduced the binding capacity of this particular antibody for both melanomas and gliomas. These results suggest that the structures recognized by some of these monoclonal antibodies are not tumor-specific antigens, but differentiation antigens present on tumor cells with a common embryologic origin.

D. AIM AND SCOPE OF THE PRESENT ARTICLE

In this chapter we will describe the characteristics of nine monoclonal antibodies secreted by hybrids obtained from five fusions between two distinct mouse myeloma cell lines [P3-NSl/Ag4 (Köhler *et al.*, 1976) and P3X63/Ag8 (Köhler and Milstein, 1975)] and spleen cells from mice immunized with membrane-enriched fractions from two melanoma cell lines (Me43 and IGR-3). It will be shown that these antibodies have a preferential reactivity for melanoma cells, as assessed by an indirect antibody binding radioimmunoassay (RIA) (Klinman, 1972; Williams, 1977). However, five of them cross-react with structures also present on some gliomas and neuroblastomas, and two of them react with Ia antigens present on some melanoma and glioma cell lines. Our results will also show that each of these antibodies recognizes different antigenic determinants expressed on melanoma cells.

We will also review the characteristics of three monoclonal antibodies secreted by hybrids obtained from three fusions between mouse myeloma cells (P3X63/Ag8) and spleen cells from mice immunized with cells from the glioma line LN-18 (Diserens *et al.*, 1981). Two of these antibodies have a preferential reactivity for glioma cells, while the product from the third hybrid displayed a unique cross-reactivity for melanoma and neuroblastoma cells (Schnegg *et al.,* 1981). By comparing the reactivity spectrum of these antibodies for the panel of 25 tumor cell lines tested, it will be apparent that they each react with a distinct antigenic determinant located on different molecules. In general, we have concentrated our effort toward a thorough evaluation of the tumor and organ specificity of the monoclonal antibodies to be selected for further immunochemical characterization of the relevant antigens.

II. Production of Somatic Cell Hybrids

A. CELL LINES

All human cell lines used in this study were grown in Roswell Park Memorial Institute Medium (RPMI) 1640 supplemented with 10% heat-inactivated fetal calf serum (FCS). The principal characteristics of the two melanoma cell lines (Me43 and IGR-3) and the glioma cell line (LN-18) used for immunization are summarized in Table I. The BALB/c myeloma

TABLE I

CHARACTERISTICS OF THE MELANOMA AND GLIOMA CELL LINES USED FOR IMMUNIZATION

Cell line	Me43	IGR-3	LN-18
Line	Established 1976 in our laboratory	Established 1973 (Aubert *et al.,* 1976)	Established 1978 (Diserens *et al.,* 1981)
Origin	Nodular melanoma from a 52-year-old Caucasian male (primary tumor)	Primary nodular-type melanoma from a 60-year-old Caucasian male	Malignant glioma from a 61-year-old Caucasian male (grade IV according to Kernohan's classification)
Cells	Grow as a monolayer in 10% FCS, melanin granules present	Grow as a monolayer in 10% FCS, melanin granules present	Grow as a monolayer in 10% FCS, GFA absent, S-100 negative, microfibrils present
Fibronectin (LETS)	Positive	Positive	Positive
Tumorigenicity in nude mice	Yes	Yes	Yes
Ia antigen(s)	Absent	DR 1.7	DR 3

cell lines used for fusion (P3-NSl/Ag4 and P3X63/Ag8) were both maintained in RPMI medium containing 10% horse serum. These two cell lines are resistant to 8-azoguanine (20 μg/ml) and do not grow in hypoxanthine–aminopterin–thymidine (HAT)-selective medium (Cowan *et al.*, 1974; Köhler and Milstein, 1975).

B. Preparation of Crude Membrane Fractions

Membrane fractions from the two melanoma lines (Me43 and IGR-3) were prepared by nitrogen cavitation (Schmidt-Ulrich *et al.*, 1974). Briefly, washed cells at a minimum concentration of 5×10^7 cells/ml in 0.075 M KCl, 0.065 M NaCl, 0.25 mM MgCl$_2$, and 0.01 mM HEPES (pH 7.4) were exposed to 10 atm N$_2$ for 20 minutes at 4°C while being stirred gently. After being returned to normal atmospheric pressure, the disrupted cells were collected and centrifuged at 400 g for 15 minutes and finally at 20,000 g for 30 minutes. The pellet obtained after the 20,000 g spin was used to immunize the recipient animals. The protein concentration in this fraction was determined by the microburet method.

C. Immunization

Three- to four-month-old BALB/c mice were immunized intraperitoneally (ip) with two injections of membrane-enriched fractions from the two melanoma cell lines (Me43 or IGR-3; 0.1 mg of membrane protein in 0.2 ml of 0.9% NaCl solution), in complete Freund's adjuvant. After 20 days, the mice were boosted intravenously (iv) with the same amount of protein in 0.9% NaCl. Three days later, the mice were killed and their spleens were used for fusion. For antiglioma fusions, BALB/c mice were injected ip with 10^7 whole cells of the established human glioma cell line (LN-18) suspended in 0.2 ml RPMI 1640 medium. These mice were boosted ip with the same number of cells 4 weeks later. Three days later, the mice were killed and their spleen cells were used for fusion.

D. Cell Fusion

Cell fusion was performed by incubating 10^7 mouse myeloma cells (P3-NSl/Ag4 or P3X63/Ag8) with 10^8 mouse spleen cells in 0.3 ml of 40% polyethylene glycol (PEG, MW 1000) for 3 minutes at 37°C (Pontecorvo,

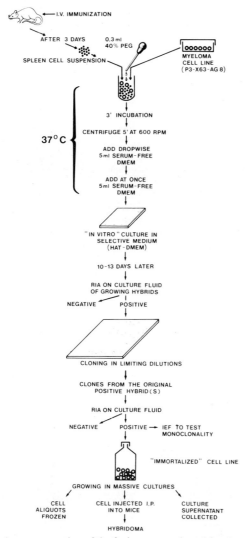

FIG. 1. Schematic representation of the fusion protocol used for the production of mono-clonal antibodies.

1975). The cells were centrifuged for 5 minutes at 200 g, then 5 ml serum-free RPMI 1640 medium was added dropwise to dilute the PEG. After fusion the cells were washed and resuspended in 100 ml of HAT medium and distributed in four 96-well plates of 0.6 cm diameter (see Fig. 1 for a schematic representation of the fusion protocol used).

E. ANTIBODY-DETECTION RADIOIMMUNOASSAY

The production of specific antibodies by HAT-selected hybrids was detected by an antibody binding assay essentially the same as that described by Williams (1977). Briefly, 5×10^4 target cells, in 100 μl of medium, were incubated for 90 minutes at 4°C with 100 μl of culture fluid from the different hybrids in U-bottomed microtest plates. The plates were centrifuged at 200 g for 3 minutes and the supernatants removed. After four washings with 100 μl of medium 100 μl of ^{125}I-labeled purified rabbit anti-mouse F(ab')$_2$ (10 ng of protein corresponding to about 100,000 cpm) was added and incubated for 90 minutes at 4°C. The cells were then washed three times with medium and transferred to tubes for gamma counting. The positive hybrids detected by this method were then cloned by a limiting dilution system (Accolla *et al.*, 1980) in a 96-well plate, and a representative clone of each specificity was chosen for further studies (see Fig. 2 for a schematic representation of the antibody binding radioimmunoassay used).

III. Screening for Antibody-Secreting Hybrids

A. SOMATIC CELL HYBRIDS FROM "ANTIMELANOMA" FUSIONS

We obtained a total of 193 growing hybrids from the five fusions between spleen cells from mice immunized with melanoma cell membranes and mouse myeloma cells. In an initial screening, 55 of these hybrids were

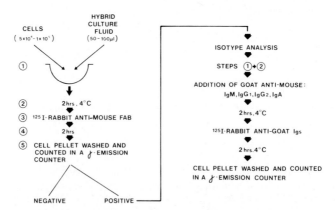

FIG. 2. Radioimmunoassay for cell surface antigens. Schematic representation of the indirect binding RIA used for the detection of monoclonal antibodies.

TABLE II

SOMATIC CELL HYBRIDS PRODUCING MONOCLONAL ANTIBODIES
AGAINST MELANOMA AND GLIOMA

Fusion code	Immunizing antigen	Myeloma strain used	Number of growing hybrids	Number of positive hybrids for the immunizing cells	Number of hybrids with restricted reactivity selected
Me-1	Me43[a]	P3-NSl/Ag4	26	7	3
Me-2	Me43[a]	P3-NSl/Ag4	8	0	0
Me-3	IGR-3[a]	P3X63/Ag8	14	4	2
Me-4	IGR-3[a]	P3X63/Ag8	87	39	3
Me-5	Me43[a]	P3X63/Ag8	58	5	1
Gl-1	LN-18[b]	P3-NSl/Ag4	3	0	0
Gl-2	LN-18[b]	P3X63/Ag8	21	0	0
Gl-3	LN-18[b]	P3X63/Ag8	345	36	3

[a] Mice immunized with membrane-enriched fractions.
[b] Mice immunized with intact cells.

found to produce antibodies binding to one of the immunizing cell lines (Table II). Twenty-six growing hybrids were obtained from the first fusion (Me-1). Seven of them produced antibodies directed against the immunizing melanoma cells (Me43). At a first screening for specificity, culture fluids from these seven hybrids were tested against two nonmelanoma control cell lines: a myeloid line (K562) (Lozzio and Lozzio, 1975) and an endometrial carcinoma cell line (END-1) (Carrel *et al.*, 1979). Four out of seven hybrids secreted antibodies which reacted with one of the two control cell lines. The reactivity of the three hybrids secreting antibodies which did not react with these two control cell lines was further investigated. From the second fusion (Me-2) we obtained eight growing hybrids, none of which secreted antibodies binding to the immunizing melanoma cell line (IGR-3).

Fourteen growing hybrids were obtained from the third fusion (Me-3) and four of them produced antibodies binding to the immunizing melanoma line (Me43). Two out of these four antibodies bound to the control nonmelanoma cell line (K562) and were discarded. The two remaining hybrids were kept for further specificity analysis. Fusion number four (Me-4) produced 87 growing hybrids; 39 of them secreted antibodies which bound to the immunizing melanoma cells (IGR-3), of which 36 hybrid products bound to one or the other of the two control cell lines and were discarded. The remaining three clones were chosen for further specificity analysis. From fusion number 5 (Me-5) we obtained a total of 58 growing hybrids, 5 of which secreted antibodies which bound to the immunizing melanoma cell line (Me43). After the first screening against the two control cell lines, four of them were discarded and the specificity of the remaining hybridoma product was further investigated. After this preliminary screening, the nine selected hybrids were cloned by limiting dilution and a representative clone from each hybrid was chosen for specificity analysis.

B. Somatic Cell Hybrids from "Antiglioma" Fusions

From the first two fusions (Gl-1 and Gl-2) we obtained a total of 24 growing hybrids; none of them secreted antibodies which bound to the immunizing glioma cell line (LN-18). A total of 345 hybrids were obtained from the third fusion (Gl-3); 36 of these hybrids secreted antibodies binding to the immunizing glioma cells. After a first screening against the two control lines, 33 hybrids were discarded since they bound to one or the other of these lines. The three hybrids secreting antibodies which did not react with either of these control cell lines were cloned by limiting dilution and representative clones for each hybrid were chosen for further specificity analysis.

IV. Specificity Analysis

A. Monoclonal Antimelanoma Antibodies

Table III summarizes the binding results obtained with the nine hybridoma products selected from 5 antimelanoma fusions and tested on 11 different melanoma cell lines. The results are expressed as a binding ratio (BR) which represents the number of counts per minute bound to tumor cells in the presence of hybrid culture fluid divided by the cell-bound counts per minute in the presence of control culture fluid using the mouse myeloma P3X63/Ag8, which produces an IgG_1 (κ) immunoglobulin of unknown specificity. The background counts obtained with control culture fluid varied for each cell line tested, ranging between 50 and 205 cpm. The binding results obtained with the nine selected antibodies tested on 15 nonmelanoma control cell lines are summarized in Table IV. The control cell lines included four colon carcinomas, two breast carcinomas, one lung carcinoma, one endometrial carcinoma, one cervical carcinoma, one rhabdomyosarcoma, one choriocarcinoma, two B-cell lines, one T-cell line, and one normal fibroblast line. The binding on glioma cell lines will be reported in Section V,A and Table VII.

TABLE III
BINDING OF HYBRIDOMA ANTIMELANOMA ANTIBODIES TO MELANOMA CELL LINES

Cell line used as target	Hybridoma product[a]								
	Me1-5	Me1-7	Me1-14	Me3-TB7	Me3-NE4	Me4-H3	Me4-F8	Me4-H4	Me5-D5
IGR-3	23	4	20	16	39	6	10	5	6
Me43	20	11	23	22	1	5	9	6	7
MP-6	13	7	12	6	12	2	2	5	5
MP-8	4	2	5	7	9	5	8	4	9
Mel-57	9	6	11	13	26	4	12	6	3
Daudel	8	9	12	21	27	5	6	4	7
Mel-67	10	3	9	7	7	6	7	14	9
Mel-2Am	12	8	15	18	16	5	10	8	5
MelEi78	25	2	24	3	2	2	4	3	7
Me8	8	3	13	9	18	2	6	7	5
SK-Mel-1	9	2	7	2	2	5	7	6	8

[a] Values are expressed as binding ratio which equals the total number of cell-bound counts divided by the number of cell-bound counts using P3X63/Ag8 culture fluid; BR ≥ 4 is considered as positive.

TABLE IV

Binding of Hybridoma Antimelanoma Antibodies to Various Nonmelanoma Cells

Cell line used as target	Hybridoma product[a]								
	Me1-5	Me1-7	Me1-14	Me3-TB7	Me3-NE4	Me4-H3	Me4-F8	Me4-H4	Me5-D5
Co-115[b]	2	2	1	2	3	2	2	2	2
Co-125[b]	2	1	2	2	2	1	2	1	2
LOVO[b]	2	2	2	2	1	2	1	2	2
HT-29[b]	2	1	2	2	2	1	2	2	2
MCF-7[c]	1	2	2	2	2	1	2	2	1
BR-3[c]	2	2	1	2	1	2	2	1	2
DMS-79[d]	2	1	1	1	2	1	2	1	1
END-1[e]	1	2	1	2	18	2	2	2	2
Me-180[f]	2	2	2	2	1	1	2	1	2
RD[g]	2	1	2	2	2	2	2	2	1
BeWo[h]	2	2	1	2	2	2	1	1	2
Raji[i]	1	2	2	1	23	2	2	2	2
6410[i]	2	1	2	2	15	1	2	2	2
8402[j]	1	2	1	2	2	2	2	2	2
FBL-239[k]	2	2	2	2	2	2	2	2	2

[a] Results are expressed as binding ratio which equals the total number of cell-bound counts divided by the number of cell-bound counts using P3X63/Ag8 culture fluid.
[b] Colon carcinoma.
[c] Breast carcinoma.
[d] Lung carcinoma.
[e] Endometrial carcinoma.
[f] Cervical carcinoma.
[g] Rhabdomyosarcoma.
[h] Choriocarcinoma.
[i] B-cell line.
[j] T-cell line.
[k] Normal skin fibroblasts.

As shown in Table III, antibodies from clone Me1-5 gave BR values of 4 or more on all 11 melanoma cell lines tested. The highest BR values were obtained for the three melanoma lines (IGR-3, Me43, and MelEi78), with values ranging from 20 to 25. Antibodies secreted by clone Me1-7 showed a restricted specificity for a limited number of melanoma cell lines with a BR ranging from 4 to 11 for 6 out of the 11 melanoma lines tested. The hybridoma product from clone Me1-14 gave a BR ranging from 5 to 24 with all of the 11 melanoma cell lines tested. The antibodies from the other six selected hybrids also gave significant binding of 8 to 10 for the 11 melanoma cell lines. The most important information is that none of these selected hybrid products (except Me3-NE4) reacted significantly with any of the 15 nonmelanoma and nonglioma control cell lines tested, as shown in Table IV. The only monoclonal antibody which reacted with control cell lines was from hybrid Me3-NE4. It gave BR values ranging from 15 to 23 with only 3 out of 15 control cell lines: END-1, Raji, and 6410, which are known to express HLA-DR antigens.

B. MONOCLONAL ANTIGLIOMA ANTIBODIES

The binding results obtained with the 3 selected clones from the antiglioma fusions tested on 13 different glioblastoma lines are summarized on Table V. Antibodies from the first clone (Gl3-BF7) bound to 10 out of 13 glioma lines with BR values ranging from 5 to 30. Antibodies from the second clone (Gl3-GE2) bound to 12 out of 13 gliomas, and antibodies from the third clone (Gl3-C6) bound to 7 out of 13 gliomas. Gl3-C6 is a subclone of the previously described CG-12 clone (Schnegg et al., 1981). Antibodies from these 3 clones were further tested on 14 nongliogenous control cell lines, including 1 endometrial carcinoma, 1 cervical carcinoma, 2 breast carcinomas, 4 colon carcinomas, 1 rhabdomyosarcoma, 1 lung carcinoma, 1 meningioma, 1 B- and 1 T-cell line, and 1 normal skin fibroblast line. Melanoma cell lines will be discussed in Section V,B. As summarized in Table VI, none of these hybridoma products bound significantly to any of the control cell lines tested.

As a control, two other monoclonal antibodies have been included in these experiments: namely, a monoclonal anti-CEA (CEA-23) (Accolla et al., 1980) and a monoclonal anti-Ia (D1-12)(Carrel et al., 1981). Monoclonal anti-CEA antibodies bound to 3 out of 4 colon carcinoma cell lines, with BR values ranging from 8 to 13, but bound to no other tumor cell lines, while monoclonal anti-Ia antibodies bound to the endometrial carcinoma line END-1, which is known to express HLA-DR antigens (Carrel et al., 1979), and to the B-cell line Raji.

TABLE V

BINDING OF HYBRIDOMA ANTIGLIOMA ANTIBODIES TO GLIOMA CELL LINES

Cell line used as target	Hybridoma product[a]				
	GI3-BF7	GI3-GE2	GI3-C6	CEA-23[b]	D1-12[c]
LN-229	2	7	8	1	13
LN-18	19	11	22	2	2
LN-121	2	5	2	2	17
LN-215	13	12	5	2	2
MG-1073	8	7	3	2	2
LN-71	30	26	9	1	1
LN-135	2	6	2	2	11
U-343	18	16	5	2	—
U-118	6	2	12	1	—
U-251	8	6	2	2	—
LN-140	7	8	3	2	—
LN-10	5	7	2	2	—
LN-40	9	14	7	2	—

[a] Results are expressed as binding ratio which equals the total number of cell-bound counts divided by the number of cell-bound counts using P3X63/Ag8 culture fluid.

[b] Monoclonal anti-CEA.

[c] Monoclonal anti-Ia.

C. QUANTITATIVE ABSORPTION EXPERIMENTS

The specificity of the various hybridoma products for melanoma and glioma cells was further demonstrated by quantitative absorption experiments. Increasing numbers of cells from different cell lines were added to 200 μl of culture fluid of a given hybrid clone and incubated for 1 hour at room temperature. The cells were then centrifuged and the remaining binding activity in the supernatant tested in the RIA. The results obtained for four different antimelanoma antibodies (Me1-5, Me1-14, Me3-TB7, and Me4-F8) are shown in Fig. 5. Increasing numbers of cells from three melanoma lines (Mel-67, Mel-57, and IGR-3) and two control lines (Co-115 and END-1) were used. Figure 3A shows that cells from the three melanoma lines absorbed the binding activity of Me1-5 culture fluid for IGR-3 melanoma target cells, while as many as 16×10^6 colon carcinoma cells (Co-115) or endometrial carcinoma cells (END-1) gave no significant binding inhibition. Similarly, Fig. 3B, C, and D show that between 1 and 2×10^6 cells from the three melanoma lines were sufficient to absorb 50% of the binding to IGR-3 of culture fluid from clones Me1-14, Me3-TB7, and Me4-F8, while no inhibition was obtained with the two control cell lines used.

TABLE VI

BINDING OF HYBRIDOMA ANTIGLIOMA ANTIBODIES TO VARIOUS NONGLIOGENOUS CELLS

Cell line used as target	Hybridoma product[a]				
	Gl3-BF7	Gl3-GE2	Gl3-C6	CEA-23[b]	D1-12[c]
END-1[d]	2	1	2	1	17
Me-180[e]	1	2	1	2	1
BR-3[f]	1	2	2	1	2
MCF-7[f]	2	2	2	2	2
HT-29[g]	2	1	2	13	2
Co-125[g]	1	2	1	3	2
Co-115[g]	2	1	2	10	3
LOVO[g]	2	2	2	8	2
RD[h]	2	1	1	2	2
DMS-79[i]	2	3	2	2	1
Men-246[j]	2	2	1	2	2
Raji[k]	1	1	1	2	21
Jurkat[l]	2	2	1	2	1
PBL[m]	2	2	2	1	3
FBL-239[n]	2	2	2	2	1

[a] Results are expressed as binding ratio which equals the total number of cell-bound counts divided by the number of cell-bound counts using P3X63/Ag8 culture fluid.
[b] Monoclonal anti-CEA.
[c] Monoclonal anti-Ia.
[d] Endometrial carcinoma.
[e] Cervical carcinoma.
[f] Breast carcinoma.
[g] Colon carcinoma.
[h] Rhabdomyosarcoma.
[i] Lung carcinoma.
[j] Meningioma .
[k] B-cell line.
[l] T-cell line.
[m] PBL (pool of five donors).
[n] Normal skin fibroblasts.

Similar experiments were performed with the three different antiglioma antibodies (Gl3-FE2, Gl3-BF7, and Gl3-C6) using the following cell lines for absorption: two gliomas (LN-215 and LN-140), one melanoma (IGR-3), one colon carcinoma (Co-115), and one endometrial carcinoma (END-1). The remaining binding activity of the hybrid supernatants was tested on the glioma cells (LN-18). Figure 4A shows that cells from the two glioma lines absorbed the binding activity of Gl3-GE2 culture fluid while as many as 1.6×10^7 melanoma cells or colon carcinoma and endo-

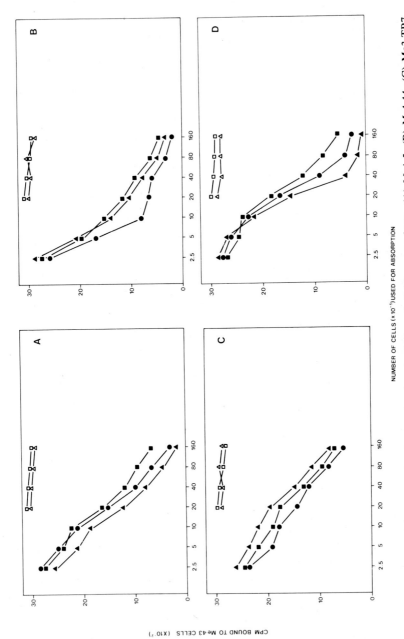

NUMBER OF CELLS (×10⁻³)USED FOR ABSORPTION

CPM BOUND TO Me43 CELLS (×10⁻²)

FIG. 3. Quantitative absorption of monoclonal antimelanoma hybridoma products. (A) Me1-5, (B) Me1-14, (C) Me3-TB7, (D) Me4-F8. Binding RIA using Me43 melanoma cells as targets. Each point represents cpm bound by the various culture fluids after absorption of 50 μl with the number of cells indicated on the abscissa. The cells used for absorption were melanoma cells (▲——▲, Mel-67; ■——■, Mel-57; ●——●, IGR-3), colon carcinoma cells (□——□, Co-115), and endometrial carcinoma cells (△——△, END-1).

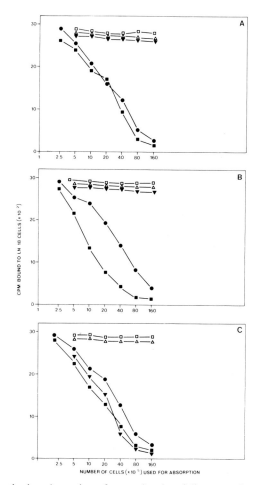

FIG. 4. Quantitative absorption of monoclonal antiglioma products. (A) Gl3-GE2, (B) Gl3-BF7, (C) Gl3-C6. Binding assay using LN-18 glioma cells as targets. Each point represents cpm bound by the various culture fluids after absorption of 50 μl with the number of cells indicated on the abscissa. The cells used for absorption were glioma cells (●——●, LN-215; ■——■, LN-140), melanoma cells (▲——▲, IGR-3), colon carcinoma cells (□——□, Co-115), and endometrial carcinoma cells (△——△, END-1).

metrial cells gave almost no inhibition of binding. Similar results were obtained for Gl3-BF7 culture fluid (Fig. 4B). For the Gl3-C6 monoclonal antibodies the results were different in the sense that not only the cells from the two glioma lines but also those from the melanoma line absorbed the reactivity for the glioma cells, while the two control carcinoma lines gave no binding inhibition. These results indicate the presence of a common antigen between gliomas and melanomas.

D. BINDING ASSAY FOR FIBRONECTIN

The two melanoma cell lines (Me43 and IGR-3) as well as the glioma line (LN-18) used for immunization were shown to produce large amounts of fibronectin (Table I). It was therefore of importance to determine if one of the various monoclonal antibodies obtained was directed against this protein. To answer this question, we used a solid-phase radioimmunoassay, essentially the same as that described by Zardi *et al.* (1980). Unlabeled fibronectin (0.01 mg/well) was adsorbed to the wells of polyvinyl plates. Culture fluid from the different hybrids was added (50 μl) and the plates were incubated for 2 hours before adding ^{125}I-labeled rabbit anti-mouse antibodies. After a second incubation for 1 hour at 37°C, the plates were washed and the wells cut in order to count their radioactivity. As shown in Fig. 5, none of the seven antimelanoma hybridoma products (Me1-5, Me1-7, Me1-14, Me3-TB7, Me4-F8, Me4-H3, or Me5-D5) and none of the three antiglioblastoma antibodies tested (Gl3-GE2, Gl3-BF7, or Gl3-C6) bound to fibronectin. As a positive control, a monoclonal anti-fibronectin antibody was used (Zardi *et al.*, 1980). It was therefore possible to rule out the possibility that our monoclonal antibodies were directed against fibronectin.

V. Common Neuroectodermal Antigens

A. MONOCLONAL ANTIMELANOMA ANTIBODIES BINDING TO GLIOMAS AND NEUROBLASTOMAS

During the specificity analysis of the nine selected clones from the five different melanoma fusions, it was observed that some of these hybridoma products cross-reacted with other neural crest-derived tissues such as gliomas and neuroblastomas. As shown in Table VII, antibodies from clone Me1-5 bound to five out of seven gliomas and to three out of three neuroblastomas tested, with BR values ranging from 7 to 16. Similarly, antibodies from Me1-14 bound also to five out of seven gliomas, but only to one neuroblastoma. A widespread cross-reactivity with these cell lines was also observed with antibodies from the hybrids Me3-TB7, Me4-F8, and Me5-D5. Of great interest is the fact that two monoclonal antimelanoma antibodies (Me1-7 and Me4-H3) did not react with any of the gliomas or neuroblastomas tested. Thus, these antibodies may be considered as having the most restricted melanoma specificity. As a control, the monoclonal anti-Ia antibodies (D1-12) were again found to bind to the three glioma cell lines which expressed HLA-DR antigens (LN-229, LN-121, and LN-135).

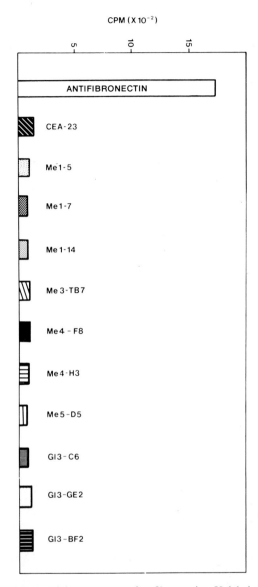

FIG. 5. Solid-phase radioimmunoassay for fibronectin. Unlabeled fibronectin (0.01 mg/well) was adsorbed to the wells of a polyvinyl plate. Culture fluid was then incubated for 2 hours before adding ^{125}I-labeled rabbit anti-mouse antibodies. Monoclonal antifibronectin (Zardi *et al.,* 1980) was used as a positive control. Monoclonal anti-CEA (Accolla *et al.,* 1980) was used as negative control. Monoclonal antimelanoma antibodies (Me1-5, Me1-7, Me1-14, Me3-TB7, Me4-F8, Me4-H3, and Me5-D5) and monoclonal antiglioma antibodies (Gl3-GE2, Gl3-BF7, and Gl3-C6) were tested. One sees that only the monoclonal anti-LETS and none of the other monoclonal antibodies gave a significant binding to insolubilized fibronectin.

TABLE VII

Binding of Hybridoma Antimelanoma Antibodies to Gliomas and Neuroblastomas

Cell line used as target	Hybridoma product[a]							
	Me1-5	Me1-7	Me1-14	Me3-TB7	Me4-H3	Me4-F8	Me5-D5	D1-12[b]
Gliomas								
LN-229	11	1	33	5	2	2	4	13
LN-18	9	1	13	1	1	2	3	1
LN-121	16	3	14	5	2	6	8	20
LN-215	12	3	7	5	2	9	7	1
MG-1073	2	1	2	6	2	1	2	2
LN-71	3	2	3	3	1	3	4	1
LN-135	16	3	12	5	1	9	8	9
Neuroblastomas								
IMR-32	8	3	10	7	2	5	11	1
SK-N-SM	7	2	3	4	1	4	5	1
SK-N-SH	7	2	2	4	1	4	9	1

[a] Results are expressed as binding ratio which equals the total number of cell-bound counts divided by the number of cell-bound counts using P3X63/Ag8 culture fluid.

[b] Monoclonal anti-Ia antibodies.

B. Monoclonal Antiglioma Antibodies Binding to Melanomas and Neuroblastomas

Table VIII summarizes the binding results obtained on nine melanoma cell lines and on three neuroblastoma cell lines with the three selected clonal products from the glioma fusion (Gl-3). Antibodies from clones Gl3-BF7 and Gl3-GE2 bound to only one out of nine melanomas, while antibodies from clone Gl3-C6 reacted with six out of nine melanomas and with one out of three neuroblastomas, with BR values ranging from 4 to 15. No reactivity with the control monoclonal anti-CEA antibodies (CEA-23) was observed, whereas the monoclonal anti-Ia antibodies (D1-12) bound to six out of nine melanoma lines.

C. Cross-reactivity of Antimelanoma and Antiglioma Antibodies for Neuroectodermal Antigens

The reactivity spectrum of the five monoclonal antimelanoma antibodies (Me1-5, Me1-14, Me3-TB7, Me4-F8, and Me5-D5) cross-reacting

TABLE VIII

Binding of Hybridoma Antiglioma Antibodies to
Melanomas and Neuroblastomas

Cell line used as target	Hybridoma product[a]				
	Gl3-BF7	Gl3-GE2	Gl3-C6	CEA-23[b]	D1-12[c]
Melanomas					
Me8	1	1	3	1	8
Me43	1	1	15	1	1
MP-6	2	5	14	1	17
Mel-67	2	2	4	2	29
MP-8	6	3	4	1	25
Mel-57	2	2	5	1	7
IGR-3	2	2	18	2	39
Mel-2Am	2	1	3	1	1
SK-Mel-1	2	2	1	1	1
Neuroblastomas					
IMR/32	3	3	8	2	1
SK-N-SM	1	2	2	1	1
SK-N-SH	1	2	1	1	1

[a] Results are expressed as binding ratio which equals the total number of cell-bound counts divided by the number of cell-bound counts using P3X63/Ag8 culture fluid.

[b] Monoclonal anti-CEA.

[c] Monoclonal anti-Ia (framework).

TABLE IX

CROSS-REACTIVITY OF MONOCLONAL ANTIMELANOMA AND ANTIGLIOMA
ANTIBODIES FOR NEUROECTODERMAL ANTIGENS

Cell line used as target	Hybridoma product[a]					
	Me1-5	Me1-14	Me3-TB7	Me4-F8	Me5-D5	Gl3-C6
Melanomas						
Me43	+++	+++	+++	+++	++	+++
IGR-3	+++	+++	+++	++	+	+++
Mel-67	++	+++	+++	+++	—	+
MP-6	+++	+++	+	—	+	+++
MP-8	+	+	+	+++	++	+
Gliomas						
LN-229	+++	+++	++	—	+	++
LN-18	++	+++	—	—	—	+++
LN-121	+++	+++	++	++	+	—
LN-215	+++	++	++	++	+	+
LN-135	+++	+++	++	—	+	—
Neuroblastomas						
IMR-32	++	+++	++	+	++	++
SK-N-SM	++	—	+	+	+	—
SK-N-SH	++	—	+	+	++	—

[a] +++, Very strong reactivity (BR ≥ 13); ++, strong reactivity (BR ≥ 9); + positive reactivity (BR ≥ 4); —, no reactivity (BR ≥ 2).

with gliomas and neuroblastomas, and of the monoclonal antiglioma antibodies (Gl3-C6) cross-reacting with melanomas and neuroblastomas has been analyzed on five melanoma cell lines, five glioma lines, and three neuroblastoma lines (Table IX). From this study it can be concluded that these six monoclonal antibodies are not directed against the same antigenic molecule present on individual cell lines, since in no instance is there a complete homology between the reactivity spectrum of each of these different antibodies for the cell lines tested. For example, Me1-5, Me1-14, and Gl3-C6 look similar in their reactivity with all five melanoma cell lines. However, Me1-5 and Me1-14 react with all gliomas, whereas Gl3-C6 reacts with only three out of five gliomas. Finally, Me1-5 reacts with all neuroblastomas while Me1-14 reacts with only one of them. Likewise, if we compare the binding capacity of Me4-F8 and Me5-D5, they both react with four out of five melanomas and with all three neuroblastomas; however Me4-F8 has no reactivity for the MP-6 melanoma line, whereas Me5-D5 has no reactivity for the Mel-67 melanoma line. In addition, both monoclonal antibodies have a completely different reactivity with the five gliomas. The conclusion from this analysis is that there might be as many as six different antigenic molecules identified by each different monoclonal antibody and which are expressed on different tumor cell lines sharing a common embryologic origin.

VI. Characterization of the Different Monoclonal Antibodies

A. Isotope Analysis

The isotope of each hybridoma product was determined by the following binding radioimmunoassay: 4×10^5 target cells were incubated with culture fluid in U plates. After centrifugation and washing, 100 μl of the appropriate dilution ($^1/_{100}$–$^1/_{1000}$) of goat antiserum specific for either IgM, IgG$_1$, IgG$_2$, or IgA (Meloy, Springfield, VA) were added. After washing, ^{125}I-labeled rabbit anti-goat IgG was added. The cells were washed again and their bound radioactivity counted. All incubation steps lasted 2 hours each and were done at 4°C. The results obtained from the isotope analysis of six antimelanoma and three antiglioblastoma monoclonal antibodies are summarized in Fig. 6. Four antimelanoma clones (Mel-14, Me3-TB7, Me3-NE4, and Me4-F8) secreted antibodies of the IgG$_2$ subclasses, whereas Mel-5 secreted antibodies of the IgG$_1$ subclass and Mel-7 of the IgM class. The isotype of two antiglioma antibodies (Gl3-GE2 and Gl3-C6) was IgG$_1$, while the third antiglioblastoma antibody (Gl3-BF7) reacted with both IgG$_1$ and IgG$_2$ antisera, indicating that it contains two heavy chains of different IgG subclasses.

B. Reciprocal Binding Inhibition Tests

To determine whether the various monoclonal antibodies were directed against identical or different antigenic determinants, a series of binding inhibition experiments was performed. In these assays, [^{3}H]leucine-labeled antibodies from the various clones were tested for their binding capacity to melanoma or glioma target cells in the presence of an excess of unlabeled (cold) antibodies from the same or from different clones. Antibodies from the various clones were internally labeled by the addition of 10 μCi of [^{3}H]leucine to cultures of 10^6 hybrid cells in 1 ml of leucine-free medium. After 24 hours of incubation at 37°C, culture fluids were harvested and 25 μl of each ^{3}H-labeled antibody was incubated for 2 hours with 5×10^4 target cells (melanoma or glioblastoma). The cells were then centrifuged and counted in a β-liquid scintillation counter. For competi-

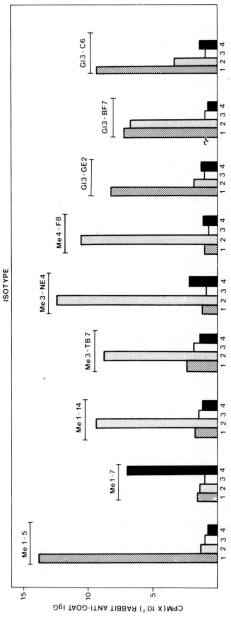

FIG. 6. Determination of the immunoglobulin classes and subclasses (isotype) of hybridoma antibodies. Monoclonal antimelanoma antibodies (Mel-15, Mel-7, Mel-14, Me3-TB7, Me3-NE4, and Me4-F8) were tested on IGR-3 melanoma cells. Monoclonal antiglioma antibodies (Gl3-GE2, Gl3-BF7, and Gl3-C6) were tested on LN-18 glioma cells. Goat antisera specific for mouse IgG$_1$, IgG$_2$, IgA, or IgM (100 μl diluted 1:500) were used in the second incubation. The results are expressed as cpm of ^{125}I-labeled rabbit antibodies against goat IgG.

tion analysis, 25 μl of unlabeled antibodies from 10-times concentrated culture fluid of different hybrids was allowed to react for 10 minutes with the target cells before the addition of 25 μl of ^{3}H-labeled antibodies. After 3 hours the cells were washed and counted.

The results obtained for four different antimelanoma antibodies (Me1-5, Me1-14, Me3-TB7, and Me4-F8) are shown in Fig. 7. The binding of ^{3}H-labeled Me1-5 antibodies for IGR-3 melanoma cells was inhibited by cold antibodies from the same clone, but not by cold Me1-14, Me3-TB7, or Me4-F8 antibodies (Fig. 7A). Figure 7B shows the converse experiment, where the binding of labeled Me1-14 antibodies was inhibited by cold Me1-14 culture fluid but not by Me1-5, Me3-TB7, or Me4-F8. Figure 7C and D show likewise that labeled Me3-TB7 antibodies competed only with cold Me3-TB7 and labeled Me4-F8 antibodies competed only with cold Me4-F8. These results clearly indicate that the antimelanoma antibodies from these four clones react with different antigenic determinants present on the same melanoma target cells.

Similar binding inhibition experiments were performed with the three selected clones from the antiglioma fusion (Gl3-GE2, Gl3-BF7, and Gl3-C6). The results obtained are presented in Fig. 8. Figure 8 shows that the binding of ^{3}H-labeled Gl3-GE2 antibodies to LN-18 glioma cells was in-

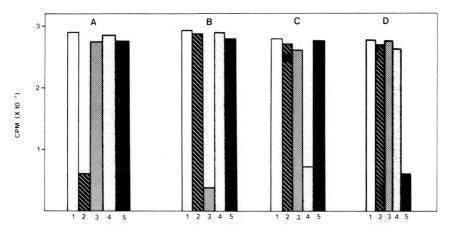

FIG. 7. Competition of binding for antimelanoma antibodies: binding inhibition experiments with ^{3}H-labeled monoclonal antimelanoma antibodies. For inhibition, 25 μl of cold antibodies in the form of 10-times concentrated culture fluids of (1) control myeloma P3X63/Ag8, (2) clone Me1-5, (3) clone Me1-14, (4) Me3-TB7, and (5) clone Me4-F8 were allowed to react for 10 minutes with Me43 melanoma target cells before the addition of 25 μl ^{3}H-labeled antibodies. After 3 hours the cells were washed and counted in a β-liquid scintillation counter. Results are expressed as cpm bound to 5×10^5 target cells. (A) ^{3}H-labeled Me1-5, (B) ^{3}H-labeled Me1-14, (C) ^{3}H-labeled Me3-TB7, (D) ^{3}H-labeled Me4-F8.

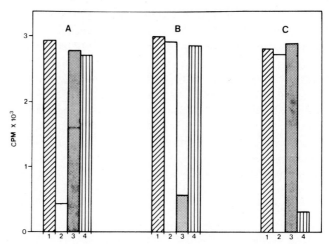

F<small>IG</small>. 8. Competition of binding for antiglioma antibodies: binding inhibition experiments with ^{3}H-labeled monoclonal antiglioma antibodies Gl3-GE2, Gl3-BF7, and Gl3-C6. For inhibition, 25 μl of cold antibodies in the form of 10-times concentrated culture fluid of (1) control myeloma P3X63/Ag8, (2) clone Gl3-GE2, (3) clone Gl3-BF7, and (4) clone Gl3-C6 were allowed to react for 10 minutes with LN-18 glioma cells before the addition of 25 μl ^{3}H-labeled antibodies obtained as described in Section VI,B. After 3 hours the cells were washed and counted in a β-liquid scintillation counter. Results are expressed as cpm bound to 5 × 10^5 target cells. (A) ^{3}H-labeled Gl3-GE2, (B) ^{3}H-labeled Gl3-BF7, (C) ^{3}H-labeled Gl3-C6.

hibited only by cold Gl3-GE2 antibodies and not by Gl3-BF7 and Gl3-C6 antibodies. Figure 8B and C show the converse experiment where the binding of labeled Gl3-BF7 and Gl3-C6 antibodies was inhibited only by cold antibodies from the same clone. The results from these experiments also show that the antibodies from the three antiglioma clones each react with a different antigenic determinant present on the same glioma cells.

VII. Cytotoxicity of Monoclonal Antibodies and Distribution of Antigens on Melanoma Cells

A. M<small>ETHODOLOGY</small>

Target cells were labeled with ^{51}Cr using a modification of the method of Brunner *et al.* (1968). Target cells were adjusted to 5 × 10^6/ml in Tris–phosphate-buffered saline containing 5% FCS. To 0.2 ml of the cell suspension (10^6 cells) 100 μCi/μg of ^{51}Cr in 150 μl was added. After incubation for 30 minutes at 37°C with occasional shaking, the labeled target cells were washed three times with 5 ml of medium plus 5% FCS. Complement-dependent cytotoxicity (CDC) was measured by a ^{51}Cr release assay as described previously (Carrel *et al.*, 1977). Briefly, 10^4 labeled target cells in 25-μl volumes were distributed into plastic tubes and incubated with 25 μl of culture fluid or ascites for 30 minutes at 37°C before adding 50 μl of fresh rabbit serum as a source of complement. The tubes were then incubated for 3 hours at 37°C. Cold medium was then added to stop the reaction, the tubes were centrifuged at 200 g for 10 minutes, and the radioactivity in the supernatant was counted. Specific lysis was determined as follows:

$$\% \text{ specific lysis} = (TR - SR)/(MR - SR) \times 100$$

where TR (test release) represents the radioactivity released by target cells incubated with hybridoma product or ascites and complement, SR (spontaneous release) represents the radioactivity released by target cells incubated with complement alone, and MR (maximum release) is the total amount of radioactivity released by incubation of target cells with 1 ml of water.

To increase the antibody titer per unit of volume, all clones have been grown as ascites tumors in mice. Pristane-primed BALB/c mice were injected intraperitoneally with 4×10^7 cells per mouse in 300 μl of medium. The ascites fluid was collected 2 weeks after tumor inoculation. It contained antibodies which in most instances bound significantly to melanoma cells up to a dilution of 1:10,000 in the RIA. The titration curves obtained with serial dilutions of these ascites fluids for binding to IGR-3 melanoma cells are shown in Fig. 3B; BR values greater than 20 were obtained for each hybridoma product at a 1:1000 dilution. No significant binding was obtained when the same ascites fluids were tested against nonmelanoma cells.

B. COMPLEMENT-DEPENDENT CYTOTOXICITY REACTIVITY OF MONOCLONAL ANTIBODIES

The reactivity of the antibodies from the nine selected hybridoma antimelanomas and from the three selected hybridoma antigliomas was tested by CDC on ^{51}Cr-labeled target cells using ascites fluid from each clone at a 1:1000 dilution in the presence of fresh rabbit serum as a source of complement. The results obtained are summarized in Table X. Each hybridoma product was tested against seven melanoma cell lines, three glioma lines, and three neuroblastoma lines. The results are expressed as percentage of specific lysis of ^{51}Cr-labeled target cells. None of the three

TABLE X
CYTOTOXIC ACTIVITY OF HYBRIDOMA ANTIMELANOMA AND ANTIGLIOMA ANTIBODIES

Cell line used as target	Hybridoma product[a]											
	Me1-5	Me1-7	Me1-14	Me3-TB7	Me3-NE4	Me4-H3	Me4-F8	Me4-H4	Me5-D5	Gl3-BF7	Gl3-GE2	Gl3-C6
Melanomas												
IGR-3	0	0	0	57	83	0	68	0	0	0	0	0
Me43	0	0	0	34	0	0	28	0	0	0	0	0
MP-8	0	0	0	14	0	0	21	0	0	0	0	0
Mel-57	0	0	0	44	38	0	31	0	0	0	0	0
Daudel	0	0	0	28	42	0	36	0	0	0	0	0
Mel-67	0	0	0	51	75	0	48	0	0	0	0	0
Mel-2Am	0	0	0	67	52	20	46	0	0	0	0	0
Gliomas												
LN-135	0	0	0	0	68	0	0	0	0	0	0	0
LN-215	0	0	0	0	0	0	0	0	0	0	0	0
LN-18	0	0	0	0	0	0	0	0	0	0	0	0
Neuroblastomas												
IMR-32	0	0	0	0	0	0	0	0	0	0	0	0
SK-N-SM	0	0	0	0	0	0	0	0	0	0	0	0
SK-N-SH	0	0	0	0	0	0	0	0	0	0	0	0

[a] Values are expressed as percentage of specific lysis of ^{51}Cr-labeled target cells.

clones selected from the first antimelanoma fusion (Me-1) secreted cyto-lytic antibodies, while antibodies from the two clones of the third fusion (Me-3) were able to lyse labeled target cells.

A significant lysis was observed with Me3-TB7 antibodies for seven out of seven melanoma lines tested, the percentage of specific lysis varying from 34 to 67%. No significant lysis was obtained for the three gliomas and the three neuroblastomas tested, despite the fact that Me3-TB7 anti-bodies bound significantly to two of the three gliomas. Antibodies from clone Me3-NE4, shown to be directed against HLA-DR antigens, were cytolytic for all cell lines expressing DR antigens. Up to 83% specific lysis was obtained for melanoma cells (IGR-3) and 68% lysis for glioblastoma cells (LN-135). Among the three selected hybridoma products from fusion number 4, Me4-F8 antibodies were also cytolytic for seven out of seven melanoma lines tested, the percentage of cells lysed varying from 31 to 68%. However, as already observed for Me3-TB7 antibodies, Me4-F8 an-tibodies were not cytolytic for the three gliomas and three neuroblas-tomas tested, despite the fact that these antibodies bound significantly to two out of three gliomas and to three out of three neuroblastomas. Sur-prisingly, antibodies from clone Me4-H3 were cytolytic only for mela-noma cells from line Mel-2Am, while they bound to all other melanomas tested. The two hybridoma products from fusion Me-5 and the three prod-ucts from the antiglioma fusion were not cytolytic.

Representative titration curves of the three cytolytic monoclonal anti-melanoma antibodies tested on IGR-3 melanoma are shown in Fig. 9A. More than 50% of the labeled target cells were lysed at a 1:1000 dilution for all ascites fluids tested, and even at 1:20,000 a significant percentage of lysed cells was obtained. The three cytolytic antimelanoma antibodies (Me3-TB7, Me3-NE4, and Me4-F8) belong to the IgG_2 subclass which is known to fix complement. However, it should be noted that two monoclo-nal antibodies, one of the IgG_2 subclass (Me1-14) and one of the IgM class (Me1-7), were not cytolytic even at high concentrations at which they gave significant binding to melanoma target cells. These results indicate that the accepted belief that IgG_2 and IgM antibodies are cytolytic in the presence of complement does not always hold for monoclonal antibodies. Furthermore, it is surprising that two monoclonal antimelanoma anti-bodies of the IgG_2 subclass (Me3-TB7 and Me4-F8) which are strongly cy-totoxic for melanoma cells are unable to lyse either glioma or neuroblas-toma cells, despite the fact that they display significant binding to several of these types of tumor cell lines (Table VII). This lack of cytotoxicity of antimelanoma antibodies for glioma cells does not seem to be due to a par-ticular resistance to lysis by complement of glioma cells, since at least one

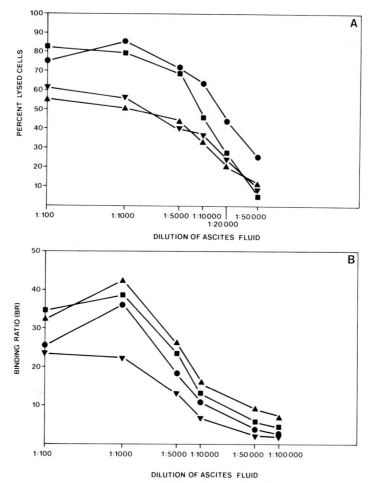

FIG. 9. (A) Cytotoxic activity of monoclonal antimelanoma antibodies against ^{51}Cr-labeled IGR-3 melanoma target cells. Ascites fluid of the different hybridomas was serially diluted with RPMI 1640 medium containing 10% FCS. Results are given as percentage specific lysis of target cells. Monoclonal antimelanoma antibodies: Me3-NE4 (■——■), Me3-TB7 (▲——▲), and Me4-F8 (▼——▼). Monoclonal anti-Ia antibodies: D1-12 (●——●). (B) Binding assay of monoclonal antimelanoma antibodies to IGR-3 target cells. Ascites fluid of the various hybridomas was serially diluted. Results are expressed as binding radio in RIA as described in Section II,E. The test was done with 5×10^4 target cells. Monoclonal antimelanoma antibodies: Me1-5 (■——■), Me1-7 (▼——▼), and Me1-14 (▲——▲). Monoclonal antiglioma antibodies: Gl3-C6 (●——●).

of these cell lines which expressed HLA-DR antigens (LN-135) was significantly lysed by the antibodies directed against this antigen (Me3-NE4).

C. ANALYSIS OF MELANOMA ANTIGENS BY FLUORESCENT-ACTIVATED CELL SORTER

The cellular expression of the antigens defined by four different anti-melanoma antibodies (Me1-5, Me1-14, Me3-TB7, and Me4-F8) has been analyzed by a fluorescent-activated cell sorter (FACS II, Becton Dickinson, Los Angeles, California). Figure 10A shows a representative fluorescence pattern obtained after reacting IGR-3 melanoma cells in suspension with Me1-5 monoclonal antibodies and a fluorescein-labeled goat anti-mouse immunoglobulin. No negative cell population could be detected, suggesting that all cells from the IGR-3 line express the antigen recognized by antibodies from the Me1-5 clone. A quite similar homogeneous antigenic distribution was observed with Me1-14, Me3-TB7, and Me4-F8 antibodies (Fig. 10B, C, and D). The cellular distribution of Ia antigens on these cells has been analyzed in parallel using two different anti-Ia antibodies (D1-12 and Me3-NE4). A representative experiment is depicted in Fig. 11A and B. A bimodal distribution of the melanoma cells bearing Ia antigens was observed for both antibodies, with a small population lack-

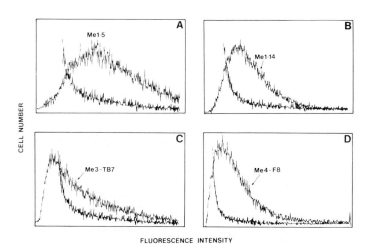

FIG. 10. Flow cytofluorometric analysis of the binding of different monoclonal antimelanoma antibodies. (A) Me1-5, (B) Me1-14, (C) Me3-TB7, (D) Me4-F8 on IGR-3 melanoma cells. The control background fluorescence staining was obtained by incubating target cells with fluorescein-labeled goat anti-mouse immunoglobulin alone. One sees that all four monoclonal antimelanoma antibodies stain the great majority of target cells.

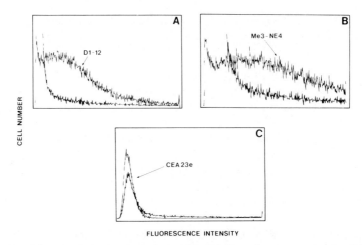

CELL NUMBER

FLUORESCENCE INTENSITY

FIG. 11. Flow cytofluorometric analysis of the binding of two monoclonal anti-Ia anti-bodies [(A) D1-12, (B) Me3-NE4] and a monoclonal anti-CEA antibody [(C) CEA-23 (negative control)] on IGR-3 melanoma cells. Background fluorescent staining was obtained by incubating cells with fluorescein-labeled goat anti-mouse immunoglobulin. One sees that there is a great heterogeneity of cell staining with anti-Ia antibodies showing a strongly positive and an entirely negative cell population.

ing expression of Ia. As a control, a monoclonal anti-CEA was included in this study. Figure 11C confirms the lack of expression of CEA on IGR-3 melanoma cells (Dent *et al.*, 1980).

VIII. Discussion

The results reported here illustrate the definite advantages of cell-fusion technology for the production of antibodies against tumor-associated antigens. While conventional xenoantisera against human tumor cells required extensive absorption to remove antibodies directed against antigens present on normal cells and contained very small amounts of antibodies with an apparent tumor specificity, our results show that the screening of a few hundred hybrids led to the selection of several clones producing antibodies with a restricted specificity for melanomas or gliomas.

Out of five fusions between spleen cells from mice immunized with crude membrane fractions of two different melanoma cell lines and cells from two different mouse myeloma cell lines, a total of 193 hybrids was obtained. Fifty-three of them secreted antibodies binding to one of the immunizing cell lines and nine of those produced antibodies reacting preferentially with melanoma cell lines. The antibodies from one of these nine selected hybrids (Me3-NE4) were also found to react with B-lymphoblastoid cell lines and were identified as having an anti-HLA-DR specificity, whereas the eight other monoclonal antibodies did not bind to the numerous nonmelanoma cell lines tested, with the notable exception of some glioma and neuroblastoma cell lines. Antibodies from six different clones (Me1-5, Me1-14, Me3-TB7, Me4-F8, Me4-H4, and Me5-D5) displayed a broad reactivity with the majority of the melanoma lines tested, indicating that they were directed against antigens widely expressed on melanoma cells corresponding to the class 2 antigens, whereas antibodies from the two other clones (Me1-7 and Me4-H3) bound to only a few melanoma lines, suggesting the existence of a second set of antigens expressed only on subpopulations of melanoma cells.

Among the 369 hybrids obtained from the three fusions of spleen cells of mice immunized with glioma cell lines, 36 hybrids produced antibodies binding to the immunizing cell line, and the antibodies from three of these hybrids reacted preferentially with glioma cells. Further specificity analysis showed that the antibodies from 2 of these clones (G13-BF7 and G13-GE2) reacted with the majority of the 13 glioma lines and with one of the nongliogenous cell lines tested, suggesting that they recognized a class 2 glioma-associated antigen. In contrast, the antibodies from the third clone (Gl3-C6) bound to only half of the glioma lines but also reacted with the majority of the melanoma and one of the neuroblastoma lines tested.

Since it is generally accepted that melanomas as well as gliomas and neuroblastomas are derived from cells originating from the neural crest, it was logical to consider that both the monoclonal antimelanoma antibodies cross-reacting with gliomas and neuroblastomas and the monoclonal antiglioma antibodies cross-reacting with melanomas were all directed against common early differentiation antigens. Therefore, the reactivity spectrum of the six monoclonal antibodies which may define these neuroectodermal antigens was the subject of a special analysis on several melanoma, glioma, and neuroblastoma cell lines. The results showed that the antibodies from each of these clones had a different pattern of reactivity toward the different cell lines, indicating that the antigenic determinants detected by these antibodies were not associated with the same antigen. These results suggest the existence of at least six different antigenic molecules expressed on several tumor cell lines of the same embryologic origin. In addition to their different patterns of reactivity toward the different tumor cell lines, each of the monoclonal antibodies was also shown by reciprocal binding experiments to be directed against a different antigenic determinant present on the cells of a given cell line. In each case, the binding of ^{3}H-labeled antibodies from one clone was inhibited only by cold antibodies from the same clone.

The close relationship between glial cells and melanocytes has also been demonstrated recently by Gaynor *et al.* (1980), who showed that a typical marker of the glial cells, the S-100 protein, was also present on cells from melanoma lines. Kennett and Gilbert (1979) showed that a monoclonal antibody against neuroblastoma cells also reacted with glioma cells and fetal brain, but there was no information about a possible reactivity of this monoclonal antibody with melanoma cells. In addition, several of the monoclonal antimelanoma antibodies described by Steplewski *et al.* (1979) and Dippold *et al.* (1980) also reacted with astrocytomas.

After the discussion of these interesting cross-reactions between melanomas, gliomas, and neuroblastomas, one should also stress some additional evidence for the tissue specificity of the different monoclonal antibodies which was obtained by quantitative adsorptions. These experiments are important since, if one relies entirely on binding tests, one could always argue that the tumor-associated antigens might be expressed on the different control cell lines but at a lower density than is detectable in the binding test. In adsorption experiments, however, we could show that up to 1.6×10^7 colon carcinoma or endometrial carcinoma cells were unable to inhibit the binding to melanoma cells of 100 μl of culture fluid from antimelanoma clones, whereas the binding of the same antibody was inhibited by 2.5×10^5 cells from different melanoma lines. Similar results were obtained with the two most specific antiglioma clones whose binding to glioma cells was inhibited only by gliomas. In addition, the antiglioma antibodies which cross-reacted with melanomas were entirely inhibited in their binding to gliomas by absorption with melanoma cells.

Concerning the cytolytic activity of the monoclonal antibodies for the tumor cells in the presence of complement, we were not surprised to observe that all the antibodies of the IgG_1 subclasses were not cytolytic and that some antibodies of the IgG_2 subclass were active in cytotoxicity tests. However, two monoclonal antimelanoma antibodies, one of the IgM class and one of the IgG_2 subclass, which were expected to be cytolytic gave entirely negative results in the complement-dependent cytotoxicity test against melanoma cells, despite the fact that in the binding assay they gave as high values as the cytolytic clone on the same target cells. This failure to induce CDC may be due to the fact that monoclonal antibodies usually react with a single antigenic determinant on each antigenic molecule. Thus, in the case of antigens with relatively low density, there is not enough IgG in close proximity to provoke the fixation of the C1q component of complement.

A more surprising observation was that two monoclonal antimelanoma antibodies, both of the IgG_2 subclass, which gave rather high binding both on melanoma and glioblastoma target cells were strongly cytolytic on melanoma cells and not cytolytic on glioma cells. Again the failure to provoke CDC on gliomas may be due to a lower density of the antigenic determinant on the glioma than on the melanoma cells. A second explanation for the discrepancy of CDC activity of the same antibodies on different tumor cells could be that the relevant antigenic determinants are localized on different carrier molecules in the two cell types. Then, one would have to assume that the carrier molecule in the glioma cells would be more external on the cell membrane, thus preventing the damage provoked by activated complement. Finally, a third explanation for this phenomenon could be that the antigenic determinants present on the different tumor cells are similar but not identical. Thus, in spite of their monoclonality, the antibodies would have more affinity for the antigenic determinants present on the immunizing tumor cells and they would only cross-react with the similar determinants present on glioma cell lines. This type of dissection of the reactivity toward unknown antigens present on different cell types has been possible only because of the use of monoclonal antibodies.

To determine which of the three proposed explanations for the cytotoxicity results is correct, the affinity of the antibodies for the different tumor cells will have to be measured and the antigens immunoprecipitated by these monoclonal antibodies will have to be characterized. Preliminary results showed that the antigens recognized by most of our monoclonal antibodies consisted of proteins, since treatment of the cells with proteolytic enzymes markedly decreased the binding of the antibodies. We also know from the specificity analysis that not one of our selected monoclonal antibodies was directed against gp95 or gp97 (Dippold *et al.*, 1980; Brown *et al.*, 1981) since our antibodies had a more restricted reactivity for melanomas and gliomas than the anti-gp95 or -gp97 antibodies. Until now, however, using most of the modern methods to radiolabel and analyze cell surface proteins, including biosynthetic labeling, we have not been able to characterize precisely the antigens detected by our monoclonal antibodies. The only proteins which were easily immunoprecipitated from the extract of some melanomas and gliomas were the two chains of the Ia antigen which served as excellent positive controls.

The analysis by the fluorescent-activated cell sorter of the antigens identified by four of our antimelanoma antibodies showed that these antigens are expressed on almost all cells from the melanoma cell line IGR-3. Despite the preliminary nature of these experiments, which should be completed with the analysis of different cell lines and cells from recently resected melanomas, these results are encouraging for those who hope to use such monoclonal antibodies for immunodiagnosis or immunotherapy. The fact that the great majority of cells from a cell line which was established 8 years ago and which has not been recloned during the last 4 years express antigens identified by four of our monoclonal antibodies suggests that these antigens are highly conserved in melanoma cells and may play an important role in the biology of these tumor cells.

ACKNOWLEDGMENTS

We thank Prof. J.-C. Cerottini for advice and suggestions, Dr. P. Sekaly for performing the cell-sorter analysis, and Dr. A. Kelso for reviewing the manuscript. The excellent technical assistance of Mrs. S. Salvi and E. Duruz is deeply appreciated.

REFERENCES

Accolla, R. S., Carrel, S., and Mach, J.-P. (1980). *Proc. Natl. Acad. Sci. U.S.A.* **77**, 563–566.
Aubert, C. H., Lagrange, C., Rorsman, H., and Rosengre, E. (1976). *Eur. J. Cancer* **12**, 441–445.
Brown, J. P., Woodburg, R. G., Hart, C. E., Hellström, I., and Hellström, K. E. (1981). *Proc. Natl. Acad. Sci. U.S.A.* **78**, 539–543.
Brunner, K. T., Mauel, J., Cerottini, J.-C., and Chapuis, B. (1968). *Immunology* **14**, 181–196.
Bystryn, J. C. (1977). *J. Natl. Cancer Inst.* **59**, 325–328.
Carey, T. E., Takahashi, T., Resnick, L. A., Oettgen, H. F., and Old, L. J. (1976). *Proc. Natl. Acad. Sci. U.S.A.* **73**, 3278–3282.
Carrel, S., and Theilkaes, L. (1973). *Nature (London)* **242**, 609–610.
Carrel, S., Delisle, M.-C., and Mach, J.-P. (1977). *Cancer Res.* **37**, 2644–2650.
Carrel, S., Gross, N., Heumann, D., and Mach, J.-P. (1979). *Transplantation* **27**, 431–433.
Carrel, S., Dent, P. B., and Liao, S. K. (1980a). *Cancer Immunol. Immunother.* **8**, 192–203.
Carrel, S., Accolla, R. S., Carmagnola, A. L., and Mach, J.-P. (1980b). *Cancer Res.* **40**, 2523–2528.
Carrel, S., Tosi, R., Gross, N., Tanigaki, N., Carmagnola, A. L., and Accolla, R. S. (1981). *Mol. Immunol.* **18**, 403–411.
Coakham, H. (1974). *Nature (London)* **250**, 328–332.
Coakham, H. R., Kornblith, P. L., Quindlen, E. A., Pollock, L. A., Wood, W. C., and Hastnett, L. C. (1980). *J. Natl. Cancer Inst.* **64**, 223–239.
Cornain, S., De Vries, J. E., Collard, J., Vennegoor, C., van Wingarden, I., and Rümke, P. H. (1975). *Int. J. Cancer* **16**, 981–997.
Cowan, N. J., Secher, D. S., and Milstein, C. (1974). *J. Mol. Biol.* **90**, 697–701.
Deng, C., El-Awar, N., Cicciarella, J., Terasaki, P. I., Billing, R., and Lagasse, L. (1981). *Lancet* **14**, 403–405.
Dent, P. B., Carrel, S., and Mach, J.-P. (1980). *J. Natl. Cancer Inst.* **64**, 309–316.
Dippold, W. G., Lloyd, K. O., Li, T. C., Ikeda, H., Oettgen, H. F., and Old, L. J. (1980). *Proc. Natl. Acad. Sci. U.S.A.* **77**, 6114–6118.
Diserens, A.-C., de Tribolet, N., Martin-Achard, A., Gaide, A. C., Schnegg, J.-F., and Carrel, S. (1981). *Acta Neuropathol.* **53**, 21–28.
Ferrone, S., and Pellegrino, M. A. (1977). *J. Natl. Cancer Inst.* **58**, 1201–1204.

Fritze, D., Kern, D. H., Drogemuller, C. R., and Pilch, Y. H. (1976). *Cancer Res.* **36,** 458–466.

Gaynor, R., Irie, R., Morton, D., and Herschman, H. R. (1980). *Nature (London)* **286,** 400–401.

Gupta, R. K., and Morton, D. L. (1975). *Cancer Res.* **35,** 58–62.

Herlyn, M., Steplewski, Z., Herlyn, D., and Koprowski, H. (1979). *Proc. Natl. Acad. Sci. U.S.A.* **76,** 1438–1442.

Hersey, P., Honeyman, M., Edwards, A., Adams, E., and McCarthy, W. H. (1976). *Int. J. Cancer* **18,** 564–573.

Imai, K., Ng, A.-K., and Ferrone, S. (1981). *J. Natl. Cancer Inst.* **66,** 489–496.

Kennett, R. H., and Gilbert, F. (1979). *Science* **203,** 1120–1121.

Klinman, N. R. (1972). *J. Exp. Med.* **136,** 241–260.

Köhler, G., and Milstein, C. (1975). *Nature (London)* **256,** 495–497.

Köhler, G., Howe, S. C., and Milstein, C. (1976). *Eur. J. Immunol.* **6,** 292–295.

Koprowski, H., Steplewski, Z., Herlyn, D., and Herlyn, M. (1978). *Proc. Natl. Acad. Sci. U.S.A.* **75,** 3405–3409.

Lewis, M. G., Ikonopisov, R. L., Nairn, R. C., Phillips, T. M., Fairley, G. H., Bodenham, D. C., and Alexander, P. (1969). *Br. Med. J.* **3,** 547–552.

Liao, S. K., Leong, S. P. L., Sutherland, C. M., Dent, P. B., Kwong, P. C., and Krementz, E. T. (1978). *Cancer Res.* **38,** 4394–4399.

Liao, S. K., Kwong, P. C., Thompson, J. C., and Dent, P. B. (1979). *Cancer Res.* **39,** 183–192.

Lozzio, C. B., and Lozzio, B. B. (1975). *Blood* **45,** 321–334.

McCabe, R. P., Ferrone, S., Pellegrino, M. A., Kern, D. H., Holmes, E. C., and Reisfeld, R. A. (1978). *J. Natl. Cancer Inst.* **60,** 773–777.

Metzgar, R. S., Bergoc, P. M., Moreno, M. Y., and Seigler, H. F. (1973). *J. Natl. Cancer Inst.* **50,** 1065–1068.

Morgan, A. C., Galloway, D. R., Imai, K., and Reisfeld, R. A. (1981). *J. Immunol.* **126,** 365–370.

Morton, D. L., Malmgreen, R. A., Holmes, E. C., and Ketcham, A. S. (1968). *Surgery* **64,** 233–240.

Muna, N. M., Marcus, S., and Smart, C. (1969). *Cancer* **23,** 88–95.

Pfreundschuh, M., Shiku, H., Takahashi, T., Ueda, R., Ransohoff, J., Oettgen, H. F., and Old, L. J. (1978). *Proc. Natl. Acad. Sci. U.S.A.* **75,** 5122–5126.

Pontecorvo, G. (1975). *Somatic Cell Genet.* **1,** 397–400.

Schlom, J., Wunderlich, D., and Teramoto, Y. A. (1980). *Proc. Natl. Acad. Sci. U.S.A.* **11,** 6841–6845.

Schmidt-Ulrich, R., Ferber, E., Knuefermann, H., Fischer, H., and Hoelzl-Wallach, D. F. (1974). *Biochim. Biophys. Acta* **332,** 175–191.

Schnegg, J. F., Diserens, A. C., Carrel, S., and de Tribolet, N. (1981). *Cancer Res.* **41,** 1209–1213.

Shiku, H., Takahashi, T., Oettgen, H. F., and Old, L. J. (1976). *J. Exp. Med.* **144,** 873–881.

Shiku, H., Takahashi, T., Oettgen, H. F., and Old, L. J. (1977). *J. Exp. Med.* **145,** 784–789.

Sorg, C., Brüggen, J., Seibert, E., and Macher, E. (1978). *Cancer Immunol. Immunother.* **3,** 259–271.

Steplewski, Z., Herlyn, M., Herlyn, D., Clark, W., and Koprowski, H. (1979). *Eur. J. Immunol.* **9,** 94–96.

Stuhlmiller, G. M., and Seigler, H. F. (1975). *Cancer Res.* **35,** 2132–2137.

Viza, D., and Phillips, J. (1975). *Int. J. Cancer* **16,** 312–317.

Williams, A. F. (1977). *Contemp. Top. Mol. Immunol.* **6,** 93–116.

Wilson, B. S., Indiveri, F., Pellegrino, M. A., and Ferrone, S. (1979). *J. Exp. Med.* **149,** 658–668.

Winchester, R. J., Wang, C., Gibofsky, A., Kunkel, H. G., Lloyd, K. O., and Old, L. J. (1978). *Proc. Natl. Acad. Sci. U.S.A.* **75,** 6235–6239.

Woodbury, R. G., Brown, J. P., Yeh, M. X., Hellström, I., and Hellström, K. E. (1980). *Proc. Natl. Acad. Sci. U.S.A.* **77,** 2183–2187.

Yeh, M. Y., Hellström, I., Brown, J. P., Warner, G. A., Hansen, J. A., and Hellström, K. E. (1979). *Proc. Natl. Acad. Sci. U.S.A.* **76,** 2927–2931.

Zardi, L., Carnemolla, B., Siri, A., Santi, L., and Accolla, R. S. (1980). *Int. J. Cancer* **25,** 325–328.

CHAPTER X

CELL SURFACE CHANGES IN MALIGNANCY

ROGER H. KENNETT, ZDENKA L. JONAK,
AND REBECCA BYRD

I. Focus on the Tumor Cell Surface

The cell surface has often been a focal point in studies of molecular changes associated with malignancy. The rationales for such studies usually include the following:

1. Molecules involved in cell–cell interactions and growth control regulation in response to external signals are likely to be expressed on cell surface membranes.

2. Certain tumor viruses identified in animal systems do affect alteration of cell surface structure and composition (De Leo *et al.*, 1979; Simrell and Klein, 1979; Strand, 1980).

3. Both qualitative and quantitative differences in cell-surface molecules have been detected in several cases in which tumor cells were compared to the normal cells from which the malignant cells were apparently derived (Weiss, 1980; Black, 1980; Hakomori, 1975).

A. TYPES OF CELL SURFACE ALTERATIONS

There are a variety of ways in which the plasma membranes of tumor cells may differ from the normal cells to which they are compared (Table

TABLE I

POSSIBLE MECHANISMS OF CELL SURFACE ALTERATIONS IN TUMOR CELLS

1. Expression of viral antigens
2. Expression of a "mutant" form of a normal molecule
3. Abnormal expression of normal differentiation antigens, such as fetal antigens. Expression out of normal context or increased expression due to increase in the number of genes or rate of transcription
4. Uncovering of "new" antigenic determinants on normal antigens resulting from a rearrangement or modification (i.e., phosphorylation) of the molecule—probably a secondary change resulting from other changes in cell surface composition
5. Alteration of a cell surface receptor so that it does not receive a message involved in control of cell growth and/or differentiation; similarly, an alteration in an enzyme active site with resulting alteration in specificity or activity[a]
6. Loss of expression of a cell surface molecule

[a] Neither of these cases would necessarily involve the appearance of new antigenic determinants.

I). These differences may be detected initially by biochemical or immunological means, with antigenic differences being detected either by serum antibodies or by cellular reactions against the tumor cells. Each of these alterations could, in fact, be a secondary effect of the malignant phenotype. They could represent changes that have taken place during the expansion of the tumor and might not necessarily be directly related to the genetic event that produced the initial tumor phenotype. They may be related to characteristics of increased metastasis or invasiveness rather than the initial stages of malignancy (Fidler and Kripke, 1977; Brunson and Nicholson, 1978). Although such ambiguity does exist initially, identifying and characterizing such changes are essential steps in understanding the molecular basis of tumor development.

One type of molecule that may initially appear to be tumor specific is a normal differentiation antigen characteristic of the stage of cellular differentiation represented by the tumor cell. This may result from the fact that normally cells at this stage of differentiation are present in extremely low numbers, and expansion of the malignant clones makes it "visible" and eventually even predominant. Detection of cell surface antigens expressed on mitotic or rapidly dividing cells would also fall into this category (Judd *et al.*, 1980).

It is only by continuing both to identify malignant–nonmalignant cell surface differences and to analyze the molecular-genetic basis for these differences that we will come to an understanding of the real significance of the cell surface changes detected in malignancy. This should make it possible to define which, if any, are really directly related to the changes that take place when a cell crosses over the boundaries of controlled growth into the category of being a malignant tumor.

B. Possible Genetic Mechanisms

For those cell surface alterations which are likely to be related to the primary cause of the malignant phenotype, there are, in general, two possible genetic mechanisms: introduction of foreign genetic material into the cell (i.e., viral infection) and alteration in the structure and/or expression of genetic material present in the germ line genome. Changes in the second category may result from classical mutations in structural or even regulatory genes which affect mechanisms of growth control, or possibly even from "mutations" that result from mistakes taking place during the rearrangement of genetic material involved in the normal expression of eukaryotic genes—similar to those described recently in the case of immunoglobulin genes (Maki *et al.*, 1980; Davis *et al.*, 1980). It is possible that such rearrangements of DNA may be involved in the expression of other families of genes during cellular differentiation and that the malfunction of normal genetic mechanisms may result in the formation of a cellular phenotype which is no longer responsive to normal control mechanisms and which continues to divide rather than to proceed down the normal differentiation pathway. Application of molecular-genetic techniques (Abelson, 1980; Maniatis, 1980), which have elucidated some mechanisms of eukaryotic gene expression, to the study of possible abnormal gene expression in malignant cells should soon make it possible to define tumor–normal cell differences at the level of the genetic material.

II. Practical Applications of Detecting Tumor–Normal Cell Differences

Definition of cell surface changes related to the malignant phenotype has implications not only for our understanding of the mechanisms involved in the induction of malignancy and of the relationship between cancer cells and immune surveillance, but also potentially for providing practical tests for detecting tumor cells at early stages of malignancy and for monitoring the effectiveness of treatment regimens. Antibodies defining antigens apparently specific for tumor cells can be applied to many procedures for the detection or treatment of tumors (Table II). In some cases it is not necessary that the antigen detected be related to the malignant phenotype or be truly tumor specific (i.e., the product of a new gene

TABLE II
POTENTIAL PRACTICAL APPLICATIONS OF ANTIBODIES TO TUMOR ANTIGENS

Application	Reference
Tumor identification	
Diagnosis	Greaves *et al.* (1980); Bradstock *et al.* (1980); Koprowski *et al.* (1981); Janossy *et al.* (1980)
Detection of metastasis	Kennett *et al.* (1980); Levine *et al.* (1980); S. Brown *et al.* (1980); Kennett *et al.* (1981)
Immunotherapy	
Cytolytic antibodies	Bernstein *et al.* (1980); Herlyn *et al.* (1980); Nadler *et al.* (1980)
Antibodies with attached drugs or cytotoxic agents	Gilliland *et al.* (1980); Krolick *et al.* (1980); Youle and Neville (1980)

not expressed in any normal cells). It is sufficient that the number of normal cells expressing the antigen be small enough, under the conditions of the test, to allow specific discrimination or treatment of the tumor cells. In the case of fetal antigens expressed by tumor cells in an adult, for example, the antigen would not be truly "tumor specific," but would in effect be "operationally tumor specific." R. Levy and his collaborators (S. Brown *et al.*, 1980) have also shown that antiidiotypic antibodies against the cell surface immunoglobulin on human B-lymphomas can be used to detect tumor cells. In this case also the molecule detected is not specific for tumor cells, but the antigenic determinants are on a limited number of normal cells and thus can be used as "tumor-specific markers." These antiidiotypic antibodies have recently been used to effectively treat a patient with B-cell lymphoma (Miller *et al.*, 1982).

III. Do Tumor-Specific Antigens Really Exist?

In spite of the large amount of work done on the characterization of "tumor-specific" or "tumor-associated" antigens, it is still not clear whether there is any direct relationship between observed cell surface changes and the primary event(s) resulting in the malignant phenotype. Of those possible mechanisms of cell surface alteration listed in Table I, only the first four would necessarily result in new antigenic determinants being expressed on the cell surface. The other two cases, on the other hand, would not be detected by experiments designed to detect tumor-associated or tumor-specific antigens. To cover this range of possible mechanisms fully will take an integrated effort involving the application of both immunological and molecular-genetic techniques to a variety of models and tumor cell systems.

Two recent advances in "biotechnology"—monoclonal antibodies and recombinant DNA—have made it potentially possible to analyze the molecular changes in gene products on the cell surface and in the genetic material from which these products are expressed. Although we will not discuss it here, the production of long-term cultures of specific T-cell lines that react against tumors (Gillis and Smith, 1977) also has great potential for defining cell surface changes in malignant cells.

Various aspects of cell surface changes in malignancy have been well reviewed (Ruddon, 1978; Hakomori, 1975; Black, 1980; Hunter, 1980; Hynes, 1980). Rather than duplicate this approach, we would like to discuss the application of these new techniques to the analysis of cell surface changes in malignancy. We will outline the exciting potential for a clearer understanding of the genetic and molecular basis of malignancy that exists now that these techniques facilitate a more discriminating and thorough analysis of genes and gene products.

IV. Application of Monoclonal Antibodies to the Analysis of Tumor Cell Surfaces

One of the difficulties in defining and characterizing antigens on the surface of tumor cells has been the inherent heterogeneity of the classical antisera by which the presence of these molecules has been detected. Antisera were often, of necessity, made in species other than that from which the tumor was derived and then rendered "specific" by absorbing out the antibodies that reacted with cells other than the tumor cells. The antibodies remaining in the antisera were often reactive against more than one antigen and, because there were antibodies of several affinities and classes present, the antisera could exhibit various specificities depending on the particular assay conditions employed. A second limiting factor was that such antisera were often available in limited amounts once they had been sufficiently absorbed and characterized.

The problems of antibody heterogeneity and limited supply have been, for the most part, alleviated by the development of methods for the production of monoclonal antibodies. Since Köhler and Milstein's (1975) original observation, this method of antibody production has been used in a wide variety of applications. The method is particularly useful for the detection of cell surface antigens because one can immunize with the complex collection of molecules that make up the cell surface and produce an antibody that detects, and that can often be used to isolate, one of the components in this mixture. Once such an antibody is produced and characterized, it can be made available to other investigators in significant quantities. They can then confirm previous results and use the standardized reagents in other experimental and clinical situations.

A. DETECTION OF TUMOR-ASSOCIATED ANTIGENS

Monoclonal antibodies made against a variety of tumors have been described (Table III). Whether any of the antigens are in a strict sense "tumor specific" remains to be determined by showing that the molecule is produced from genetic material present in the tumor cells but not in the normal cells from the same individual. An even more stringent criterion would be that the expression of the antigen is directly related to the malignant phenotype and not simply a secondary result of the neoplasia. The possibility that the antigen detected on the tumor cells is expressed on

TABLE III
MONOCLONAL ANTIBODIES AGAINST TUMOR-ASSOCIATED ANTIGENS

Species	Tumor	Reference
Human	Melanoma	Koprowski *et al.* (1978); Imai *et al.* (1980); J. P. Brown *et al.* (1980); Carrel *et al.* (1980); Dippold *et al.* (1980); Mitchell *et al.* (1980); Burk *et al.* (1980)
	Colon carcinoma	Koprowski *et al.* (1979, 1981)
	Neuroblastoma	Kennett and Gilbert (1979)
	Leukemia	Levy *et al.* (1978); Ritz *et al.* (1980); Janossy *et al.* (1980); Bradstock *et al.* (1980); Morstyn *et al.* (1981); Kersey *et al.* (1981)
	Lymphoma	S. Brown *et al.* (1980); Nadler *et al.* (1980)
	Lung cancer cells	Cuttitta *et al.* (1981)
	Glioma	Schnegg *et al.* (1981)
	Mammary carcinoma	Schlom *et al.* (1980) (human antibody)
	α-Fetoprotein	Tsung *et al.* (1980); Votila and Ruoslahti (1980)
	Carcinoembryonic antigen	Mitchell (1980); Accolla *et al.* (1980)
Rodent	Teratocarcinoma	Goodfellow *et al.* (1979)
	Fibrosarcoma	Simrell and Klein (1979)
	Sarcoma	Lennox *et al.* (1980)
	Mammary carcinoma	Gunn *et al.* (1980); Tax and Manson (1980)
	DBA-2 lymphoma	Fuji (1980)
	SV40 tumor antigen	Martinis and Croce (1978)
	RNA tumor-virus antigens	Strand (1980)

fetal cells or on some minor population of normal cells at some state of tissue differentiation is not easily excluded in most cases.

In our laboratory we developed a monoclonal antibody, PI153/3, against human neuroblastoma cells (Kennett and Gilbert, 1979). Initial screening against a panel of human cell types indicated that the antigen was expressed on tumors derived from neuroectoderm and on fetal brain, but was not detectable on other normal human tissues, including adult brain. The antigenic distribution suggested that the antibody could be used to detect neuroblastoma cells in bone marrow aspirates. In the process of detecting antigen-positive cells in marrow, it was determined in a control marrow that the PI153/3 antibody also reacted with leukemic cells (Kennett *et al.*, 1980). Further analysis indicated that the antigenic determinant was expressed on B-cell and null-cell, but not on T-cell leukemias. This makes it a useful reagent for classifying leukemia cells, an important factor in determining what course of antileukemia therapy to employ (Greaves *et al.*, 1980). Since the antibody reacted with leukemia cells, it also suggested that detection of neuroblastoma cells could possibly be complicated by reactions of PI153/3 with lymphocytes at some stages of lymphoid differentiation. To be certain that cells detected in the marrow of neuroblastoma patients were truly tumor cells, we employed a second antibody that reacts with lymphocytes but not neuroblastoma cells. We thus could distinguish between neuroblastomas (PI153/3 positive/anti-lymphocyte negative) and immature lymphocytes (PI153/3[+]/anti-lymphocyte[+]) (Kennett *et al.*, 1981). Biochemical analysis of the antigen detected by PI153/3 indicated that it is a glycoprotein (Momoi *et al.*, 1980). Whether the glycoprotein is the same on both neuroblastoma and leukemia cells has not been determined. It could be two different molecules sharing a similar or identical antigenic determinant.

Because monoclonal antibodies react with single antigenic determinants, and such determinants can appear on different molecules, one cannot assume that on a given cell type only one molecule is being detected or that reaction with different cell types indicates that the same molecule is expressed on both cell types. Such conclusions must be based on isolation of the antigen(s) involved and biochemical characterization of the molecules. Even with these cautions and reservations in mind, this new technology has made it possible to detect tumor antigens which, for all practical purposes with regard to the detection of tumor cells, are tumor specific. Some of the antibodies referenced in Table III appear, at this point, to be tumor specific. Koprowski *et al.* (1981) have defined a colon carcinoma antigen which is a monosialoganglioside expressed on the surface of the tumor cells and which can be detected in the serum of patients with colon carcinoma (Magnani *et al.*, 1981). Several groups

(Table III) have detected antigens on human melanoma cells which have not been detected on other normal cells tested. Although any or all of these may, upon further testing, turn out to be differentiation antigens detected because of clonal expansion of the tumor cells, it is clear that some of these antibodies will be useful for the detection of tumor cells. Continued application of hybridoma technology to the analysis of antigens on tumor cell surfaces will certainly facilitate the detection of those alterations of tumor cell surfaces that fall into categories 1–4 in Table I.

Recent reports indicate that human monoclonal antibodies can be generated by fusion of human lymphocytes with mouse or human plasmacytoma lines (Schlom *et al.*, 1980; Nowinski *et al.*, 1980; Olson and Kaplan, 1980; Croce *et al.*, 1980). This makes it likely that in the near future it will be possible to analyze the humoral immune response against tumor cells by fusing a patient's normal lymphocytes with a plasmacytoma line. Production of human monoclonal antibodies should also facilitate the use of antibodies for therapy *in vivo*, even taking into consideration, of course, the potential dangers of injecting a patient with the product of a malignant cell line. Adaptation of *in vitro* mouse immunization–hybridoma-production techniques (Luben and Mohler, 1980) to human lymphocyte systems should also facilitate the production of human monoclonal antibodies against human tumor cell antigens.

B. ANALYSIS OF ALTERED CELL SURFACE RECEPTORS OR ENZYMES

It is possible that there may be alterations in cell surface molecules not recognized as tumor–normal antigenic differences even when antibodies are made in a species other than that of the tumor's origin. For example, the active site of a cell surface receptor or of an enzyme could be altered by a mutation that affects its function without producing a significant change in the configuration of the amino acid residues at the surface of the protein; any antibodies made against the molecule on the tumor cells would react with the molecules on the corresponding normal cells. Making antibodies against the tumor and screening on normal cells would not, in this case, indicate which molecules on the surface would possibly be related to the malignant phenotype. Nevertheless, the ability to make monoclonal antibodies that react with individual determinants provides a way to identify cell surface molecules involved in the regulation of growth control and which therefore possibly play a role in the mechanisms of malignant cell growth.

One can propose a model in which a cell surface receptor normally receives a molecular signal telling a cell to "stop dividing and differentiate." On the tumor cell, this receptor could be modified so that it does not receive this message properly. If one makes monoclonal antibodies against the full array of molecules on the tumor cell in question, some of these may react with this receptor and mimic the effect of the normal growth control messenger.

Such an approach can be based on the observation that antibodies against insulin receptors can mimic the effects of insulin (Kahn *et al.*, 1977; Kasuga *et al.*, 1978). Beachy and Czech (1980) have shown that this effect can be produced with monoclonal antibodies. The advantage of using monoclonal antibodies rather than antisera is that one can be more certain that the antibody is reacting with a single cell surface molecule and that the effect is not a secondary result of an antibody reacting with, and aggregating combinations of, molecules on the cell surface. Also, there will be enough of the antibody to do sufficient characterization of the effect on cell proliferation and for isolation of the cell surface molecule involved.

Our initial screenings of monoclonal antibodies against the non-B, non-T acute lymphoblastic leukemia cell line Reh has shown that monoclonal antibodies can be detected that inhibit the proliferation of these cells, as measured by [^{3}H]thymidine incorporation (Kennett *et al.*, 1981).

McGrath *et al.* (1980) have also reported monoclonal antibodies that inhibit the proliferation of a mouse lymphoma cell line. They interpreted this on the basis of a model involving the antibody inhibiting the attachment of a virus to cell surface antigens.

The initial results in both of these cases indicate that monoclonal antibodies against tumor cell surface molecules that are not tumor specific may, in fact, be against cell surface molecules that play a role in tumor cell proliferation. Further investigation along these lines could result in a better understanding of the role of certain cell surface molecules in either normal or abnormal cell growth and/or differentiation.

A second type of molecule that could be affected by the same type of structural change—a change in a binding site structure without a significant change in surface antigenic determinants—is a cell surface enzyme. An alternative mechanism that is possible in both cases is that the normal receptor or enzyme is produced, but in much larger quantities in tumor cells as opposed to normal cells. In this case there would again be no new antigenic determinants detected but only a difference in the amount of antigen present in the normal and tumor cells.

It is now clear that certain RNA tumor viruses may produce malignant changes through the action of protein kinases—enzymes which phosphorylate proteins (Hunter, 1980; Hynes, 1980). Whether the increase in phosphorylation results from an increase in the amount of the enzyme present (which does take place in some cases) or from a slight alteration in the specificity of the enzyme is not determined. In either case, since there are similar or identical protein kinases in uninfected cells, the enzyme would not necessarily be detected as a tumor-specific product. In some cases, additional phosphorylated proteins on the surface of the tumor cells may be detected as new antigenic determinants (Crawford *et al.*, 1981). These altered proteins would be "tumor-specific" antigens that would likely appear on several types of tumors but would be secondary alterations resulting from a primary change that could not easily be detected as an antigenic difference. Although there is less precedence for this case, it is possible that antibodies against the enzyme would alter or inhibit the activity of the enzyme and return the cell to a nonmalignant phenotype.

Either of the above models—receptor- or enzyme-mediated malignancy—would provide a reasonable basis for not excluding antibodies that react with normal cell surface antigens from further analysis. It may be useful to determine their effects and specificities on tumor cells. Analysis of the qualitative and quantitative distribution of "normal" molecules on tumor cells using monoclonal antibodies may, in fact, lead to further insight into how some of these molecules may be involved in abnormal and normal growth control.

C. Detection of Oncogene Products

One of the most exciting potential applications of monoclonal antibodies in the study of gene products associated with oncogenesis is a result of recent reports that human oncogenes can be transferred to NIH/3T3 mouse fibroblasts (Weinberg, 1981). DNA obtained from several human tumors has been used to transfect these mouse cells to a malignant phenotype. A small amount of human DNA can be detected in these transformed mouse cells. This provides an ideal situation for immunizing mice with these cells so that antibodies will be made against the human gene products produced by this oncogenic DNA. This system provides great potential for detecting gene products which are responsible for the property of malignancy.

V. Application of Molecular-Genetic Techniques to the Analysis of the Genetic Basis of Malignancy

It is evident that in some cases malignancy is in some way associated with the *loss* of genetic material. Most human retinoblastomas, for example, exhibit a deletion of part of chromosome 13 (Francke, 1976). Some tumors which sometimes occur in more than one member of the same family show frequencies and characteristics that indicate that two mutations are necessary for the development of a clone of tumor cells (Knudson, 1977). A simple explanation would be that it is an illustration of a recessive mutation in which the function of the alleles from both homologous chromosomes must be removed before the phenotype can be expressed. This would also be consistent with the loss of a gene product resulting in malignancy. In such cases, there would not necessarily be any new molecules expressed in tumors that were not present in normal cells. It is likely that in at least some cases the primary genetic event resulting in malignancy does correspond to the deletion or loss of expression of a normal gene product without the appearance of any new gene products.

Approaching the study of this type of tumor by characterizing the cell surface antigens is not likely to be fruitful. The only effective way would be to make antibodies against the corresponding normal cells and to characterize the loss of the gene product. Since it is often not possible to define clearly the state of normal cellular differentiation represented by the tumor and to define the molecules that would normally be present, this is not likely to be a productive approach toward describing specific changes related to malignancy. In such a situation it would probably be more useful to use molecular-genetic techniques to compare tumor cell DNA to DNA from normal cells of the same individual. One could, thus, define the specific DNA change(s) that have taken place in the tumor cells.

In this approach several precautions would have to be taken to reduce the chances of artifacts. One should use DNA from tumor cells which are at as early a stage as possible, and from normal cells (such as peripheral blood lymphocytes or fibroblasts) that have spent a minimal amount of time in culture. This is to avoid changes in the DNA that are not directly related to the change(s) that have produced the malignant phenotype. Another consideration is that, taking the expression of immunoglobulins as an example, there may be rearrangements of DNA related to the expression of differentiated gene products that result in detectable differences in DNA structure (Maki *et al.*, 1980). With this in mind, one should perhaps choose normal and tumor cells that are as closely related, with regard to differentiated phenotype, as possible, so that differences in DNA structure would be more likely related to malignancy.

The manipulation of DNA with restriction endonucleases (Nathans and Smith, 1975) has made it possible to perform analyses of DNA structure that were inconceivable a short time ago. In the past few years many laboratories have isolated segments of eukaryotic genomes by cloning them in various plasmid and phage vectors (Maniatis, 1980). Using clones of genes that are present in the haploid genome in single or a limited number of copies, it is possible to identify the fragments of DNA within a mixture of fragments of the total genome which contain the gene locus corresponding to the cloned DNA. This is usually accomplished by digesting cellular DNA with a restriction endonuclease and separating fragments of the genome by size on a gel. The cloned gene is labeled with radioactivity by nick translation (Alwine *et al.*, 1977) and is added to the fragments of DNA which have been transferred to nitrocellulose paper. The labeled, cloned DNA binds to the fragment(s) of DNA in the total digest that are complementary in structure and, after removing the unhybridized DNA, autoradiography detects the position of the DNA fragment on the paper containing the cloned gene (modified from Southern, 1975) (Fig. 1A). There are now available at least two libraries of human genomic DNA which should contain clones of all of the human genes present in the genome (Maniatis *et al.*, 1978).

As work progresses in many laboratories, the proportion of the human genome detectable by specific probes continues to increase. It has been suggested that a collection of such probes can be used to detect polymorphic variation in DNA structure between one individual and another in a population (Botstein *et al.*, 1980). Any change in DNA structure resulting in a change in the distribution of cleavage sites for a restriction endonuclease changes the size of the DNA fragments generated by the enzyme. If such a restriction site change affects the size of the DNA fragment containing the DNA for the genes corresponding to the cloned gene used as a probe, the pattern of bands in the autoradiograph will be altered (Fig. 1B). Botstein *et al.* (1980) describe how the analysis of restriction fragment length polymorphisms (RFLP) can be used to analyze polymorphic differences in DNA, as well as how these RFLPs can be used as molecular markers for other genes which are linked to them. In their discussion they calculate that it would take approximately 150 different RFLP markers chosen at random to cover the whole human genome.

Similarly, one could use cloned molecular probes representing as much of the genome as possible to compare restriction fragment digests of DNA from tumor and normal cells of the same individual. Any differences in RFLP pattern would indicate that DNA rearrangements had taken place within that region of DNA. This could be a result of mutation or of DNA rearrangements involved in gene expression during cellular differentiation. One should, of course, determine the RFLP pattern for the same probe in DNA from normal cells from some other tissue to see if the difference in the pattern was generated by a change in DNA structure in the tumor cells. Having established this the next step would be to characterize the change in the DNA and to attempt to define whether a specific gene product is produced by the affected region. This method would be

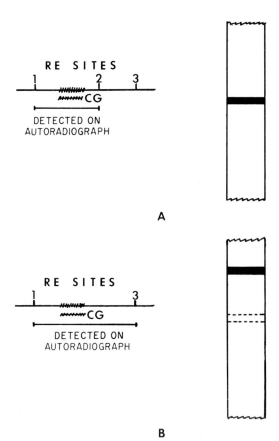

A

B

Fɪɢ. 1. Detection of changes in DNA structure by changes in the length of restriction fragments. To detect changes in specific fragments of genomic DNA one can use a combination of restriction endonucleases (RE), which cleave strands of DNA at specific sequences, and cloned genes (CG), which can be radioactively labeled and used as specific probes. The left of each figure represents the structure of the genomic DNA in the region of the cloned gene locus. The restriction enzyme cuts the DNA at various specific sites, including those near the genomic locus equivalent to the cloned gene. In the normal DNA (A) the restriction fragment detected by the CG probe is produced by cutting at sites 1 and 2. The DNA is separated by size on a gel, transferred to nitrocellulose paper, and the fragment containing the CG locus is detected by hybridizing radioactively labeled cDNA and then detecting the hybrid molecule by autoradiography. If the genomic DNA is altered near the site of the CG so that the restriction fragment is changed in size, the same experiment with altered DNA (B) will show a new radioactive band. In this example the restriction fragment is larger because a RE site (2) was removed by whatever change took place in the DNA. Alternatively, the change could have produced a smaller fragment by inserting a new restriction site between 1 and 2. If either of these took place in one eukaryotic chromosome and not in the other, then both the new (y) and the old (x) restriction fragments would be detected in the second DNA separation. By using a library of specific probes as they become available and a collection of restriction enzymes which cut at various sites, one could increase the sensitivity of the procedure so that a thorough analysis would be likely to detect tumor–normal differences as well as changes that may result from gene rearrangements during differentiation.

useful both for cases where the molecular change leading to the malignant phenotype is the loss of expression of a gene product and for cases where other types of molecular changes, as discussed previously, have taken place.

To approach the question of what cell surface changes take place in malignancy and to discover their real significance will certainly take an integrated effort. The techniques that are now available for the molecular analysis of gene expression, at both the level of the gene and at the level of specific gene products, makes it likely that we will see significant progress in this area within the next few years.

REFERENCES

Abelson, J. (1980). *Science* **209,** 1319–1321.
Accolla, R. S., Carrel, S., and Mach, J. P. (1980). *Proc. Natl. Acad. Sci. U.S.A.* **77,** 563–566.
Alwine, J. C., Kemp, D. J., and Stark, G. R. (1977). *Proc. Natl. Acad. Sci. U.S.A.* **74,** 5350–5354.
Beachy, J. C., and Czech, M. P. (1980). *J. Supramol. Struct.* **13,** 447–456.
Berstein, I. D., Tam, M. R., and Nowinski, R. C. (1980). *Science* **207,** 68–71.
Black, P. H. (1980). *Adv. Cancer Res.* **32,** 75–199.
Botstein, D., White, R. L., Skolnick, M., and Davis, R. W. (1980). *Am. J. Hum. Genet.* **32,** 314–331.
Bradstock, K. F., Janssy, G., Pizzolo, G., Hoffbrand, A. V., McMicheal, A., Pilch, J. R., Milstein, C., Beverly, P., Bollum, F. J. (1980). *J. Natl. Cancer Inst.* **65,** 33–42.
Brown, J. P., Wright, P. W., Hart, C. E., Woodbury, R. G., Hellstrom, K. E., and Hellstrom, I. (1980). *J. Biol. Chem.* **255,** 4980–4983.
Brown, S., Dilley, J., and Levy, R. (1980). *J. Immunol.* **125,** 1037–1043.
Brunson, K. W., and Nicholson, G. L. (1978). *J. Natl. Cancer Inst.* **61,** 1499–1503.
Burk, M. W., Saxton, R., Meier, S. J., and Morton, D. L. (1980). *Surg. Forum* **31,** 427–428.
Carrel, S., Accolla, R. S., Carmagnola, A. L., and Mach, J. P. (1980). *Cancer Res.* **40,** 2523–2528.
Crawford, L. V., Pim, D. C., Gurney, E. G., Goodfellow, P. N., and Taylor-Papadimitriou, J. (1981). *Proc. Natl. Acad. Sci. U.S.A.* **78,** 41–45.
Croce, C. M., Linnenbach, A., Hall, W., Steplewski, Z., and Koprowski, H. (1980). *Nature (London)* **288,** 488–489.
Cuttitta, F., Rosen, S., Gazdar, A. F., and Minna, J. D. (1981). *Proc. Natl. Acad. Sci. U.S.A.* **78,** 4591–4595.
Davis, M. M., Kim, S. K., and Hood, L. E. (1980). *Science* **209,** 1360–1365.
De Leo, A. B., Jay, G., Appella, E., Dubois, G. C., Law, L. W., and Old, L. S. (1979). *Proc. Natl. Acad. Sci. U.S.A.* **76,** 2420–2424.
Dippold, W. G., Lloyd, K. O., Li, L. T. C., Ikeda, H., Oettgen, H. F., and Old, L. J. (1980). *Proc. Natl. Acad. Sci. U.S.A.* **77,** 6114–6118.
Fidler, I. J., and Kripke, M. L. (1977). *Science* **197,** 893–895.
Francke, U. (1976). *Cytogenet. Cell Genet.* **14,** 131–134.
Fuji, H. (1980). *Transplant. Proc.* **12,** 388–390.
Gilliland, D. G., Steplewski, Z., Collier, R. J., Mitchell, K. F., Chang, T. H., and Koprowski, H. (1980). *Proc. Natl. Acad. Sci. U.S.A.* **77,** 4539–4543.

Gillis, S., and Smith, K. A. (1977). *Nature (London)*, **268**, 154–156.

Goodfellow, P. N., Levinson, J. R., Williams II, V. E., and McDevitt, H. O., (1979). *Proc. Natl. Acad. Sci. U.S.A.* **76**, 377–380.

Greaves, M., Verbi, W., Kemshead, J., and Kennett, R. (1980). *Blood* **56**, 1141–1144.

Gunn, B., Embelton, M. J., Middle, J. G., and Baldwin, R. W. (1980). *Int. J. Cancer* **26**, 325–330.

Hakomori, S. (1975). *Biochim. Biophys. Acta* **417**, 55–89.

Herlyn, D. M., Steplewski, Z., Herlyn, M. F., and Koprowski, H. (1980). *Cancer Res.* **40**, 717–721.

Hunter, T. (1980). *Cell* **22**, 647–648.

Hynes, R. O., (1980). *Cell* **21**, 601–602.

Imai, K., Molinaro, G. A., and Ferrone, S. (1980). *Transplant. Proc.* **12**, 380–383.

Janossy, G., Thomas, J. A., Pizzolo, G., Granger, S. M., McLaughlin, J., Habeshaw, J. A., Stansfeld, A. G., and Sloane, J. (1980). *Br. J. Cancer* **42**, 224–242.

Judd, W., Poodry, C. A., and Strominger, J. L. (1980). *J. Exp. Med.* **152**, 1430–1435.

Kahn, C. R., Baird, K., Flier, J. S., and Jarrett, D. B. (1977). *J. Clin. Invest.* **60**, 1094–1106.

Kasuga, M., Akanoma, Y., Tsushima, T., Suzuki, K., and Kosaka, K. (1978). *J. Clin. Endocrinol. Metab.* **47**, 66–77.

Kennett, R. H., and Gilbert, F. (1979). *Science* **203**, 1120–1121.

Kennett, R. H., Jonak, Z. L., and Bechtol, K. B. (1980). *In* "Monoclonal Antibodies" (R. H. Kennett, T. J. McKearn, and K. B. Bechtol, eds.), pp. 155–168. Plenum, New York.

Kennett, R. H., Jonak, Z. L., Bechtol, K. B., and Byrd, R. (1981). *In* "Fundamental Mechanisms in Cancer Immunology" (J. P. Saunders, J. C. Daniels, B. Serrou, C. Rosenfeld, and C. B. Denny, eds.), pp. 331–348. Elsevier, Amsterdam.

Kersey, J. H., Lebien, T. W., Abramson, C. S., Newman, R., Sutherland, R., and Greaves, M. (1981). *J. Exp. Med.* **153**, 726–731.

Knudson, A. G. (1977). *Adv. Hum. Genet.* **8**, 1–16.

Köhler, G., and Milstein, C. (1975). *Nature (London)* **256**, 495–497.

Koprowski, H., Steplewski, Z., Herlyn, D., and Herlyn, M. (1978). *Proc. Natl. Acad. Sci. U.S.A.* **75**, 3405–3409.

Koprowski, H., Steplewski, Z., Mitchell, K., Herlyn, M., Herlyn, D., and Fuhrer, P. (1979). *Somatic Cell Genet.* **5**, 957–972.

Koprowski, H., Herlyn, J., Steplewski, Z., and Sears, H. F. (1981). *Science* **212**, 53–55.

Krolick, K. A., Villemez, C., Isakson, P., Uhr, J. W., and Vitetta, E. S. (1980). *Proc. Natl. Acad. Sci. U.S.A.* **77**, 5419–5423.

Lennox, E., Cohn, J., and Lowe, T. (1980). *Transplant. Proc.* **12**, 95–98.

Levine, G., Ballou, B., Reiland, J., Solter, D., Gumerman, L., and Hakala, T. (1980). *J. Nucl. Med.* **21**, 570–573.

Levy, R., Dilley, J., and Lampson, L. A. (1978). *Curr. Top. Microbiol. Immunol.* **81**, 164–169.

Luben, R. A., and Mohler, M. A. (1980). *Mol. Immunol.* **17**, 635–639.

McGrath, M. S., Pallimer, E., and Weissman, I. L. (1980). *Nature (London)* **285**, 259–261.

Magnani, J. L., Brockhaus, M., Smith, D. F., Ginsburg, V., Blaszczyk, M., Mitchell, K. F., Steplewski, Z., and Koprowski, H. (1981). *Science* **212**, 55–56.

Maki, R., Kearney, J., Paige, C., and Tonegawa, S. (1980). *Science* **209**, 1366–1369.

Maniatis, T. (1980). *In* "Cell Biology" (L. Goldstein and D. M. Prescott, eds.), Vol. III, pp. 563–608. Academic Press, New York.

Maniatis, T., Hardison, R. C., Lacy, E., Lauer, J., O'Connell, C., Quon, D., Sim, G. K., and Efstradiadis, A. (1978). *Cell* **15**, 687–701.

Martinis, J., and Croce, C. (1978). *Proc. Natl. Acad. Sci. U.S.A.* **75**, 2320–2323.

Miller, R. A., Maloney, D. G., Warnke, R., and Levy, R. (1982). *N. Engl. J. Med.* **306**, 517–522.

Mitchell, K. F. (1980). *Cancer Immunol.* **10**, 1–5.

Mitchell, K. F., Fuhrer, J. P., Steplewski, Z., and Koprowski, H. (1980). *Proc. Natl. Acad. Sci. U.S.A.* **77**, 7287–7291.

Momoi, M., Kennett, R. H., and Glick, M. C. (1980). *J. Biol. Chem.* **255**, 11914–11921.

Morstyn, G., Metcalf, D., Burgess, A., and Fabre, J. W. (1981). *Scand. J. Haematol.* **26**, 19–30.

Nadler, L. M., Stashenko, P. H., Hardy, R., Kaplan, W. D., Button, L., Kufe, D. W., Antman, K. H., and Schlossman, S. F. (1980). *Cancer Res.* **40**, 3147–3154.

Nathans, D., and Smith, H. O. (1975). *Annu. Rev. Biochem.* **44**, 273–293.

Nowinski, R., Berglund, C., Lane, J., Lostrom, M., Bernstein, I., Young, W., and Hakomori, S. I. (1980). *Science* **210**, 537–539.

Olson, L., and Kaplan, H. S. (1980). *Proc. Natl. Acad. Sci. U.S.A.* **77**, 5429–5431.

Ritz, J., Pesando, J. M., Notis-McConarty, J., Lazarus, H., and Schlossman, S. F. (1980). *Nature (London)* **283**, 583–585.

Ruddon, R. W., ed. (1978). *In* "Biological Markers of Neoplasia: Basic and Applied Aspects." Elsevier, Amsterdam.

Schlom, J., Wunderlich, D., and Teramoto, Y. O. (1980). *Proc. Natl. Acad. Sci. U.S.A.* **77**, 6841–6845.

Schnegg, J. F., Diserens, A. C., Carrel, S., Accolla, R. S., and Detribol, N. (1981). *Cancer Res.* **41**, 1209–1213.

Simrell, C. R., and Klein, P. A. (1979). *J. Immunol.* **123**, 2386–2394.

Southern, E. M. (1975). *J. Mol. Biol.* **98**, 503–517.

Strand, M. (1980). *Proc. Natl. Acad. Sci. U.S.A.* **77**, 3234–3238.

Tax, A., and Manson, L. A. (1981). *Proc. Natl. Acad. Sci. U.S.A.* **78**, 529–533.

Tsung, Y., Milonsky, A., and Alpert, E. (1980). *N. Engl. J. Med.* **302**, 180.

Votila, M., and Ruoslahti, E. (1980). *Mol. Immunol.* **17**, 791–794.

Weinberg, R., (1981). *Biochim. Biophys. Acta* **651**, 25–35.

Weiss, D. W. (1980). *Curr. Top. Microbiol. Immunol.* **89**, 1–83.

Youle, R. J., and Neville, D. M. (1980). *Proc. Natl. Acad. Sci. U.S.A.* **77**, 5483–5486.

INDEX